CLINICAL ARTHROGRAPHY

CLINICAL ARTHROGRAPHY

ROLF-D. ARNDT, M.D.

Radiologist, St. John's Hospital and Health Center,
Santa Monica, California.

Assistant Clinical Professor of Radiology,
University of California Los Angeles,
Center for Health Sciences.

JOHN W. HORNS, M.D.

Radiologist, St. John's Hospital and Health Center,
Santa Monica, California.

Assistant Clinical Professor of Radiology,
University of California Los Angeles,
Center for Health Sciences.

RICHARD H. GOLD, M.D.

Professor of Radiology, Chief of Skeletal Radiology,
University of California Los Angeles,
Center for Health Sciences.

With a Special Contribution on
Temporomandibular Joint Arthrography by

DONALD D. BLASCHKE, D.D.S.

Assistant Professor, Section of Oral Radiology,
University of California Los Angeles,
School of Dentistry.

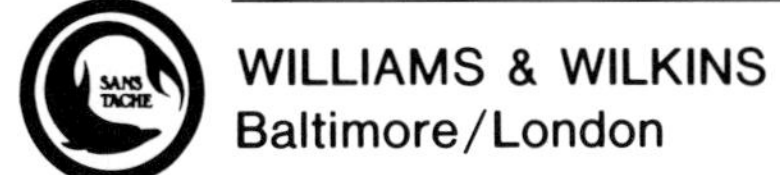

WILLIAMS & WILKINS
Baltimore/London

Copyright ©, 1981
Williams & Wilkins
428 E. Preston Street
Baltimore, Md. 21202, U.S.A.

Made in The United States of America

Library of Congress Cataloging in Publication Data

Main entry under title:

Arndt, Rolf-D.
   Clinical arthrography.

   Includes index.
   1. Joints—Radiography. I. Horns, John Willard, 1931-   joint author. II. Gold,
Richard H., joint author. III. Title. [DNLM: 1. Joints—Radiography. WE300 A747c]
RC932.A76   616.7'207572   80-14230
ISBN 0-683-00253-8

Composed and printed at
Waverly Press, Inc.
Mt. Royal and Guilford Aves.
Baltimore, Md. 21202, U.S.A.

Dedication

This book is dedicated to the memory of
Leo G. Rigler, M.D.,
inspiring teacher and friend.

Preface

There are few books on arthrography. Yet, arthrography is a regular part of daily practice for most radiologists. Arthrography is not technically difficult, but considerable knowledge and experience is required for interpretation.
This book deals with the method and interpretation of arthrography of the shoulder, knee, ankle, elbow, hip, wrist, metacarpophalangeal, interphalangeal, and temporomandibular joints. The emphasis is on orthopedic disorders, usually of traumatic origin, which is in keeping with the application of arthrography in clinical practice. Other conditions such as inflammatory and degenerative diseases, congenital disorders, and, in the case of the hip, arthrography of reconstructive joint surgery are included.
Each chapter is devoted to one joint and provides a comprehensive discussion on the method of arthrography including single and double contrast techniques where applicable, normal radiographic anatomy, and finally, the interpretation of the normal and abnormal arthrogram.
Considerable effort has been expended to provide a concise yet comprehensive text with carefully selected figures, in keeping with our philosophy to make this book a useful and practical tool for the radiologist who performs and interprets the arthrogram. It is our hope that the emphasis and scope of this book will also make it valuable to the orthopedic surgeon. It was in the radiological support of their diagnostic and therapeutic efforts that this project originated.

R. D. Arndt, M.D.
J. W. Horns, M.D.
R. H. Gold, M.D.

Acknowledgments

We would like to offer our special thanks and pay tribute to the skill and patience of Gwynne M. Gloege, medical illustrator, and Paul E. Stout and Kim Willis, photographers, for their indispensable help in preparing this book.

We gratefully acknowledge the generosity of the following physicians: Robert Watanabe, M.D., Donald Resnick, M.D., Ross T. Eto, M.D., Jerrold Mink, M.D., Lawrence W. Bassett, M.D., Darwood Hance, M.D., and W. J. Weston, M.D., for providing us with interesting cases from their practices.

Most of the material for this book was accumulated from the Radiology departments at St. John's Hospital and Health Center, Santa Monica, California, and University of California, Los Angeles Center for the Health Sciences, Los Angeles, California. We express our gratitude to the hospital administrations at both these centers.

Finally, a large measure of thanks is due to our clinical colleagues and to their patients. It is in the interest of better service to them that this entire project was carried out.

R. D. Arndt, M.D.
J. W. Horns, M. D.
R. H. Gold, M.D.

Contents

1

Arthrography of the Knee

J. W. Horns, M.D.

Knee arthrography is most often performed to detect clinically suspected meniscal lesions. However, it is also useful in the evaluation of many other knee disorders as will be shown. Some patients are referred for arthrography, although no significant abnormality is suspected after clinical evaluation. These patients usually have persistent symptoms following a vehicular or industrial accident and the arthrogram is performed to help exclude significant joint injury. The yield of positive findings at arthrography is high compared with most other radiological studies. This helps maintain the interest of the radiologist in the procedure. If the studies are to be accurate, the radiologist must remain attentive to technical details.

NORMAL GROSS ANATOMY

The knee joint, the most complex joint of the body, has three separate components: the medial femoral-tibial articulation, the lateral femoral-tibial articulation, and the patello-femoral articulation. We will discuss the articular surfaces of the bones, menisci, the ligaments, and the synovium of the knee joint. Most of the muscles, nerves, and blood vessels of the knee can be ignored for our purposes.

The condyles of the femur are in the shape of rollers. The medial and lateral condyles are separated behind by the intercondylar notch and are joined in front by the patellar articular surface of the femur. The combined articular surfaces of the femur, therefore, have the shape of an inverted "U." The articular surface of the medial condyle is longer from front to back than that of the lateral condyle. The medial condyle projects lower than the lateral condyle in relationship to the femoral axis and causes the normal slight valgus condition of the knee. The patellar articular surface of the femur has the shape of a saddle with a longitudinal groove and is also known as the trochlear surface. The lateral side of the saddle is broader than the medial side. The patellar articular surface of the femur is demarcated from the tibial articular surfaces of the femur by the faint condylo-patellar grooves. The anterior portions of the menisci occupy these grooves when the knee is fully extended.

The patella is a large sesamoid bone embedded in the tendon of the quadriceps muscle and provides a significant mechanical advantage during quadriceps contraction. Its superior border is curved, and its inferior border is shaped like the apex of a triangle. On its posterior surface is an oval articular area which is divided into medial and lateral facets by a longitudinal ridge. The lateral facet is broader than the medial. The articular area does not extend down as far as the apex.

The upper end of the tibia is expanded to form medial and lateral tibial condyles (plateaus). The medial surface has an oval outline while the lateral surface is nearly circular. The intercondylar area of the upper end of the tibia is raised in its center to form the intercondylar eminence. Projections of the eminence constitute the medial and lateral intercondylar tubercles or spines. The anterior and posterior intercondylar areas are wider than the eminence. The central attachments of the menisci and attachments of the cruciate ligaments to the tibia are in the intercondylar area and are shown in Figure 1.1. The top of each tibial condyle is flattened at its periphery where it is in contact with a meniscus and is slightly concave at its center to adapt to the adjacent femoral condyle.

The fibrocartilaginous menisci rest on top of the articulating surfaces of the tibia and cover approximately the peripheral two-thirds of each tibial condyle. They are also known as the semilunar cartilages because of their crescent shape. Each meniscus tapers from a thick convex outer border to a thin concave inner border. The lower (tibial) surface of each meniscus is flattened and the upper surface is slightly concave to accommodate the corresponding femoral condyle. The menisci are attached to the tibia and move with it in relationship to the femur. The menisci broaden those areas of the tibia that support the body weight as it is transmitted from the femoral condyles.

The medial meniscus is nearly a semicircle. Its posterior portion is wider than its anterior or middle portions. The width of the middle portion may be slightly less or slightly greater than that of the anterior portion. The width of the lateral meniscus is more uniform, usually decreasing slightly in the posterior segment. The height of both menisci at their periphery is 3 to 5 mm. The lateral meniscus forms almost a complete ring and has a shorter radius of curvature than the medial meniscus.

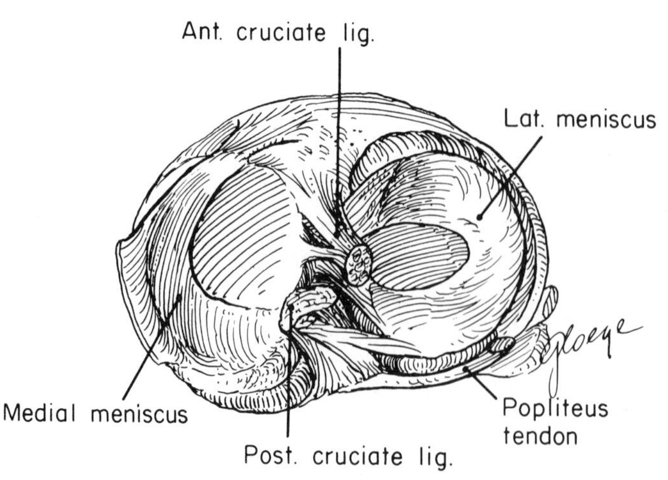

Figure 1.1. Relationships and attachments of the menisci and ligaments to the upper end of the tibia. (Modified from Grant, J.C.B., *An Atlas of Anatomy*, Ed. 5. Williams & Wilkins, Baltimore, 1962.)

There is a variation in the size of the menisci between individuals depending somewhat on body size. If one meniscus is smaller than average, then the other meniscus will also be small. Lindblom examined 200 knees at autopsy and measured the width of each meniscus at its midpoint, 45° anteriorly and 45° posteriorly. His average measurements are shown in Table 1.1 followed by the approximate range.

The anterior and posterior extremities of each meniscus are attached to the adjacent intercondylar area of the tibia. Throughout the circumference of the medial meniscus its peripheral edge is firmly adherent to the joint capsule with minor exceptions: there is commonly a shallow recess between the posterior-superior margin of the medial meniscus and the joint capsule; occasionally there are shallow recesses elsewhere between the capsule and the superior or inferior margins of the medial meniscus. These are called the meniscosynovial recesses. Often there is a transverse ligament connecting the anterior ends of the medial and lateral menisci and, occasionally, the anterior end of the medial meniscus is attached to the anterior cruciate ligament. The posterior portion of the lateral meniscus is separated from the joint capsule by the popliteus tendon and its bursa. The remainder of the lateral meniscus is attached to the capsule. In the anterior region there is usually a prominent inferior meniscosynovial recess and a smaller superior recess. In the midzone there is only an inferior recess.

The femoral and tibial condylar surfaces, the patellar surface of the femur, and the posterior surface of the patella are covered with a smooth layer of hyaline articular cartilage. The thickness of the articular cartilage is 2.6 to 3.2 mm maximum on the femoral condyles and 3.5 mm in the middle of the trochlear surface, according to Morris. The cartilage is slightly thicker on the lateral femoral condyle than on the medial condyle. The patellar cartilage is thickest at the ridge where it measures 5.4 to 6.4 mm.

The ligaments of the knee can be divided into internal and external sets. The cruciate ligaments are the major internal ligaments. The anterior cruciate ligament is fixed to the medial half of the anterior intercondylar area of the tibia. It extends upwards, backwards, and laterally to attach onto the medial part of the lateral femoral condyle. The posterior cruciate ligament is fixed to the posterior intercondylar area of the tibia and posterior horn of the lateral meniscus. It passes upward, anteriorly, and medially to attach onto the lateral aspect of the medial femoral condyle. The posterior cruciate is shorter and more vertical than the anterior cruciate.

The important external ligaments are the joint capsule and the collateral ligaments. The fibrous joint capsule is a complicated structure which encloses the knee joint like a loose sack. Over most of the circumference of the knee the capsule is attached above near the margins of the femoral condyles and below near the margins of the tibial condyles. It extends higher anteriorly than

Table 1.1
Average Measurements of Knee Menisci

	Anterior	Middle	Posterior
Medial meniscus	6 mm (4–9)	6 mm (4–9)	14 mm (10–20)
Lateral meniscus	10 mm (7–13)	10 mm (6–13)	9 mm (6–12)

posteriorly, and has an opening above the patella allowing the joint space to communicate with the suprapatellar bursa. On the lateral side the popliteus tendon passes down to the posterior aspect of the tibia through a defect in the capsule. The anterior part of the capsule is formed by the medial and lateral patellar retinacula. They are fibrous membranes derived from the quadriceps tendon and located on the medial and lateral sides of the patella and patellar ligament. The inner surface of the capsule is attached to the periphery of each meniscus and connects the menisci to the margin of the head of the tibia. This connecting portion of the capsule is called the "coronary ligament."

The tibial (medial) collateral ligament is a strong flat triangular band with apex attached to the medial epicondyle of the femur and base attached to the medial and posterior borders of the tibial condyle. Its anterior border merges with the medial patellar retinaculum, and its posterior border is continuous with the posterior joint capsule. The deep portion of the ligament is formed by the joint capsule and is adherent to the medial meniscus.

The fibular (lateral) collateral ligament is a strong cord extending from the lateral epicondyle of the femur to the head of the fibula. It is outside the joint capsule and is not attached to the capsule or the lateral meniscus.

The anatomy of the synovial membrane of the knee is complex. Most of the interior of the fibrous joint capsule is lined with synovium (Fig. 1.2 and 1.3). The synovium ends at the margins of the articular cartilage of the femur, tibia, and patella, and at the attachment of the capsule to the menisci. Beneath the peripheral edge of each meniscus there are usually shallow synovial-lined

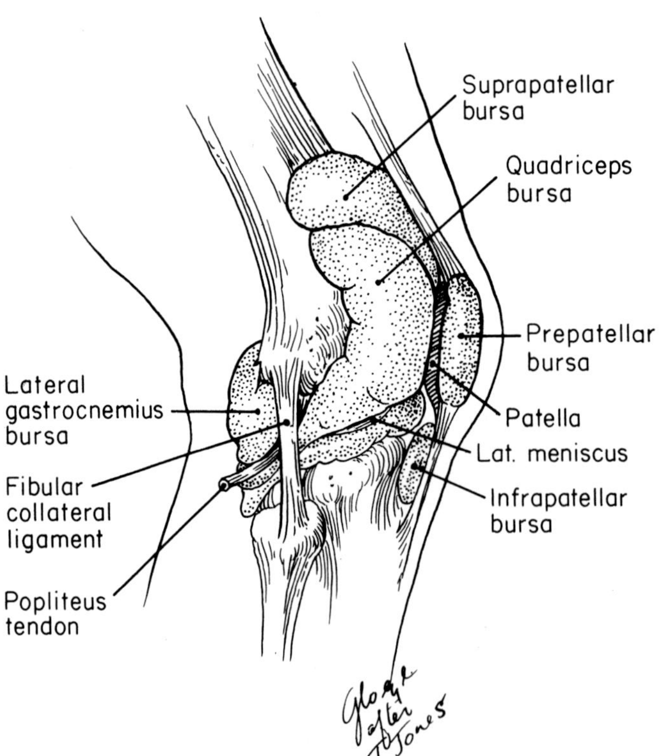

Figure 1.2. Distended knee joint, lateral view. (Modified from Grant, J.C.B., *An Atlas of Anatomy,* Ed. 5. Williams & Wilkins, Baltimore, 1962.)

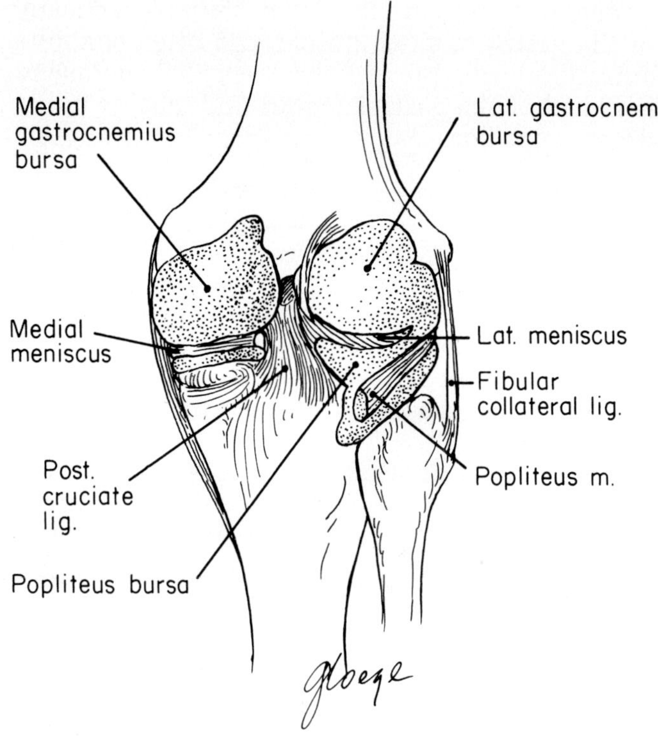

Figure 1.3. Distended knee joint, posterior view. (Modified from Grant, J.C.B., *An Atlas of Anatomy,* Ed. 5. Williams & Wilkins, Baltimore, 1962.)

capsular recesses surrounding the margins of the tibial condyles. The synovium covers the front of the anterior cruciate ligament, extends back along both sides of the cruciate ligaments, and is reflected onto the posterior joint capsule instead of covering the posterior margin of the posterior cruciate ligament. Therefore, the cruciate ligaments are not completely enclosed by the synovial sac, and are considered to be intracapsular but extrasynovial in location.

The infrapatellar synovial fold (ligamentum mucosum) is a band extending between the fat pad and the intercondylar area of the femur. It is in front of the anterior cruciate ligament and approximately parallel to it. The medial and lateral alar folds or patellar synovial folds (plicae) project into the joint on each side of the patella and run down to the sides of the infrapatellar fat pad. The medial patellar plica is often thicker than the lateral plica and may form a band between the edge of the patella and medial femoral condyle. It is sometimes continuous above with the suprapatellar synovial fold.

Of the numerous synovial-lined bursae about the knee, the five which communicate with the joint space are most significant to the arthrographer. Anteriorly, the suprapatellar bursa extends upward from the joint cavity and is located between the femur and deep surface of the quadriceps tendon. In about 70% of knees there is a suprapatellar synovial fold at the junction of the bursa and joint cavity proper, and occasionally a complete transverse septum separates the bursa from the joint. Posterolaterally the popliteus bursa surrounds the popliteus tendon and separates the tendon, joint capsule, and fibular collateral ligament from the lateral meniscus. Usually the bursa does not completely surround the tendon and the tendon is located at the lateral margin of the bursa.

The medial and lateral gastrocnemius bursae are located posteriorly, beneath the medial and lateral heads of the gastrocnemius muscle, and often communicate with the joint. The semimembranosus bursa is between the semimembranosus muscle and the medial head of the gastrocnemius and may communicate with the underlying gastrocnemius bursa.

METHOD OF ARTHROGRAPHY

Both positive contrast and double contrast arthrography of the knee have had their proponents. With either method, most arthrographers now prefer to use fluoroscopy and "spot films" which permit orthograde projections of the menisci, rather than radiography without fluoroscopy. We will give instructions for either positive contrast or double contrast arthrography and also for a combined method.

Lindblom's extensive experience was with nonfluoroscopic positive contrast arthrography. Turner and Budin and also Leven used positive contrast arthrography with fluoroscopic spot films. Double contrast arthrography with horizontal beam radiography was popularized by Andren and Wehlin and by Freiberger et al. An early report on the double contrast method with fluoroscopic spot filming was by Butt and McIntyre; now most authors advocate this method.

Tegtmeyer et al. recently compared fluoroscopic single and double contrast techniques for examination of menisci and found them to be equally effective diagnostically. The two methods were used alternately in 951 patients. The medial meniscus was assessed accurately in 97% of the cases by either method. Assessment of the lateral meniscus was accurate in 96% of single contrast studies and in 93% of double contrast studies. The difference was not statistically significant.

Our method of arthrography is a combination of single contrast and double contrast techniques. We have chosen this because abnormalities of the knee in some patients are shown better by positive single contrast while in other patients the double contrast study is more revealing. Also, if one technique yields equivocal findings, comparison with the other technique will usually lead to a decision as to whether or not there is an abnormality present. Assessment of the articular cartilages is definitely superior by double contrast.

Preliminary to the arthrogram, radiography of the knee should be obtained in the frontal, both oblique and lateral projections. These films may disclose abnormalities which might be obscured later by the contrast medium such as osteochondritis dissecans, osteochondral fracture, chondrocalcinosis, calcified intraarticular loose bodies, and signs of rheumatoid arthritis or degenerative joint disease.

The needle puncture is performed with the patient supine. A small support behind the knee flexes the joint slightly and allows the patient to relax the quadriceps femoris. Tension in this muscle forces the patella against the femur, making it difficult or impossible to insert the needle into the joint space between the patella and femur. The puncture can be made either on the lateral or medial side of the knee although the lateral puncture is usually more convenient (Fig. 1.4). The puncture site is chosen at the widest part of the patella just behind the posterior patellar surface. If necessary, the skin is shaved in this vicinity.

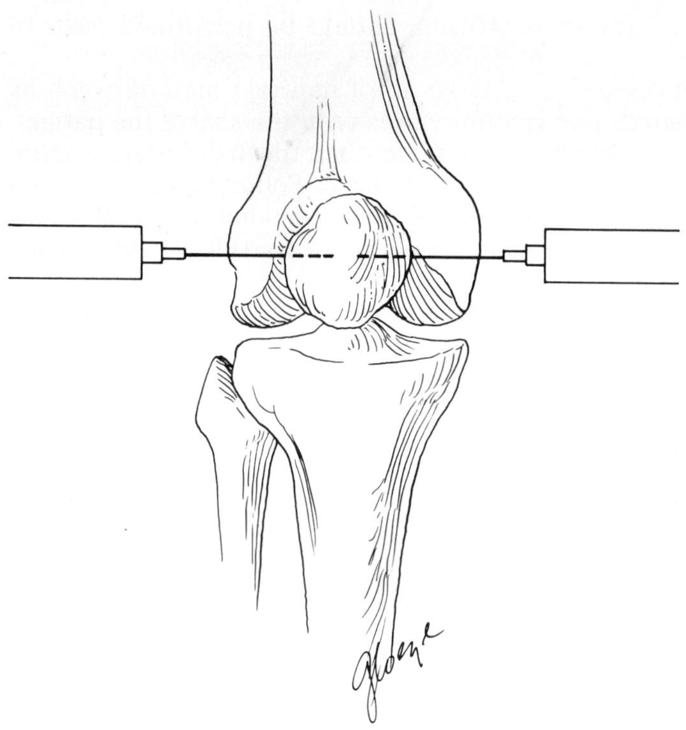

Figure 1.4. Sites of arthrocentesis for knee arthrography.

Preparation of the skin is then performed with an antiseptic agent. A sterile drape is applied, and the skin and subcutaneous tissues are anesthetized with a local anesthetic agent such as Xylocaine which is injected through a 25-gauge needle. A larger needle is then used to puncture the joint. We have found it most convenient to use a 21-gauge butterfly needle which is attached to a small caliber polyethylene tube. This needle is approximately 2 cm in length and is long enough to enter the joint space in all but the most obese patients. Usually the butterfly needle is inserted almost to the hub before it enters the joint space, so that the needle when fully inserted extends only a short distance into the joint. It produces less damage to the articular cartilage than a longer needle might if inserted further. If a conventional hypodermic needle is used for the joint puncture, it is convenient to attach a polyethylene connector tube between the Xylocaine-filled syringe and the needle. As the puncture needle is advanced through the skin and into the joint space behind the patella, the operator's opposite hand is used to displace the patella toward the puncture needle. When the depth of the needle insertion indicates that the joint space has been entered, about 5 ml of anesthetic solution are injected. If the needle has actually entered the joint space, the injection of the anesthetic material will meet with no resistance, whereas there will be resistance if the injection is being made into the tissues outside of the joint space. However, this is not the most reliable indicator of the needle position. If most of the anesthetic agent which has been injected can be aspirated back through the needle this is a more definite indication that the needle is within the joint, as is the aspiration of a joint effusion if present. In order to avoid dilution of the contrast material by residual fluid, thorough aspiration of any joint effusion should be performed prior to contrast injection.

For positive contrast arthrography, 12 to 20 ml of contrast material such as Renografin 60 or 76 are injected. The amount varies with the size of the patient. Occasionally, if a large effusion has been aspirated, then the arthrogram is more satisfactory if 25 to 30 ml of contrast material are used. Following the injection of contrast material, the knee is rapidly flexed and extended about 30 times, and then the patient is encouraged to take a few steps with full weight bearing on the affected leg. These maneuvers are necessary to disperse the contrast material throughout the joint space and give optimum demonstration of meniscus tears, ligament ruptures, and articular cartilage defects. The accuracy of the arthrogram is impaired if there is severe restriction in motion of the knee.

An optional step is tightly wrapping the knee with an elastic bandage beginning in the suprapatellar area and continuing down around the joint. Wrapping displaces contrast from the suprapatellar bursa and posterior recesses into the articular regions. The radiographs are then obtained with the patient supine on the fluoroscopic table. The knee to be examined is elevated approximately 12 in above the table top by a large radiolucent sponge. First, a set of films of the entire knee is obtained in the frontal projection, with internal rotation, and with external rotation. These exposures can be made on a single film. The fluoroscopic field of view is then reduced by collimation to about 4 cm by 2 cm and then each meniscus is examined separately. The entire length of each meniscus must be studied fluoroscopically in profile by rotation of the leg, and with appropriate stress to permit an orthograde projection of the meniscus during each exposure. Each meniscus can be positioned more accurately if the examination is begun at the midpoint with the knee in the neutral position. The knee is then rotated approximately 10° between each exposure so that four views of the anterior portion and four views of the posterior portion of the meniscus are eventually obtained. On most machines the nine exposures of each meniscus can be recorded on a single spot film with proper use of the spot film selector. If there is equivocal evidence of a meniscus lesion at fluoroscopy or on review of the films, then multiple films can be taken of the suspicious area of the meniscus with only slight amounts of rotation between exposures. By this additional examination, the arthrographer can almost always resolve the question of a meniscus lesion.

Our spot films are taken with manual setting of the exposure factors. Photo-timing might be satisfactory on some machines, but we have had unacceptable variation in film density when phototiming was used for the small radiographs of the menisci. Typical exposure factors are 60 kVP, 200 mA, and 0.25 sec. A higher milliampere would be preferred, if it were available, so the time could be shortened and possible motion artifact reduced. The technique that is chosen is used for the scout films. They are viewed prior to the arthrogram so that adjustment may be made if necessary. The smallest available focal spot should be used for the radiographs, and this must be under 1 mm in order that details be shown adequately.

The use of a grid is not necessary because scatter is adequately reduced by the collimation. The advantage of nongrid technique is that less exposure is required and the time can be shortened further.

The final film of the positive contrast arthrogram is taken in the lateral projection with the knee flexed at almost a right angle and with overpenetration so that the cruciate ligaments are visualized through the contrast material in the joint space. Particular attention is paid to the anterior cruciate ligament because it is torn much more frequently than the posterior cruciate. If the anterior cruciate ligament is not seen on this radiograph, then a repeat lateral view can be obtained with anterior stress applied to the upper tibia in order to make the anterior cruciate ligament taut. Again, the knee should be flexed to almost a right angle. A slight degree of rotation in either direction from the straight lateral view will sometimes make the anterior cruciate ligament more visible.

For a double contrast arthrogram the joint puncture is made as described above. For an adult 50 to 80 ml of air are injected into the joint space. The room air to be injected may be filtered through a sterile gauze as it is being drawn into the syringe. If a butterfly needle is used the tubing can be pinched whenever the syringe is disconnected to prevent escape of air from the joint space. Three to 5 ml of contrast agent such as Renografin 60 or 76 is then injected; 0.1 to 0.3 ml of 1:1000 epinephrine may be added to delay absorption of contrast agent by the synovium. This is not necessary if the radiographs can be quickly obtained. After removal of the needle the joint is exercised to distribute the contrast agent. The fluoroscopic spot films are taken with the patient prone on the x-ray table. Each meniscus is studied separately as appropriate abduction or adduction stress is applied to spread apart the condyles in that half of the joint being studied. The stress may be applied with one hand of the examiner holding the patient's thigh and the other hand holding his ankle. Alternatively, the stress may be applied if the examiner holds only the patient's ankle and a rigid restraint or fabric band immobilizes the thigh. Several suitable restraints are now available commercially. They would allow the examiner to increase his distance from the x-ray beam if an assistant positioned the fluoroscope and exposed the radiographs. Either a tableside fluoroscope or remote control unit could be used. As previously described the leg is turned during the examination, and multiple exposures of the meniscus are made so that eventually it is examined throughout its circumference. These films also demonstrate the articular cartilage of the femur and tibia in the half of the joint being studied.

After each meniscus is examined, the articular cartilage of the patella is then examined by means of lateral and near-lateral spot films with the patient lying on his side and the affected knee closest to the radiographic table. In the straight lateral view the beam is tangential to the central posterior ridge of the patella. Slight external rotation of the leg brings the lateral facet of the patella into view. The medial facet is seen with moderate internal rotation. The medial facet usually forms a steeper angle with the coronal plane of the knee than does the lateral facet. For this reason more internal rotation of the knee is required to see the medial facet as compared to the amount of external rotation required to see the lateral facet of the patella. With most x-ray machines, six exposures of the patella can be recorded on one film. Six views are usually sufficient for a complete study of the patella. If there is a questionable abnormality of the patella or poor visualization of one region, due to superimposed densities, then six more exposures are made of this area with slight differences in the degree of rotation of the knee.

The patella can also be radiographed in the axial projection. The most satisfactory method is to have the patient supine on the table with the knee flexed no more than 30° and supported from behind. Greater flexion than this would pull the patella more firmly into the notch of the femur and interfere with the demonstration of the patellar cartilage. The patient can hold the film. The x-ray tube is beyond the foot of the table. The x-ray beam is directed along the longitudinal axis of the patella, and an attempt is made to superimpose the inferior and superior poles of the patella. The beam makes an angle of about 10° with the tibia. An axial view of a normal patella is shown in Figure 1.9C. Both the medial and lateral facets are seen. Abnormalities of the patellar cartilage can be seen better on the lateral views than in the axial view. Therefore, axial views are not required if the patella is normal on the routine lateral views. If a localized abnormality is seen in the lateral views of the patella, then an axial view can be useful in determining the transverse diameter of the cartilage lesion. The axial view also shows the alignment of the patella with the patellar surface of the femur. The examination is completed by taking a lateral radiograph with the knee joint flexed to almost 90°.

Before the patient leaves we aspirate the residual air from the joint. A common practice is to dismiss the patient without aspirating the air. However, it may take a few days for the air to dissipate and some patients find this unpleasant.

We prefer a combination method of positive contrast and double contrast arthrography. First, a complete positive contrast arthrogram is performed as described above. Then the knee is immediately unwrapped, scrubbed with antiseptic solution and repunctured at the site that was previously anesthetized. This puncture usually causes no pain. Complete aspiration of the previously injected contrast agent is then attempted. This will leave a thin coating of contrast material on the synovium, the menisci, and articular cartilages. Fifty to 80 cc of filtered room air is then injected. The double contrast study is conducted immediately in the prone position as previously described. The contrast material is already distributed within the joint so that no exercising of the knee is required. When the study has been completed, a third puncture is made at the same site for aspiration of air from the joint.

Possible complications of arthrography include syncope, allergic reaction, sterile effusion, and infections. During the early years we had five patients who had vasovagal reactions with temporary unconsciousness after they stood erect to exercise the knee following the injection. They all happened to be robust adult males. Patients are now monitored carefully after the injection. If they have any feeling of "faintness" they remain supine and the knee is passively exercised over the side of the radiographic table. Of approximately 4000 patients, three have had mild urticaria and there have been no serious allergic reactions. In four patients who gave histories of severe reactions to contrast agent, arthrograms were performed with air only. The images obtained were of reduced quality, but a lateral meniscus tear was correctly diagnosed in one case.

A sterile effusion has occurred in an occasional patient within one day following the arthrogram. No effusion has recurred after it was aspirated once. No knee joint infections have been caused by our arthrograms in the series of approximately 4000 examinations.

Note. We have recently found that 105-mm camera spot films with phototiming are satisfactory for knee arthrography. By this means the entire arthrogram, except for the axial view of the patella, can be recorded on the camera films. Radiation exposure of patient and person manipulating the knee is reduced.

NORMAL RADIOGRAPHIC ANATOMY

On the arthrogram, each meniscus is projected in triangular cross section with its apex directed toward the center of the joint. The inner edge is sharp and the surfaces are smooth. Slight concavity or convexity of the surfaces may be seen. On the positive contrast study there should be contrast material between each meniscus and the articular cartilage of the femoral and tibial condyles and between the patella and femur. With the double contrast technique the upper and lower meniscal surfaces should be covered by a thin layer of contrast and surrounded by air in the joint space. An attempt should be made to distract the joint sufficiently to completely separate the menisci from the articular cartilage. This is not always possible, particularly at the posterior horns of the menisci.

The meniscosynovial recesses at the capsular attachments of the menisci fill with contrast material on the positive contrast arthrogram, while on the double contrast study they are filled with air and have a surface coating of contrast (Fig. 1.5). By either method of arthrography, the recess in front of or behind the tangent point will be superimposed on the section of the meniscus seen in profile. This appearance may simulate contrast material within a meniscus tear, particularly a horizontal fissure. The study of multiple projections of the questionable area will be helpful. Freiberger and Kaye have described two radiographic features of these capsular attachment recesses. The "choppy sea" sign is due to the uneven wavy contours of the meniscosynovial junction within the recess. The contour of the recess is often more irregular than a horizontal tear. The "end sign" is his second sign. This refers to the continuation between the superimposed recess and the recess located at the tangent point where the meniscus is seen in profile.

Sometimes there are clefts between the ligaments that arise from the anterior horn of the medial meniscus (Fig. 1.6). They are seen on the near-lateral views of the knee and can usually, but not always be differentiated from meniscal tears by their extreme anterior location. These clefts may appear quite different on the positive and double contrast studies, or may not be seen on both studies. This will help in differentiating between a normal finding and a tear. Also, superimposition of the infrapatellar fat pad on the anterior horn of a meniscus can simulate a tear. The superimposed margin of a fat pad should continue beyond the meniscus outline and have a different appearance than a tear. It must be remembered that isolated anterior horn tears of the medial meniscus are rare.

In the examination of the menisci, the most difficult area is the posterior-lateral region. There the popliteus tendon sheath communicates with the joint and is superimposed on the posterior horn of the lateral meniscus in certain projections. The tendon usually produces a bulge in the outer aspect of the

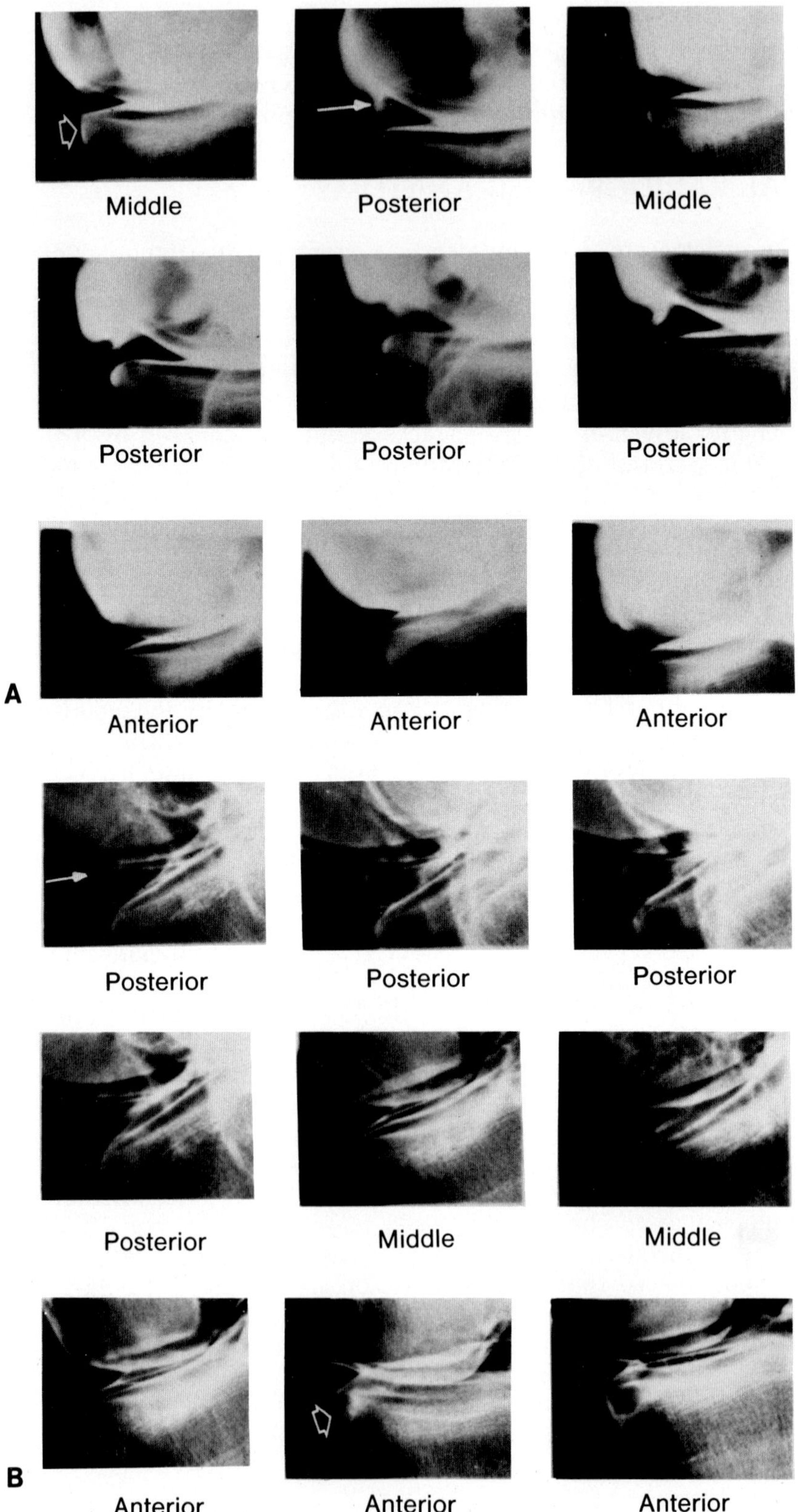

Figure 1.5. Normal medial meniscus. Examination of the entire meniscus by nine exposures on a single film. Note the posterior-superior meniscosynovial recess (*arrow*) and tibial capsular attachment recess (*open arrow*). A, Positive single contrast. B, Double contrast.

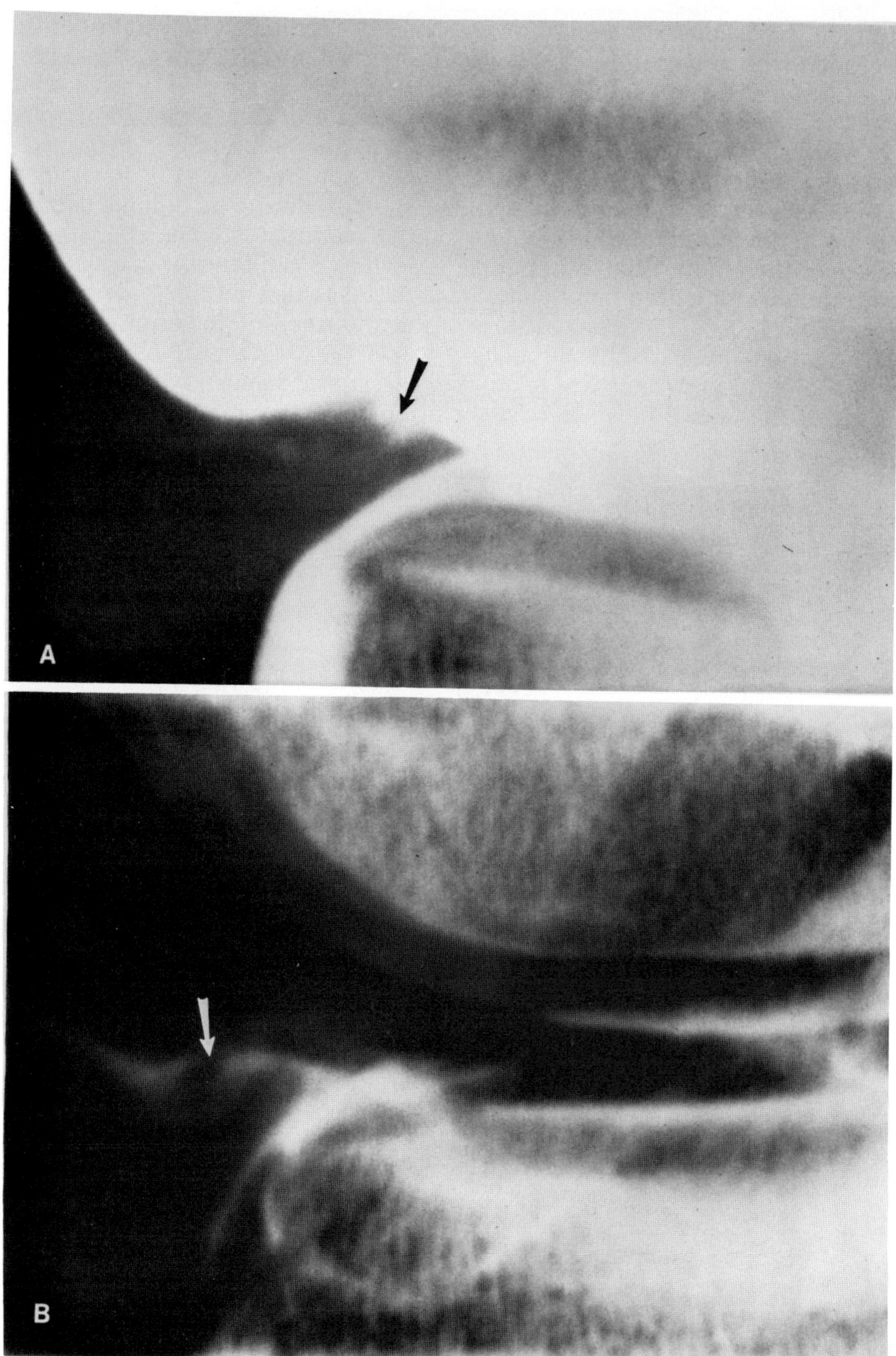

Figure 1.6. Normal cleft at anterior horn of medial meniscus (*arrow*). *A,* Positive single contrast. *B,* Double contrast.

sheath, but occasionally the tendon is seen as a round defect within the sheath. The tendon causes a shallow groove in the free outer surface of the meniscus. In this region there are thin bridges of tissue called struts or fascicles which connect the superior and inferior margins of the lateral meniscus to the capsule above and below the popliteus tendon and form the roof and floor of the recess around the tendon (Fig. 1.7). Defects normally occur in the struts, particularly where they are interrupted by the popliteus tendon during its oblique course.

On both the positive contrast and double contrast studies the articular cartilage of the femur, tibia, and patella is seen as a radiolucent zone between the subchondral bone and the contrast material which outlines the cartilage surface (Figs. 1.8 and 1.9). The cartilage of the anterior and posterior portions of the femoral condyles is not completely visualized on the arthrogram unless multiple lateral tomograms are taken. On the lateral views of the patella, the cartilage of the lateral facet and ridge can be projected anterior to the femur,

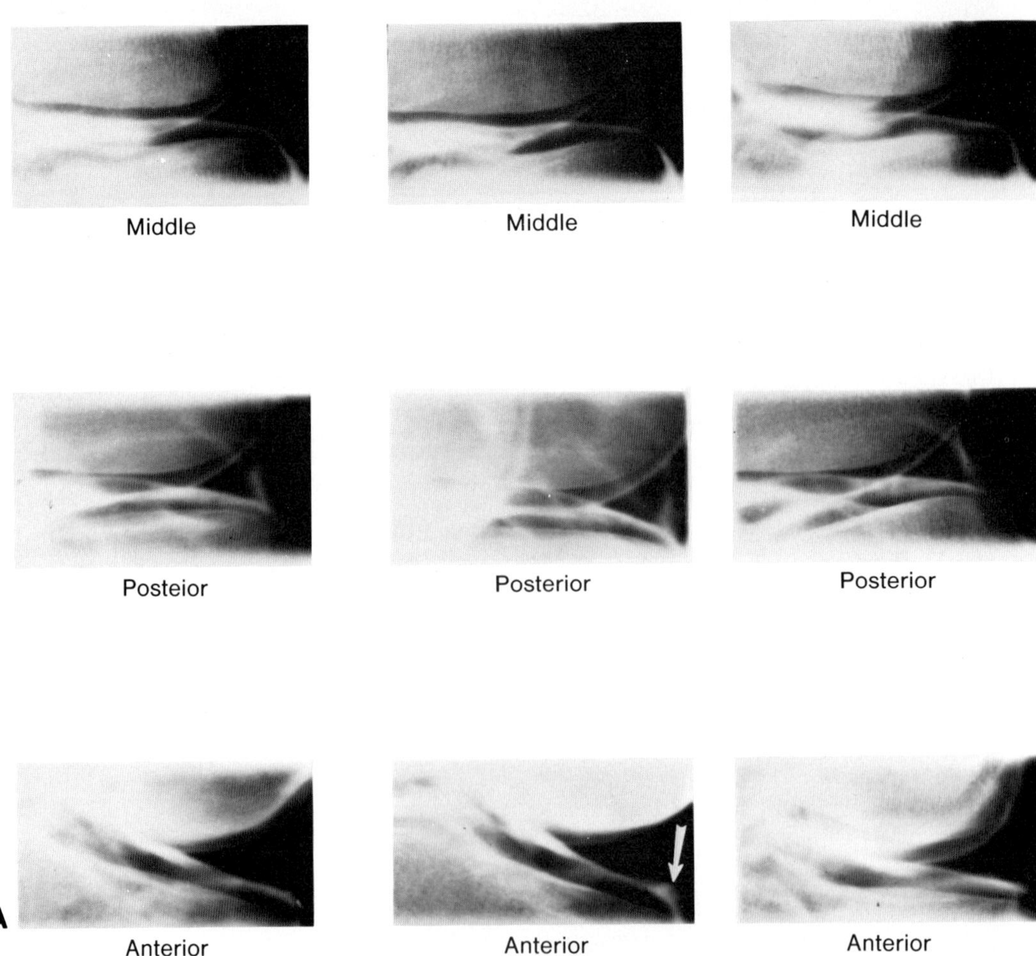

Figure 1.7. Normal lateral meniscus. *A*, Positive single contrast. *B*, Double contrast. Note anterior-inferior meniscosynovial recess (*arrow*) and struts (*open arrows*) attached to posterior segment seen only with double contrast.

whereas the cartilage of the medial facet is usually superimposed on the femur.

The synovial surfaces lining the joint capsule and communicating bursae appear smooth on the arthrogram, except that the margin of the fat pad may be irregular. The synovial covering of the cruciate ligaments, rather than the ligaments themselves, is seen on the arthrogram (Fig. 1.10).

The four synovial folds (plicae) can be shown by arthrography. On the lateral view the infrapatellar synovial fold (ligamentum mucosum) is in front of the anterior cruciate ligament. Its posterior-inferior margin may appear similar to the anterior margin of the anterior cruciate. The suprapatellar synovial fold, if present, will be seen as a transverse septum near the upper pole of the patella. The medial and lateral patellar synovial folds (alar folds) are partially demonstrated on the axial view of the patella. They project into the joint on each side of the patella (Fig. 1.9C).

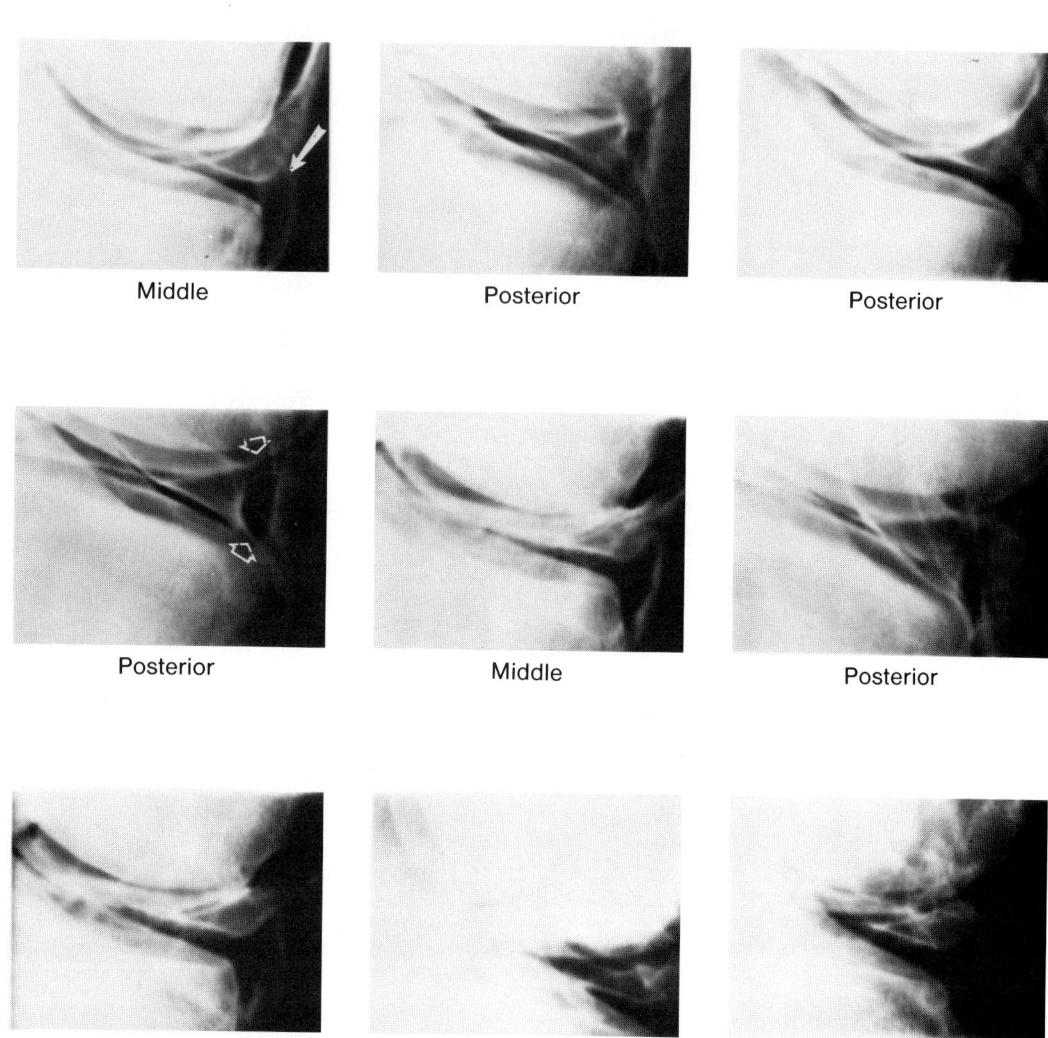

Figure 1.7*B*

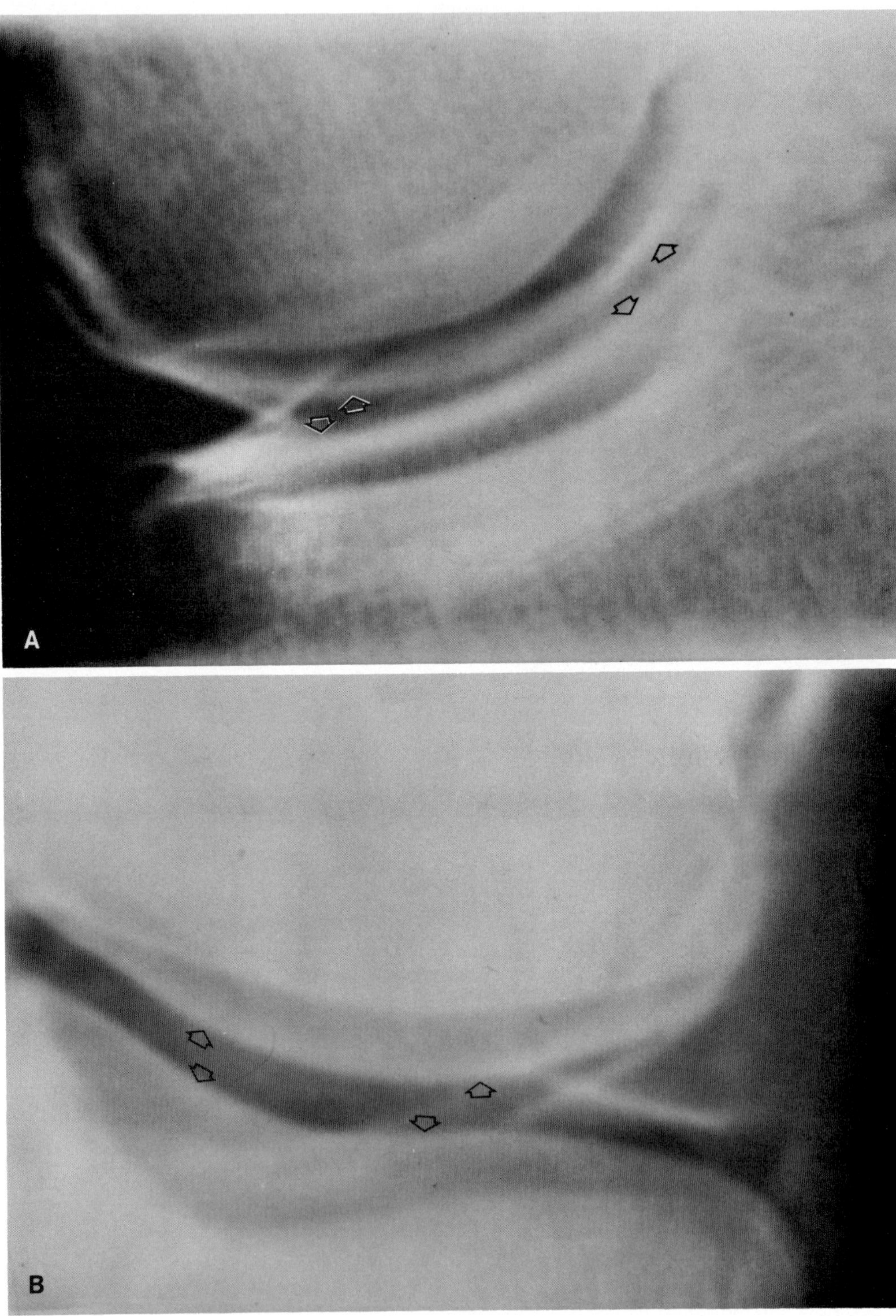

Figure 1.8. Condylar articular cartilage. Femoral and tibial articular cartilage is shown best by double contrast and is located between the layer of contrast on cartilage surface (*open arrows*) and subchondral bone. *A*, Medial joint space. *B*, Lateral joint space. Because of delay in obtaining *A* there has been a normal imbibition of contrast agent into superficial layers of the cartilage.

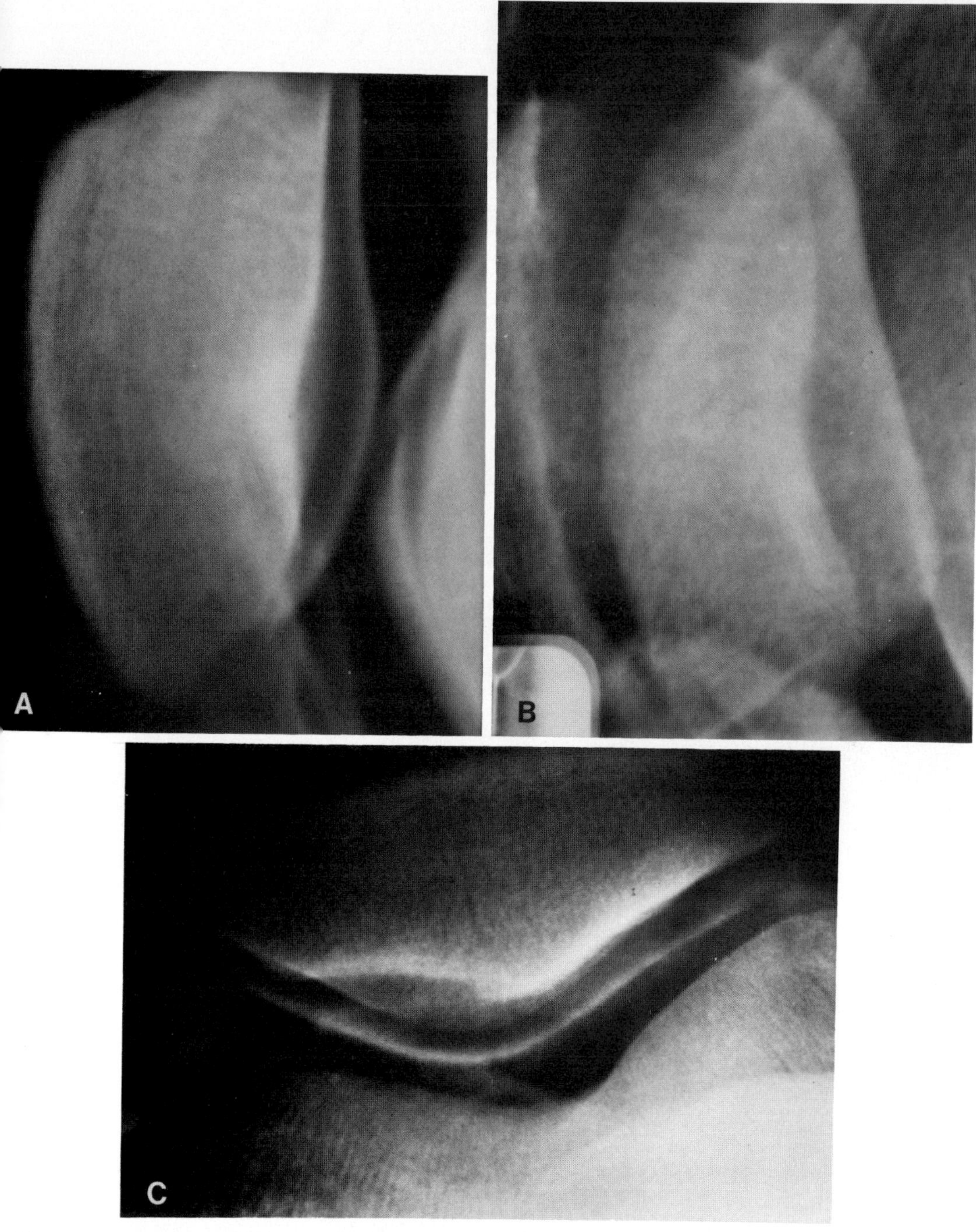

Figure 1.9. Patellar cartilage. Cartilage surface is coated with contrast. *A,* Lateral view of lateral facet. *B,* Lateral view of medial facet. *C,* Axial view shows both facets and ridge.

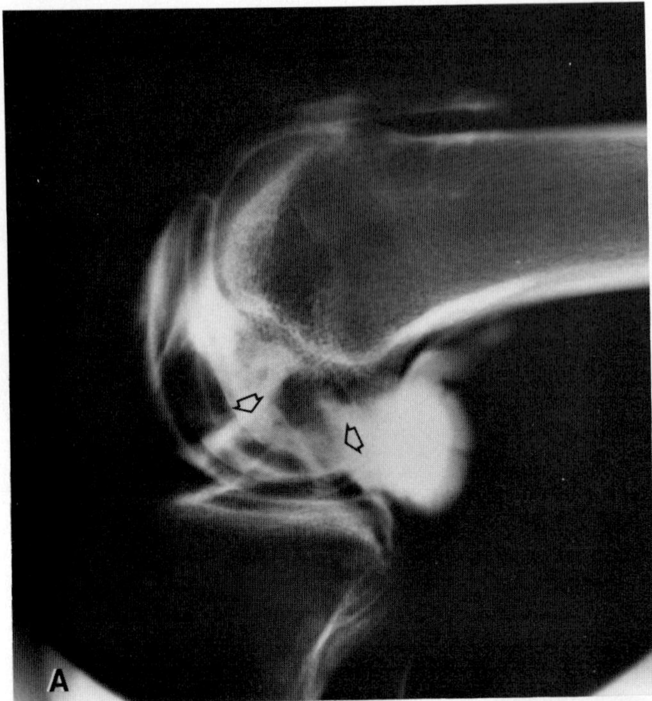
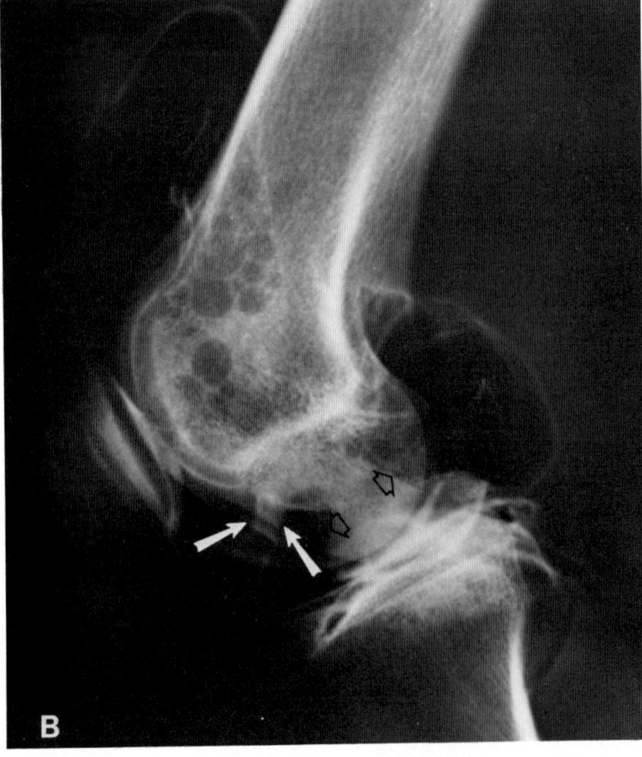

Figure 1.10. Normal cruciate ligaments. *A,* Positive single contrast. *B,* Double contrast. Anterior margin of anterior cruciate (*open arrow*) and posterior margin of posterior cruciate (*open arrow*). The ligamentum mucosum (*arrows*) extends from the infrapatellar fat pad to the intercondylar notch of the femur.

There should be no unexplained filling defects within the joint space which is opacified on the single contrast study and filled with air on the double contrast study. However, bubbles of air coated with contrast may occasionally be seen on a normal double contrast study.

Note. All of the normal and abnormal arthrograms in this chapter are shown with the medial aspect of the joint on the left side of the illustration and the lateral aspect of the joint on the right side. This convention is followed on full views of the knee, separate studies of the menisci, and axial projections of the patella. In most of the cases that are shown here the menisci are illustrated with both positive contrast and double contrast because our clinical studies are conducted by the combined method. The extrameniscal abnormalities are illustrated by the technique that gives the best demonstration.

ABNORMAL KNEE ARTHROGRAM

Meniscal Tears

Meniscal tears can be classified, according to their direction, into three types: longitudinal, transverse, and horizontal. Longitudinal tears are also called concentric tears, and transverse tears are also called radial tears. Longitudinal and transverse tears may be oblique or vertical. In actuality, tears are often complicated, consisting of a combination of the three idealized types, although one type usually predominates. Tears can also be classified according to the region of the meniscus involved. Tears may be confined to the anterior, middle, or posterior zone or may extend into more than one zone. The tear may be at the capsular attachment rather than within the substance of the meniscus. Vertical and oblique tears may extend completely through the meniscus from one surface to the other or may be incomplete and involve only the superior or inferior surface.

In most reported series, tears of the medial meniscus predominate. Smillie reported the incidence of various types of tears and other meniscal lesions in 4500 patients undergoing menisectomy. There were 3198 medial meniscus tears and 671 lateral meniscus tears for a ratio of almost 5 to 1 of medial to lateral tears. Lindblom, in a smaller series, reported a ratio of 3.8 to 1 for medial to lateral tears. Smillie found that a horizontal tear in the posterior segment was the most frequent type of medial meniscus tear (60%), and second most common (26%) was a complete longitudinal tear (the "bucket handle" or "bowstring-type tear"). Tears confined to the anterior segment are unusual and had an incidence of 1% in Smillie's series. The most common (30%) of the lateral meniscus tears is the "parrot beak" tear of the middle third. This is primarily a radial tear beginning at the inner edge, and may also have a longitudinal or horizontal component.

Meniscus lesions in children are often associated with developmental abnormalities. Discoid menisci in particular are prone to tear and may cause symptoms even if intact. In early adulthood, ruptures of the menisci are caused by trauma. In later life degenerative changes in the menisci occur naturally and are not necessarily symptomatic. Recent autopsy studies have shown a high inci-

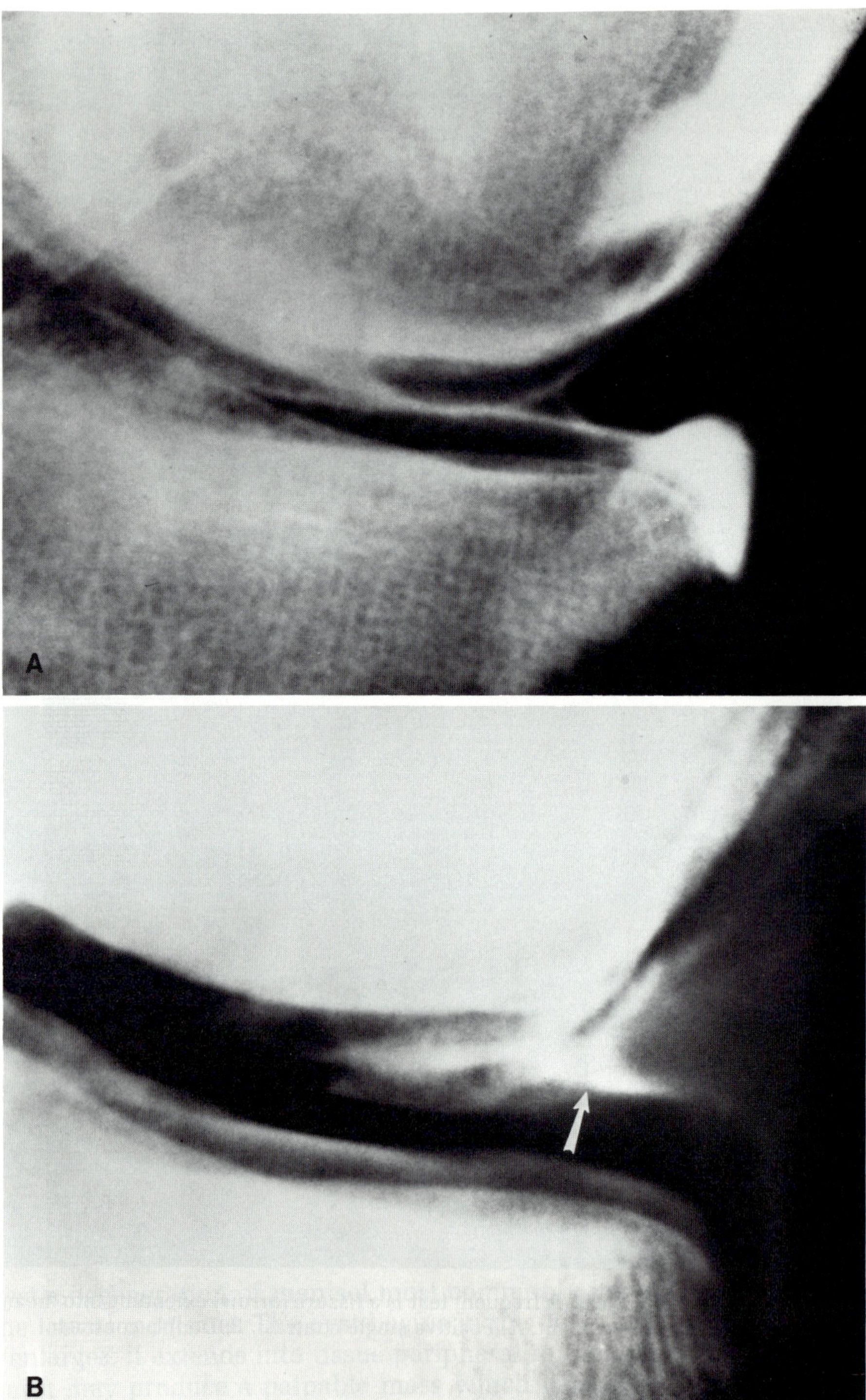

Figure 1.12. Lateral meniscus tear. Vertical tear of lateral meniscus, anteriorly, near inner edge shown on positive contrast (*A*). On the double contrast study (*B*) the inner fragment is white due to imbibed contrast agent (*arrow*).

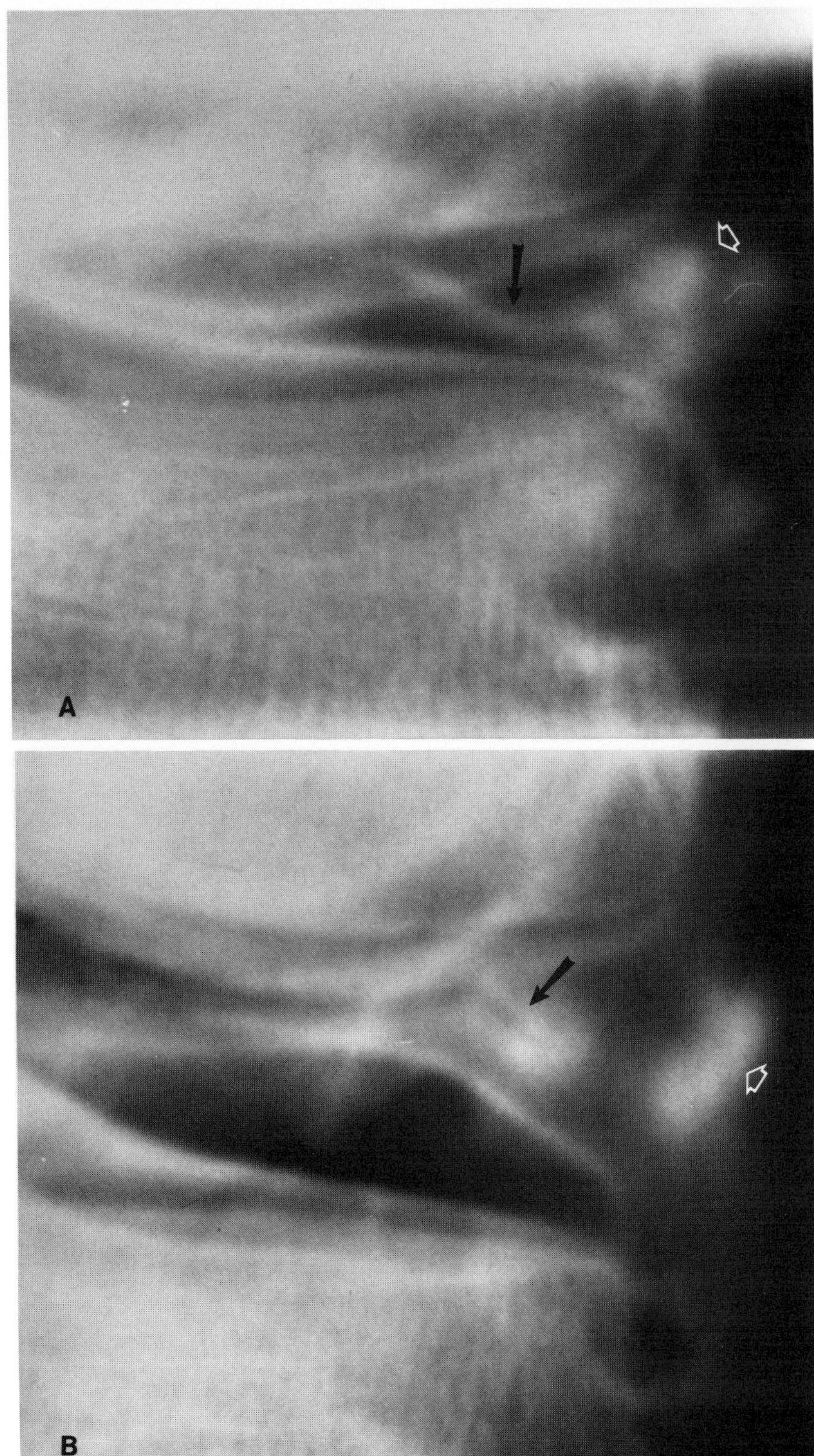

Figure 1.13. Lateral meniscus tear and meniscal cyst. Horizontal tear in midzone (*arrow*) communicates with cyst (*open arrow*) that extends peripheral to the meniscus. *A*, Positive single contrast. *B*, Double contrast.

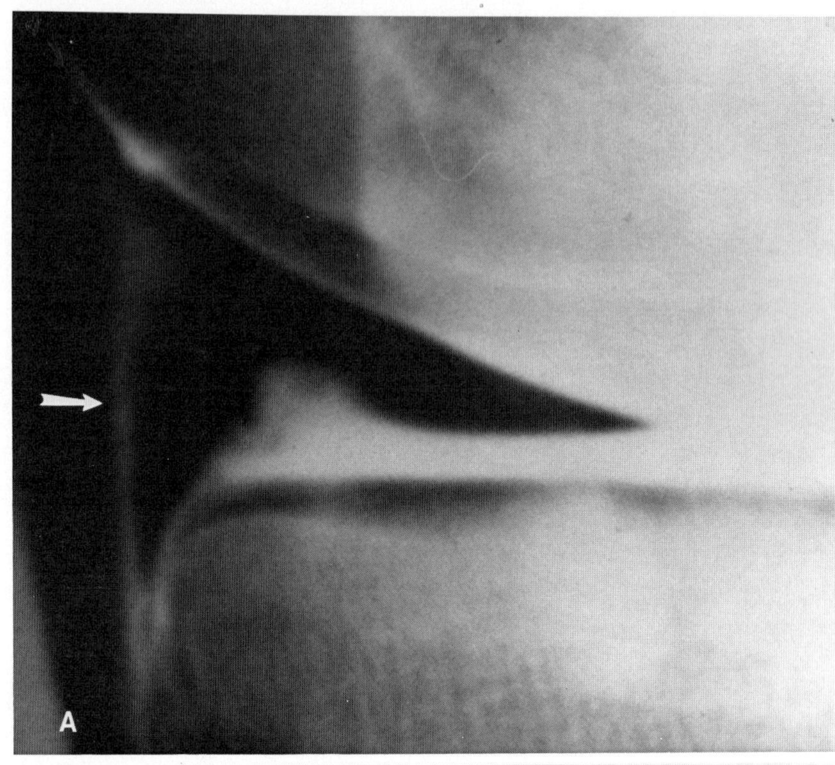

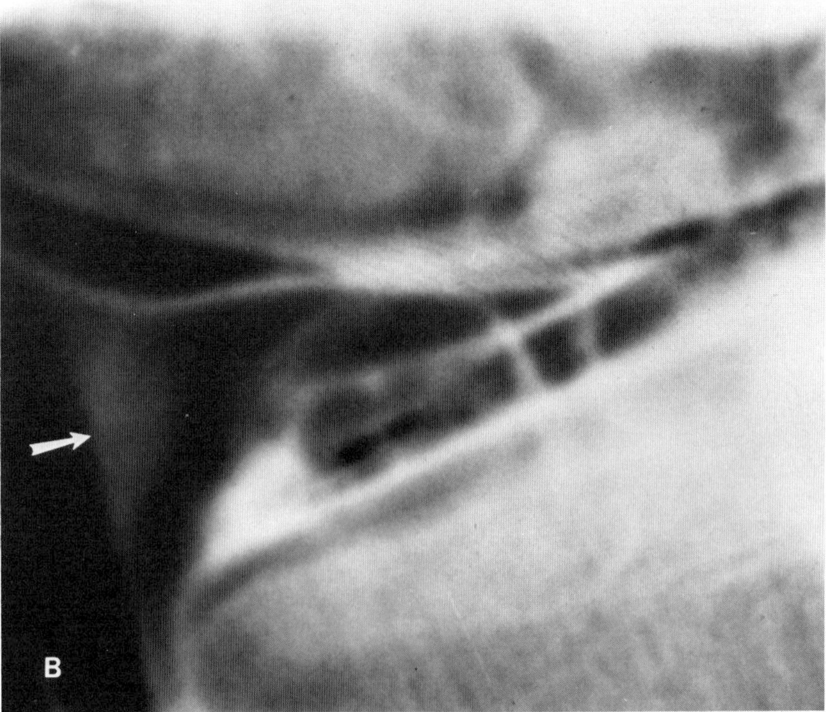

Figure 1.14. Medial meniscus tear. Broad tear of undersurface of medial meniscus, posterior segment. *A,* Positive single contrast. *B,* Double contrast. Note also extravasation of contrast agent indicating medial collateral ligament tear (*arrow*).

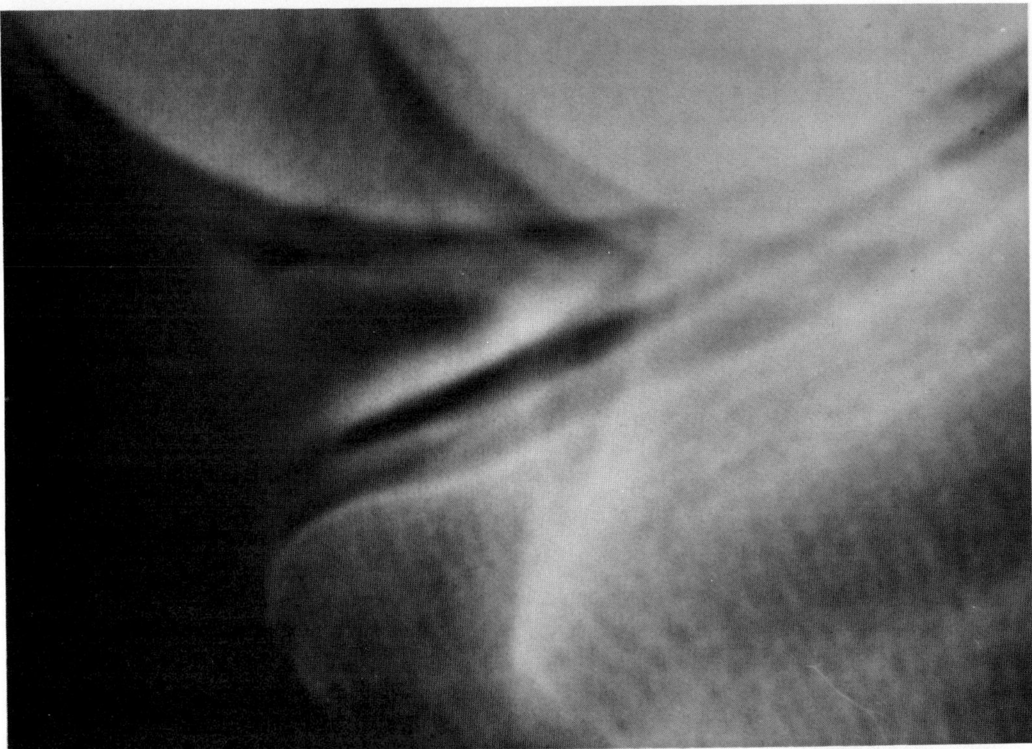

Figure 1.15. Degeneration of medial meniscus, old injury. Undersurface of the degenerated cartilage has imbibed contrast agent. Double contrast study.

extension of the meniscus between the opposing femoral and tibial condyles (Fig. 1.20). A complete discoid meniscus fills the central area where there is normally contact between the femur and the tibia. In cross section it may not taper to a thin inner edge the way a normal meniscus does. An incomplete discoid meniscus is broader than a normal meniscus, particularly in the middle zone, but is less massive than a complete discoid meniscus (Fig. 1.21). The incomplete type has a thin central zone with a tendency to taper toward the inner edge. In 8000 menisectomies, Smillie found discoid menisci in 4% of operated males and 12% of operated females. The abnormality most commonly involves the lateral meniscus. Smillie reported 375 discoid lateral menisci and only five discoid medial menisci.

Ligament Tears

Most ligament tears are capable of being diagnosed by arthrography, so the arthrographer must understand the various types of injuries that may occur. Ligament tears may be either complete or incomplete. Complete rupture of a ligament may be obvious on physical examination. However, the clinical diagnosis of ligament tears is often difficult, leading Smillie to state: "Of the major injuries of the knee those of which concern the ligaments are the most frequently missed or misdiagnosed." The medial collateral and anterior cruciate are the most commonly torn ligaments. Ligament tears are often multiple and the most frequent combination is medial collateral and anterior cruciate. Lateral collateral

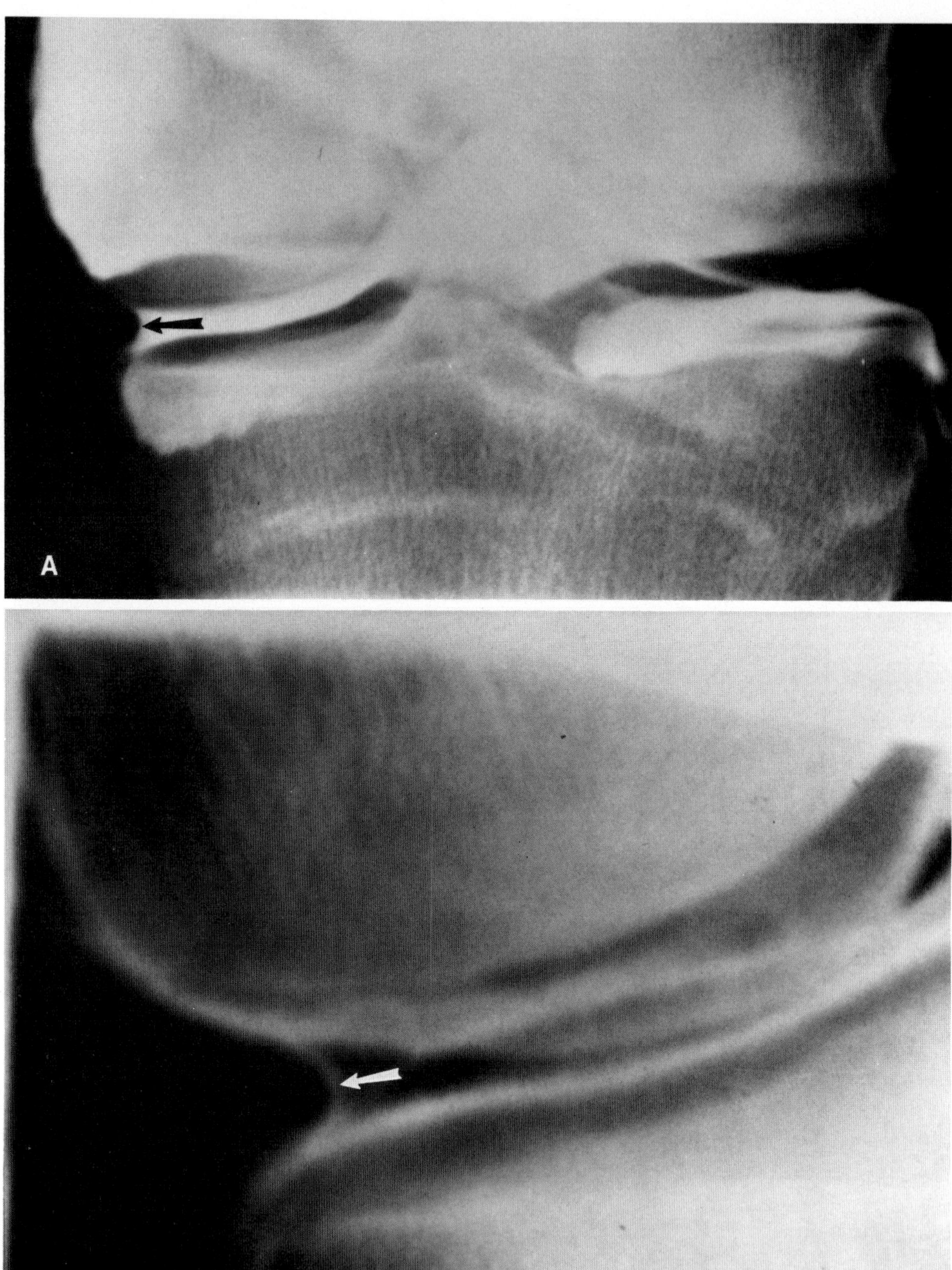

Figure 1.16. Medial meniscus tear. Vertical tear with loss of inner aspect of midzone of meniscus. Displaced meniscus fragment not seen. Blunt edge of the remaining meniscus (*arrow*) is outlined by contrast agent on positive contrast study (*A*) and by air in joint space on double contrast study (*B*).

and posterior cruciate ligament tears may also occur simultaneously. The medial collateral and anterior cruciate ligaments tend to tear at their femoral attachments, whereas tears of the posterior cruciate and fibular collateral ligaments most often occur at their lower attachments. Tears at ligament insertions sometimes result in avulsion of a bone fragment. A tear within the ligament substance can be at one level or at multiple levels. Multiple "microtears" producing a stretching of the ligament are particularly common in the anterior cruciate.

The usual radiographic sign of a complete collateral ligament tear is widening of the affected half of the joint upon the application of stress. With a partial medial collateral ligament tear, contrast leaks from the joint in the vicinity of the ligament usually superior to the joint line. The extravasated contrast travels along the deep fibers of the ligament or may opacify a space between the deep and superficial portions of the ligament. Lateral collateral ligament tears are rarely diagnosed by arthrography.

With complete anterior cruciate ligament tear, the normal anterior margin may be absent on the arthrogram (Fig. 1.22). However, if the synovial covering over the anterior surface of a torn ligament remains intact, then a distinct anterior margin of the ligament will be visible. Despite this, in most cases where the ligament is significantly torn, the arthrogram will show a posterior bowing or concavity of its anterior margin that persists when stress is applied to distract the tibia from the femur (Fig. 1.23). The application of such stress to a normal cruciate ligament causes its anterior synovial covering to become taut and straight. A posterior cruciate tear is difficult to diagnose because even a normal ligament may be indistinct on the arthrogram.

The so-called coronary ligament tear is a rupture of the capsule inferior to a meniscus, usually the medial. The attachment of the meniscus to the tibia is loosened (Fig. 1.24). Immobilization of the knee facilitates healing, and may allow spontaneous reattachment of the meniscus to the tibia. If arthrography were performed immediately following the injury, there might be a leak of contrast from the joint into the capsular tear. However, the usual arthrographic finding when the coronary ligament of the medial meniscus is torn is an obliteration of the normally occurring shallow capsular recess located at the edge of the tibial condyle beneath the meniscus. This is due to filling of the recess by granulation tissue arising from the injured synovium and capsule. The examiner must be aware that a normal capsular recess may fail to opacify if there is inadequate dispersal of contrast agent beneath the meniscus.

An extensive tear of the posterior capsule may lead to hyperextensibility of the knee and require surgical repair. Other ligament tears are usually associated with this lesion. Traumatic dislocation of the patella tears the medial patellar retinaculum, faulty healing of which can lead to recurrent dislocation. If the capsule is torn and the synovial defect has not yet sealed, then the arthrogram will show an extravasation of contrast material. However, extravasation is sometimes due to overfilling of the joint with the positive contrast agent or air during the arthrogram rather than being due to previous trauma.

Chondromalacia of Patella

In the early stage of this condition there is a localized softening and edema of the articular cartilage with fissuring of its surface. This shows on the double

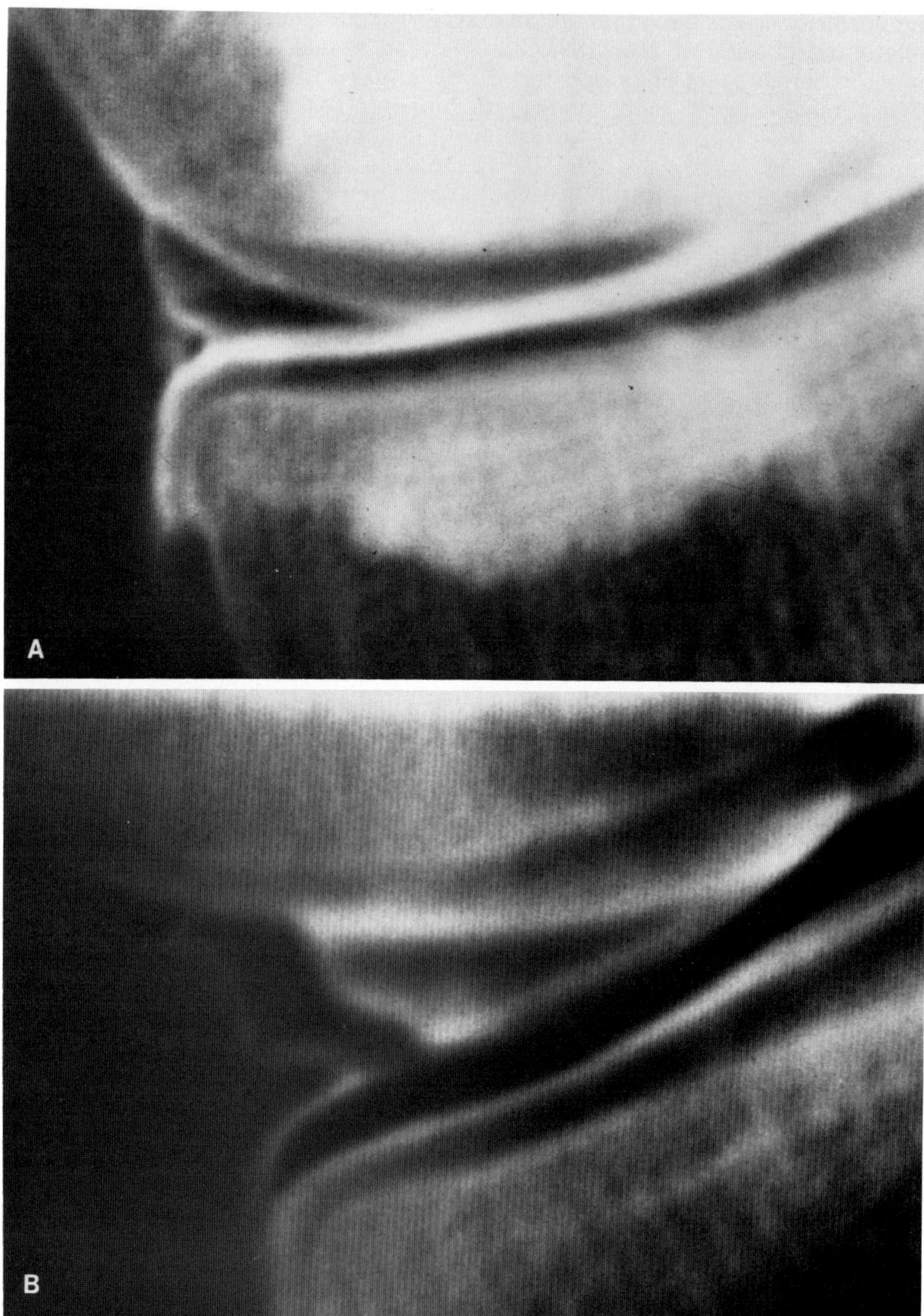

Figure 1.17. Medial meniscus Bucket handle tears. Comparison of positive single contrast (*A*) and double contrast (*B*) of the same case with separation of fragments only on double contrast study. Different case in which the torn edge of the peripheral fragment (*arrow*) is seen with double contrast (*C*) and the displaced fragment (*open arrows*) is seen best on notch view (*D*).

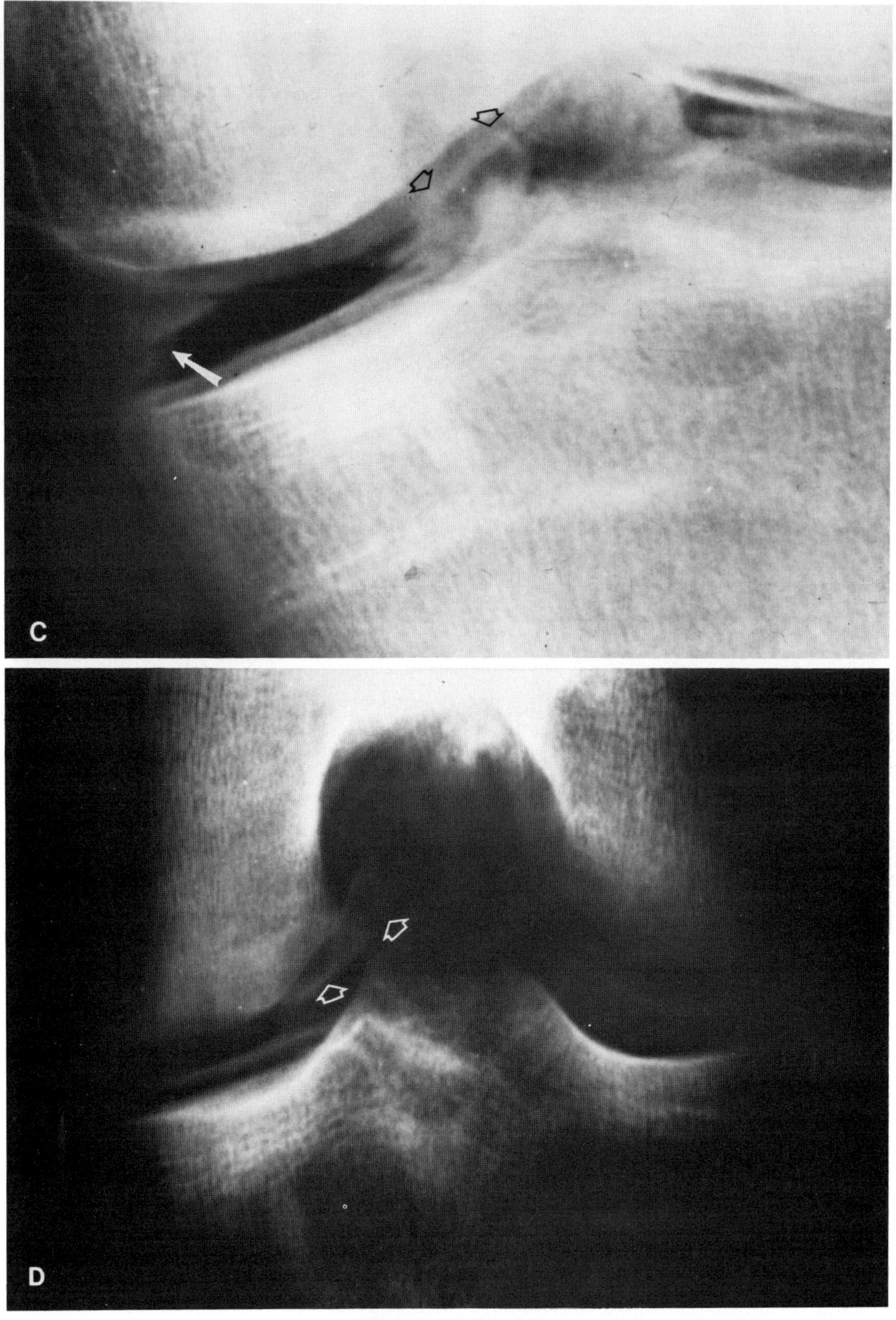

Figure 1.17 *C* and *D*

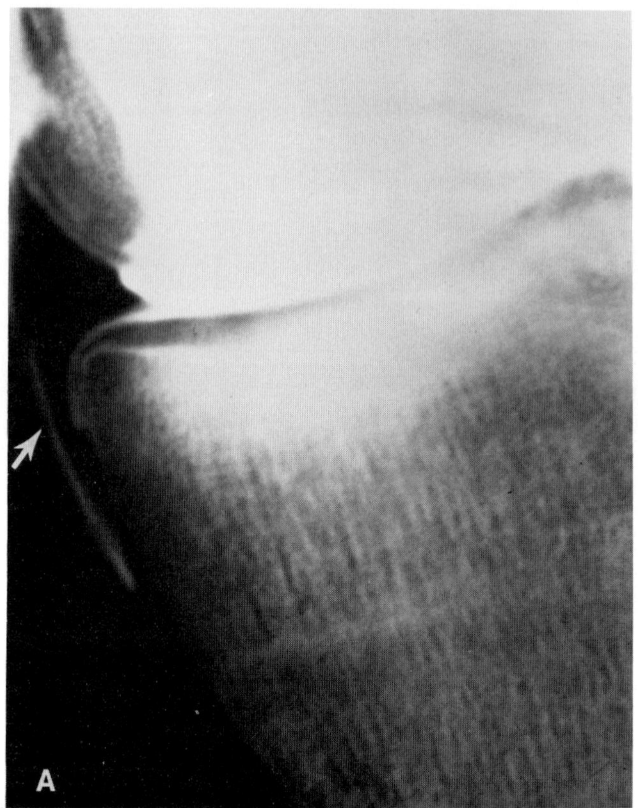

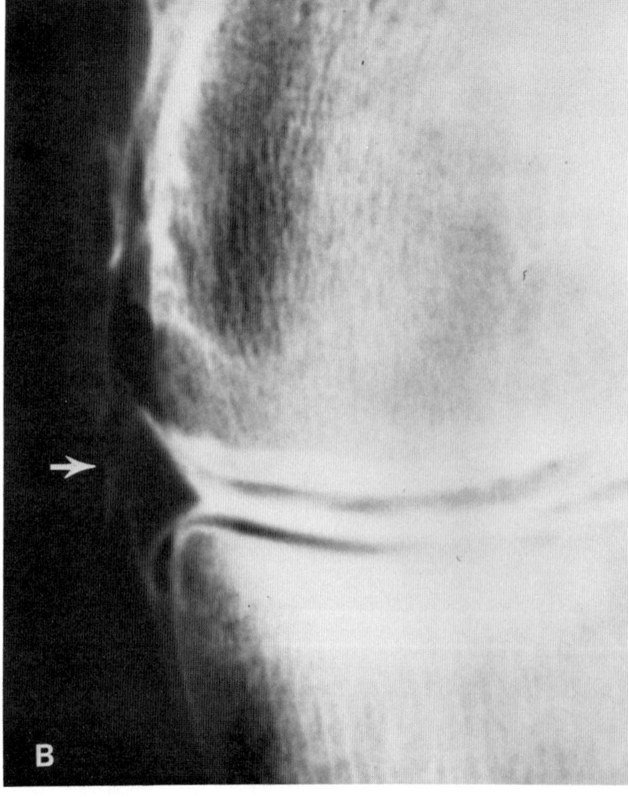

Figure 1.18. Peripheral tear of medial meniscus. Meniscus is detached from the capsule and there is extravasation (*arrow*) along the medial collateral ligament. *A*, Positive single contrast. *B*, Double contrast.

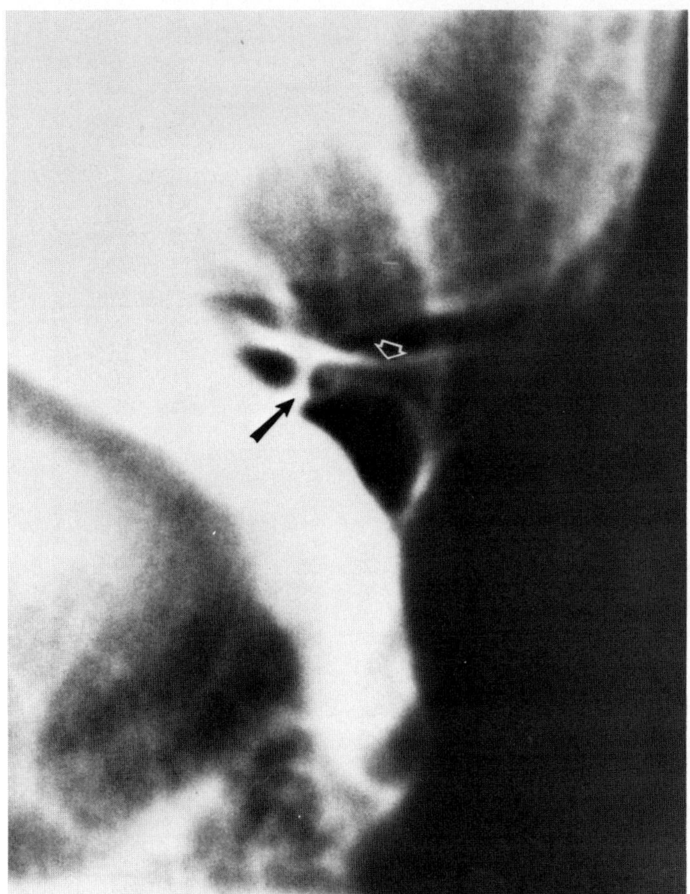

Figure 1.19. Lateral meniscus tear with partial peripheral detachment. On double contrast study note vertical meniscus tear filled with contrast agent (*arrow*) intact superior strut (*open arrow*) and absence of inferior strut due to rupture.

contrast arthrogram as localized surface irregularity and imbibition of contrast by the superficial layer of the cartilage. The early lesions are usually confined to only one facet. With progression the extent of the lesion increases, and flaking of the cartilage produces more irregularity and imbibition. Sometimes marked thickening of the cartilage occurs. Finally, the cartilage becomes worn thin (Figs. 1.25, 1.26, and 1.27). In a severe case the bone of the patella may be exposed. In degenerative joint disease there may be thinning of the patellar cartilage accompanying the condylar cartilage erosions (Fig. 1.28).

Condylar Articular Cartilage Degeneration

Degeneration of the femoral or tibial articular cartilage is a process similar to chondromalacia of the patella. Softening and fissuring of the cartilage is followed by erosion. Arthrography shows surface irregularity, contrast imbibition, and thinning of the affected cartilage on the condylar surface (Fig. 1.29). Swelling of affected cartilage is rarely seen on the condyles. Subchondral bone sclerosis and hypertrophic bony spurs are frequent, and subchondral cysts may be present. Articular cartilage degeneration and erosion are the beginning stages of osteoarthritis of the knee. This process can be caused by chronic trauma to

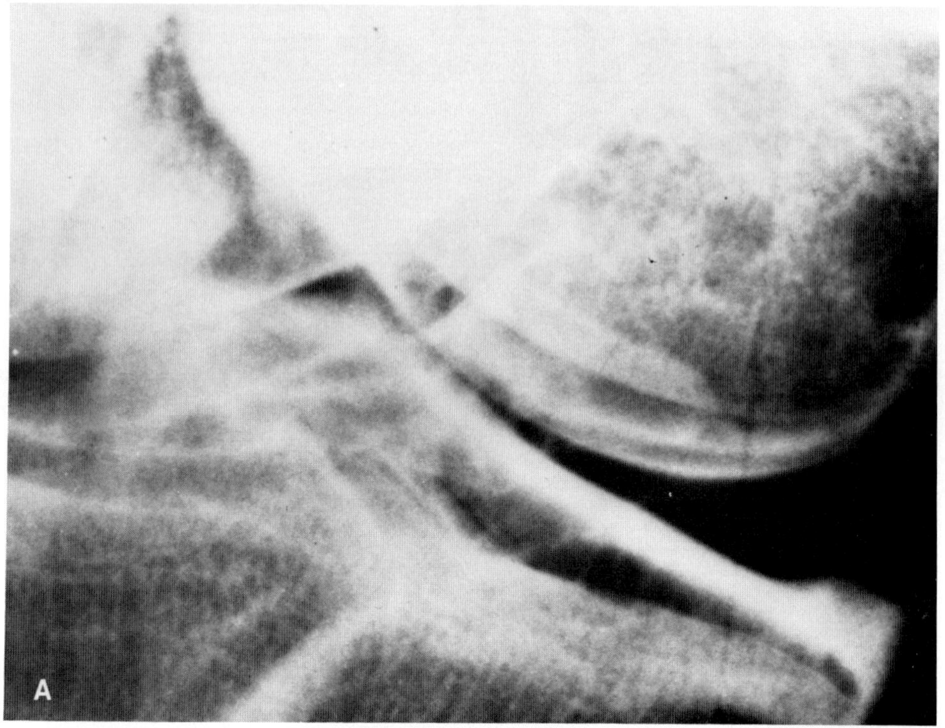

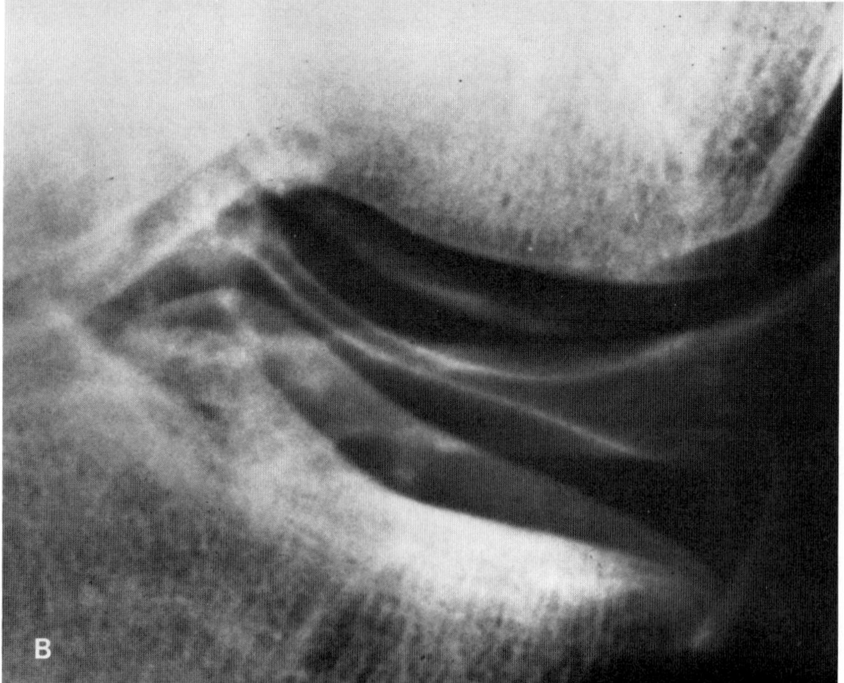

Figure 1.20. Discoid lateral meniscus. *A,* Positive single contrast study. *B,* Double contrast.

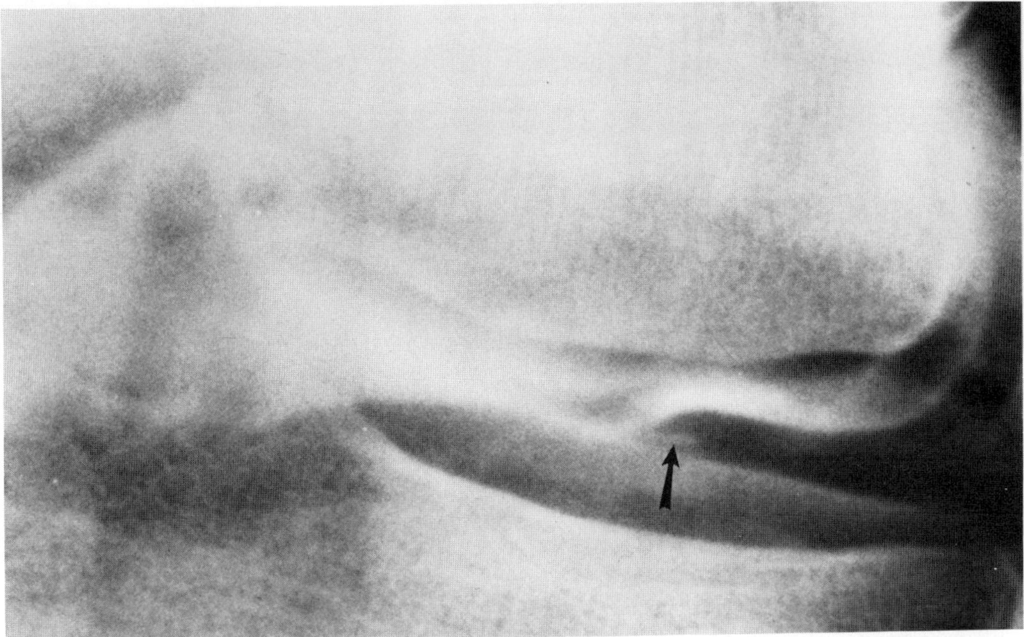

Figure 1.21. Incomplete discoid lateral meniscus with tear. Single contrast study shows blunt abnormally wide meniscus with small horizontal tear (*arrow*).

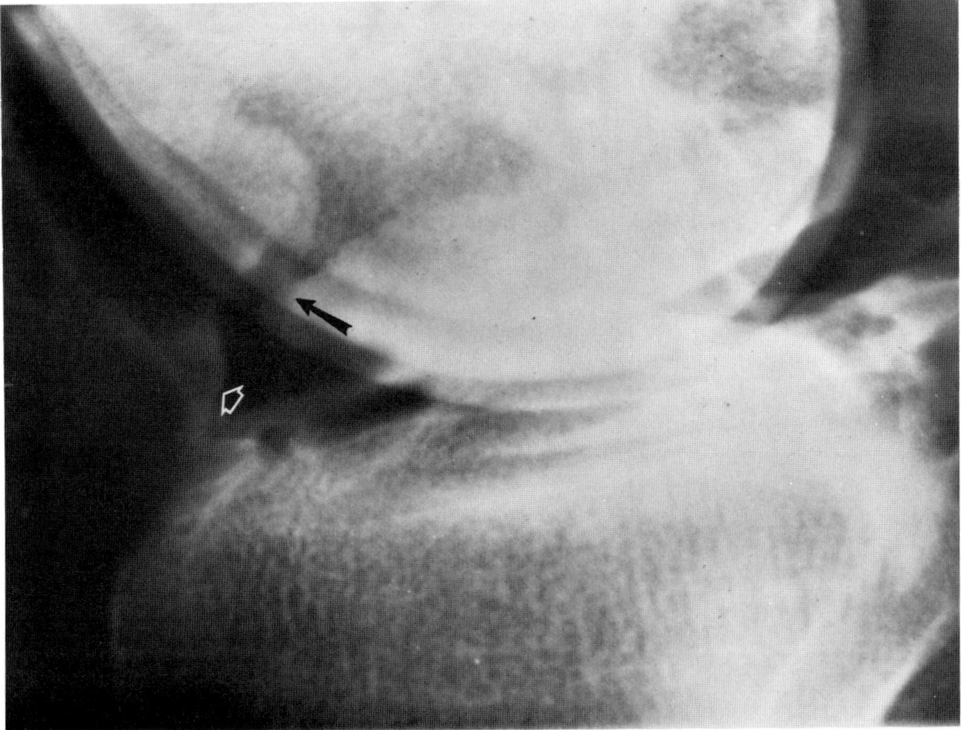

Figure 1.22. Anterior cruciate tear. Loss of normal straight margin of the ligament. Note the irregular edge of the retracted torn ligament (*arrow*). The infrapatellar fat pad is seen (*open arrow*).

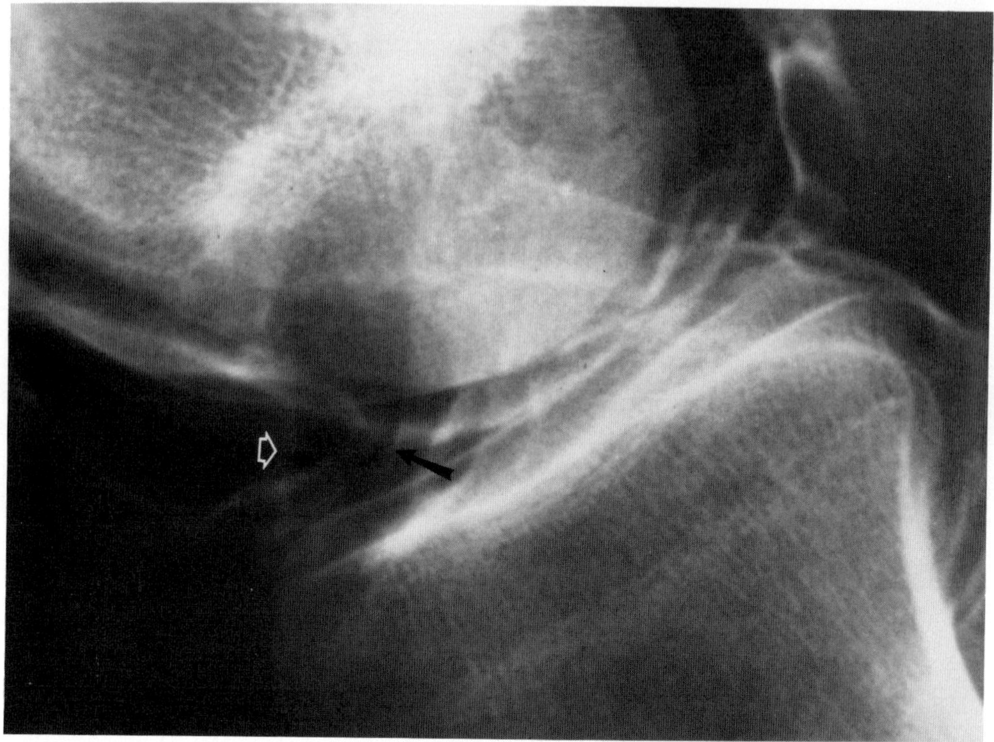

Figure 1.23. Anterior cruciate tear. Posterior bowing of the ligament (*arrow*). Note posterior margin of ligamentum mucosum (*open arrow*).

the articular cartilage from a torn meniscus. Abnormal mechanical stresses on the condylar surfaces due to ligamentous instability, with varus or valgus deformities of the knee, or following meniscectomy can cause articular cartilage degeneration and osteoarthritis. There is individual variation in the naturally occurring articular cartilage degeneration that accompanies aging.

Osteochondral Fracture

Fracture of an articular surface can involve the cartilage only (Fig. 1.30) or the cartilage and underlying bone. These fractures are often unrecognized. If a free fragment is produced it may consist of cartilage alone or cartilage attached to a small piece of bone. Plain radiographs will not show a pure cartilage fracture. Even in osteochondral fractures, a small piece of loose subchondral bone and the defect in the articular cortex are often difficult to see on plain films. However, the defect in the articular cartilage and bone is usually visible on the arthrogram. The free fragment may be seen within the joint space, and the size of the cartilaginous component of the fragment may be estimated (Fig. 1.31).

Osteochondritis Dissecans

This condition is an aseptic necrosis, probably of traumatic origin, that affects an articular surface. The lesion may remain confined to the bone and may be

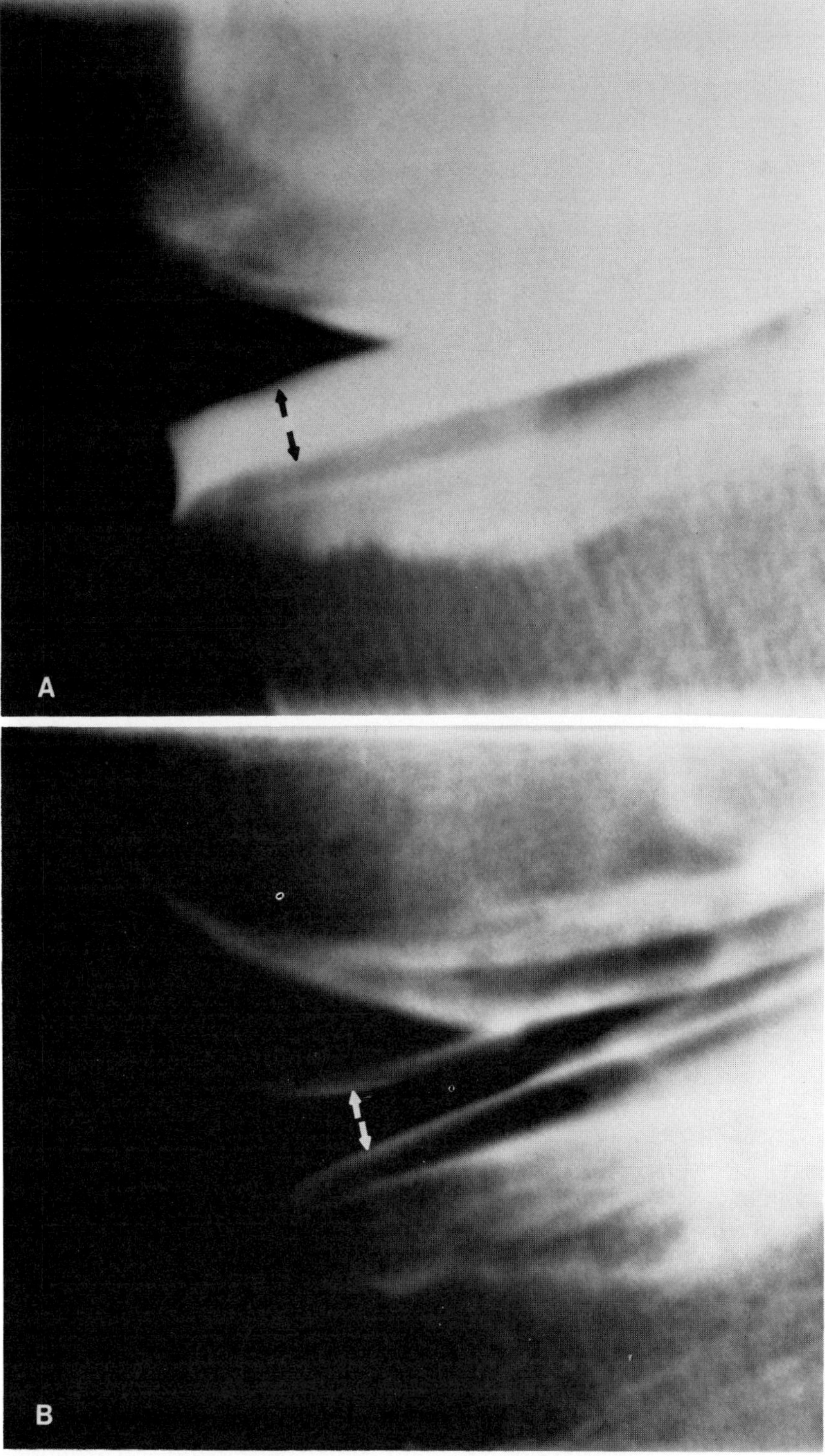

Figure 1.24. Coronary ligament tear. There is abnormal separation between the medial meniscus and the tibial surface due to laxity of capsular attachment of the meniscus to the tibia (*arrows*). *A*, Positive single contrast. *B*, Double contrast.

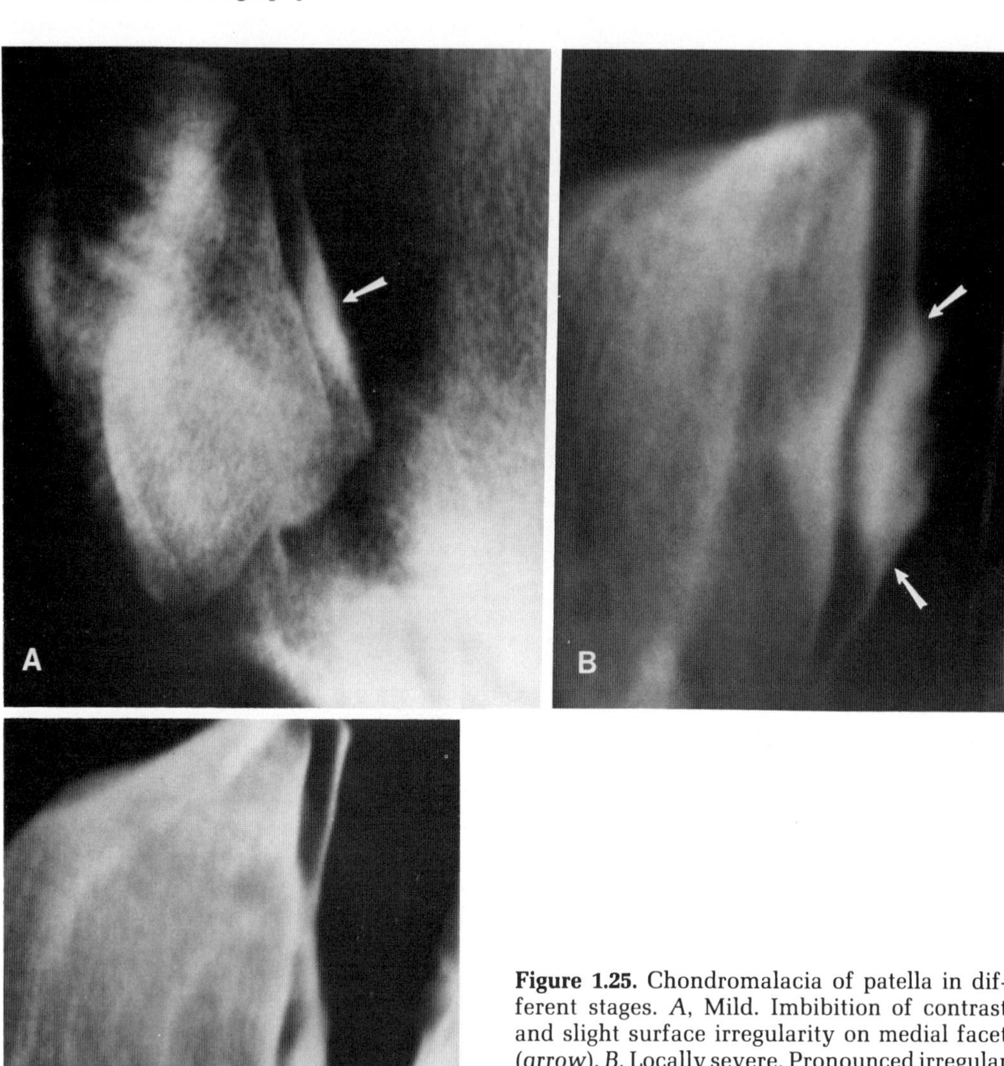

Figure 1.25. Chondromalacia of patella in different stages. *A,* Mild. Imbibition of contrast and slight surface irregularity on medial facet (*arrow*). *B,* Locally severe. Pronounced irregular thickening and imbibition of contrast (*between arrows*) on lateral facet. *C,* Moderately advanced. Cartilage of lateral facet is thin, irregular and stained with contrast. Cartilage remains normal at top of patella.

covered by intact articular cartilage. More often the affected bone becomes separated along with its attached cartilage. This osteochondral fragment may remain as a plug in the resultant crater in the articular surface, or complete detachment may occur, with a resultant intraarticular loose body (joint mouse).

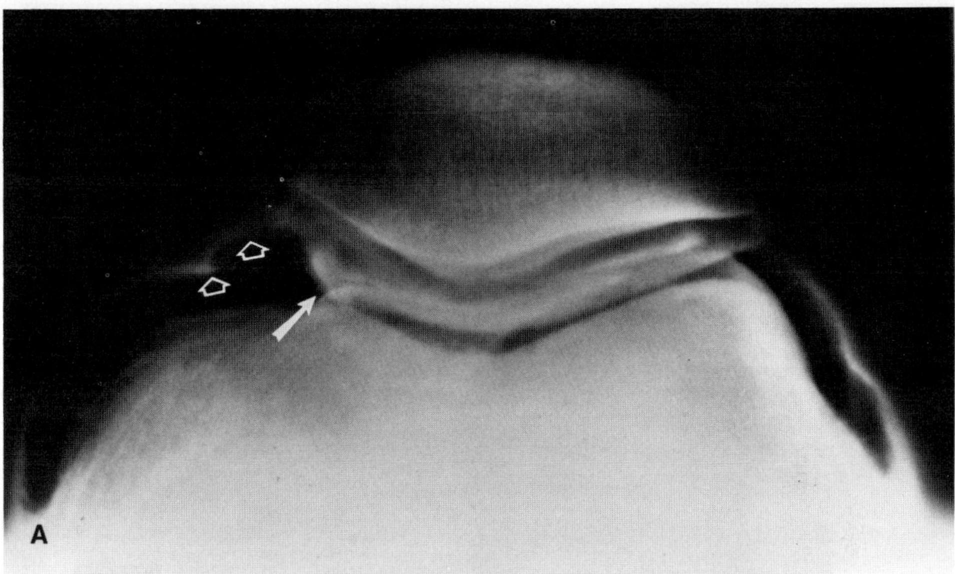

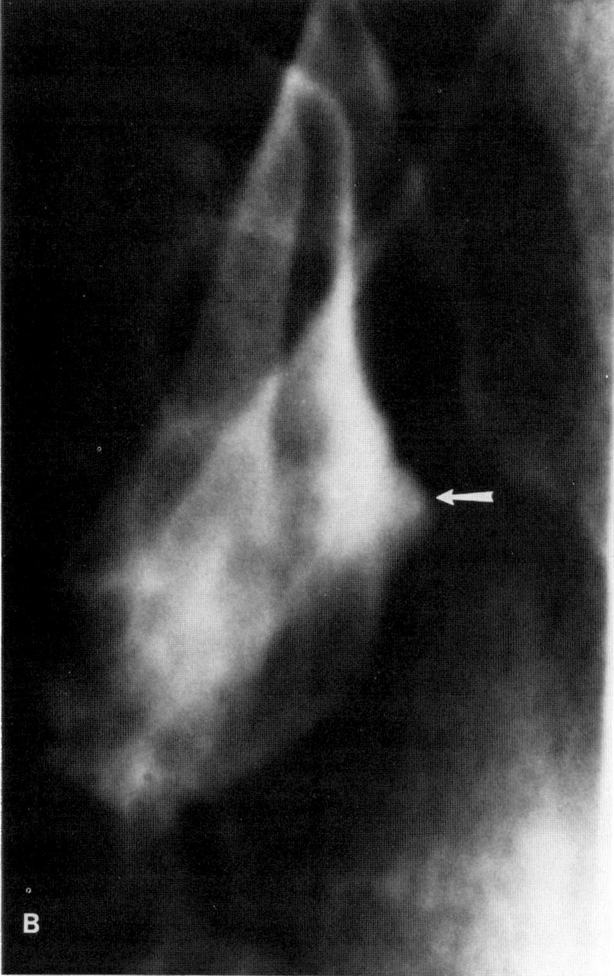

Figure 1.26. Chondromalacia of patella, same case in different projections. Localized contrast imbibition and thickening of cartilage on medial facet (*arrow*) seen in axial view (*A*) and lateral view (*B*). Note normal lateral patellar synovial fold and irregularity of medial fold (*open arrows*).

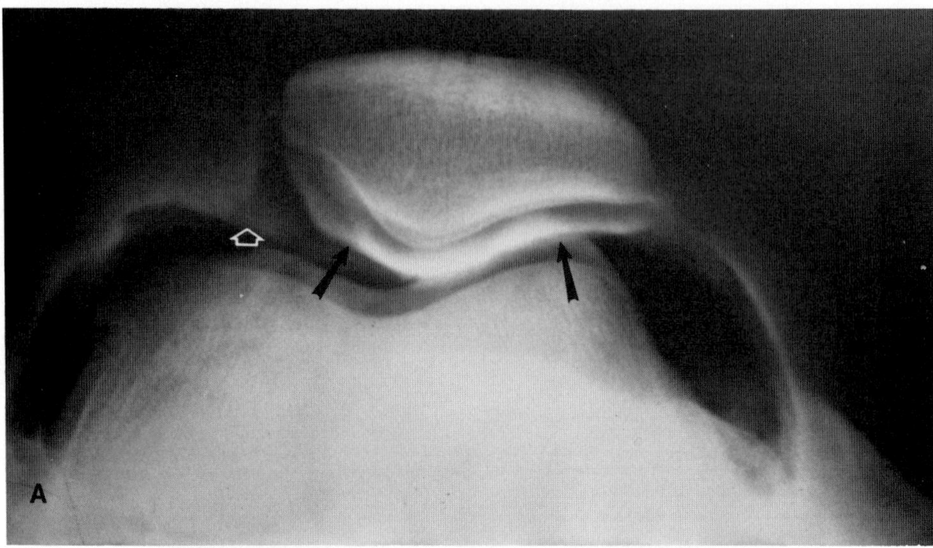

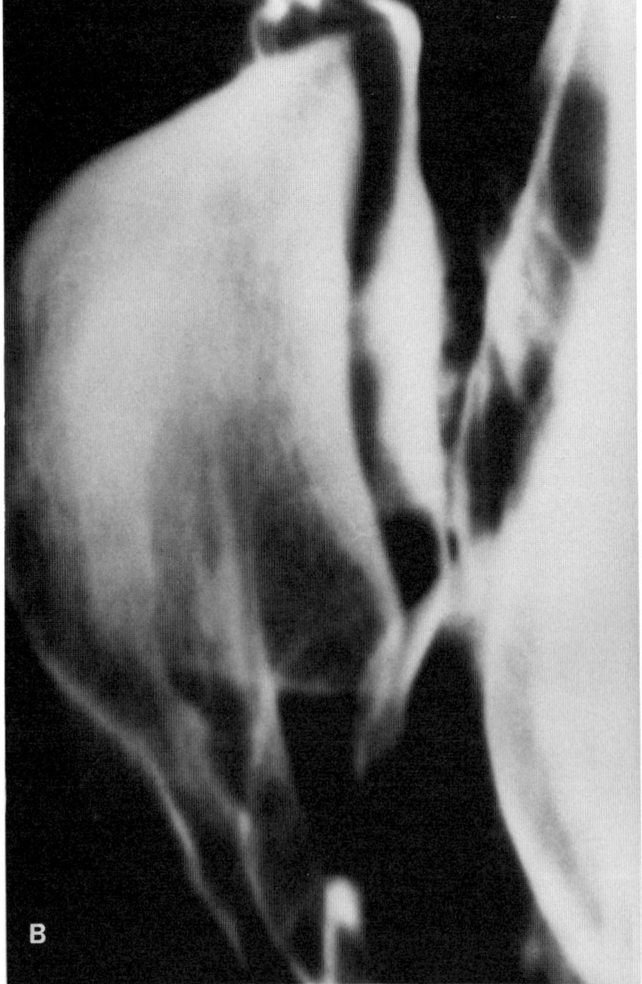

Figure 1.27. Chondromalacia of patella, same case in different projections. *A,* Axial view demonstrates that the cartilage of the ridge and lateral facet has imbibed contrast agent (*between arrows*). *B,* Lateral view of lateral facet demonstrates irregularity of cartilage with imbibition. In (*A*) note the malalignment of patella, the thick medial patellar synovial fold (*open arrow*), and the normal femoral cartilage.

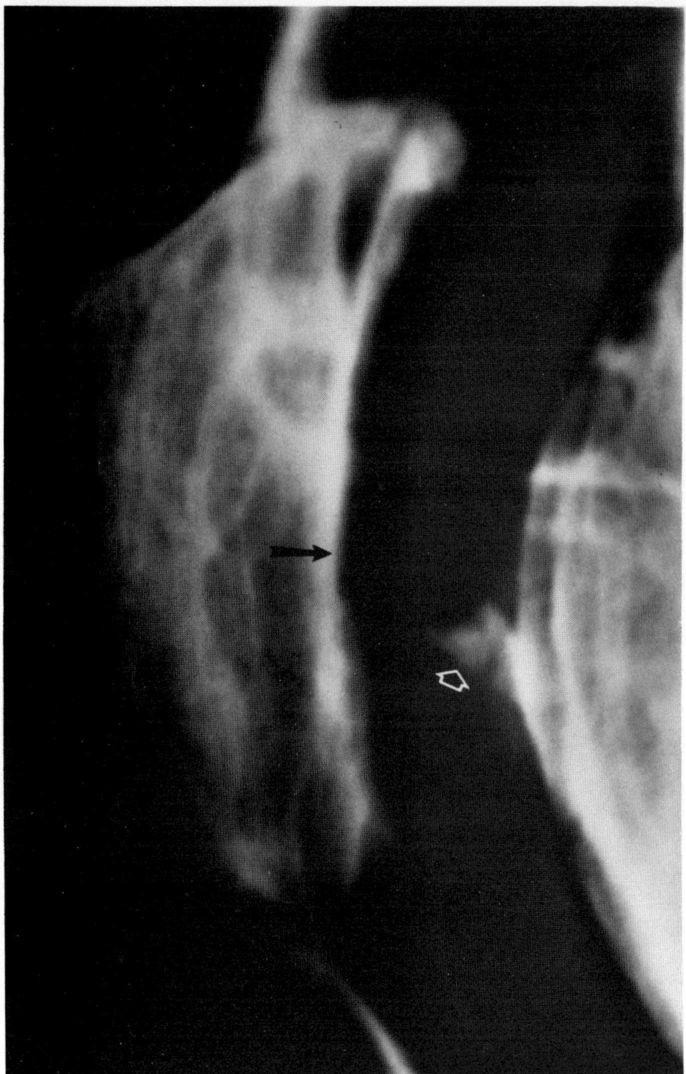

Figure 1.28. Severe erosion of patellar cartilage in degenerative joint disease. Almost complete loss of cartilage with exposure of bone (*arrow*) and small amount of residual cartilage near top and bottom of patella. Note loose cartilage fragment in joint space (*open arrow*).

The most common site of the disease is the lateral aspect of the medial condyle.

The arthrogram gives valuable information regarding the condition of the articular surface in the affected area. It may show that the cartilage overlying the lesion remains intact or that the surface has been restored because the defect has filled with scar tissue or fibrocartilage (Fig. 1.32). A defect in the articular surface will be visible if projected in profile (Fig. 1.33A). If the osteocartilaginous fragment remains in situ, then the arthrogram may help determine the extent of its attachment to the walls of the defect (Fig. 1.33B).

Loose Bodies

There are many causes of intraarticular loose bodies: osteochondritis dissecans (Fig. 1.33B), osteochondral fractures (Fig. 1.31), and degenerative joint disease (Fig. 1.28) are frequently responsible. Chondromalacia, meniscal tears,

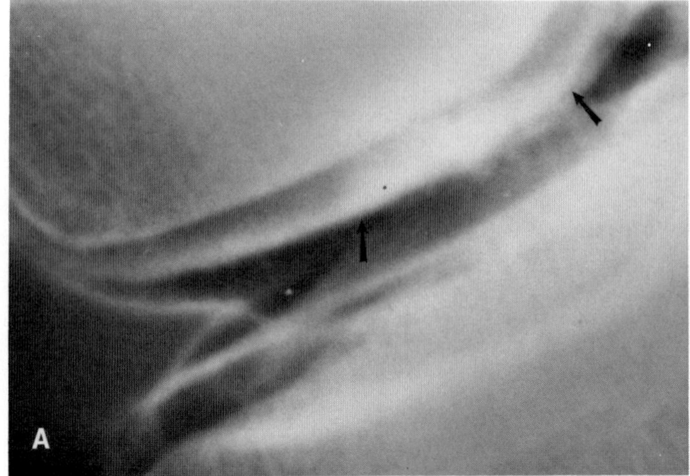

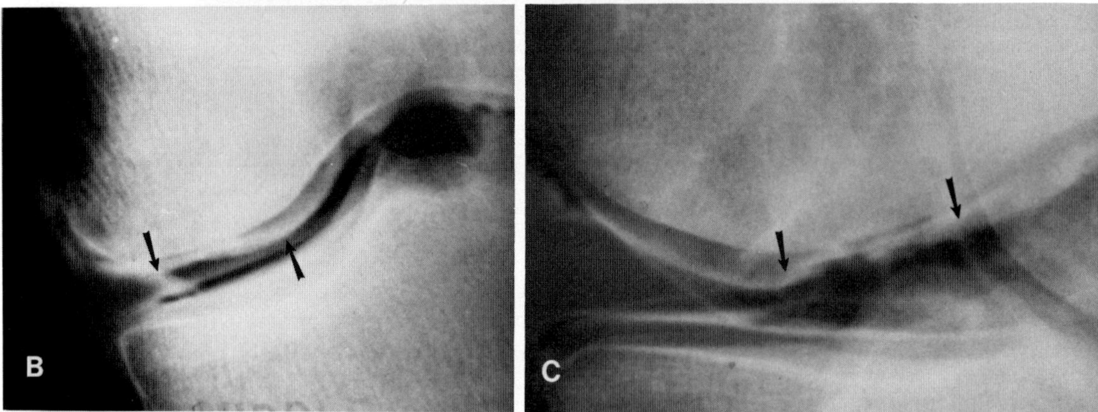

Figure 1.29. Condylar articular cartilage degeneration. *A,* Chondromalacia causing imbibition of contrast (*between arrows*). *B,* Chondromalacia and thinning of cartilage (*between arrows*). *C,* Large defect in cartilage (*between arrows*) due to either fracture or degeneration with erosion.

and synovial chondromatosis are other possible causes. Some loose bodies are calcified while others, consisting of only cartilage, may originally be uncalcified and in time may undergo calcification or ossification. Plain films are valuable in detection of calcified joint bodies. With positive contrast or double contrast arthrography, joint bodies appear as free filling defects within the joint space. The common sites of joint bodies are the intercondylar notch, suprapatellar recess, and medial and lateral gutters. Small bodies are frequently found at the periphery of the inferior joint line, wedged between the meniscus and tibia, particularly at the anterior horn of the lateral meniscus. Occasionally air arthrography is useful in the detection of small joint bodies that may be obscured on the positive contrast study or confused with bubbles on the double contrast study.

Synovial Diseases

Many conditions that affect the synovium of the knee do not produce characteristic arthrographic findings. These include acute infective arthritis and

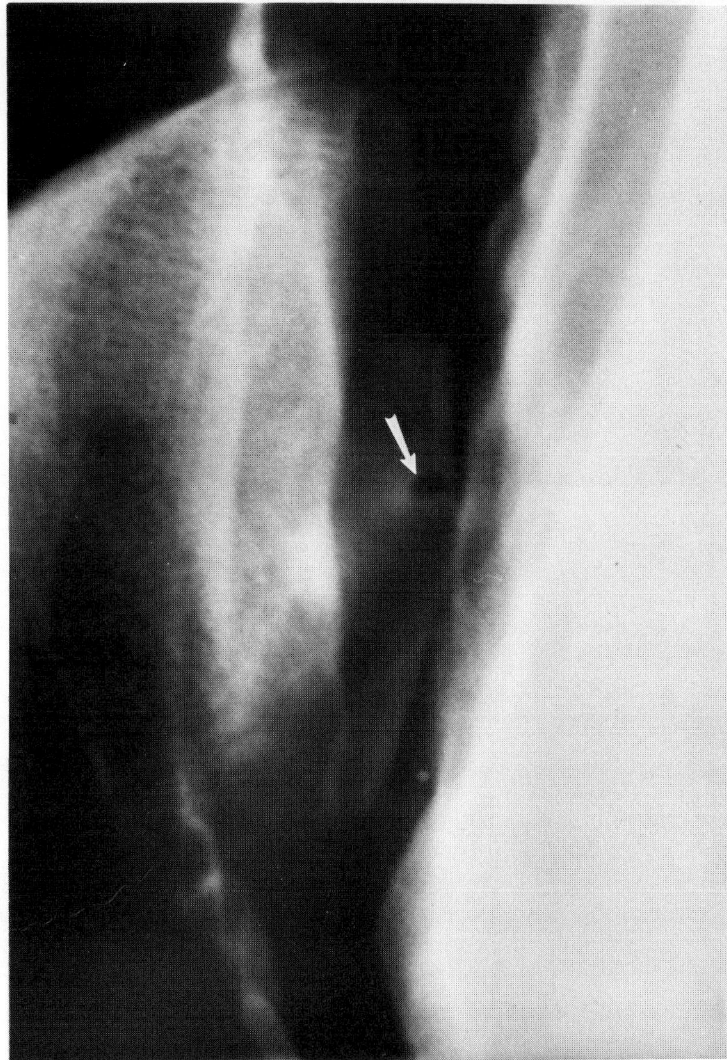

Figure 1.30. Chondral fracture. Fissure in patellar cartilage caused by a blow to the patella (*arrow*).

posttraumatic effusion. In some diseases of the synovium the plain film findings are more helpful, *i.e.,* rheumatoid arthritis, gout, and calcium pyrophosphate deposition disease.

There are some rare diseases affecting the synovium of which the arthrographer should be aware: chronic synovitis due to *tuberculosis* or *fungal disease* may cause marked irregular synovial thickening. In *pigmented villonodular synovitis* or nonpigmented *villous synovitis* there may be local or diffuse synovial thickening. In the pigmented disease there is iron deposition and the knee and tendon sheaths of the fingers are the usual sites. *Synovial chondromatosis* is a benign condition due to cartilage metaplasia of the synovium and subsynovial tissue. It most commonly affects the bursae about the knee, producing multiple raised nodules of cartilage that often calcify and may become

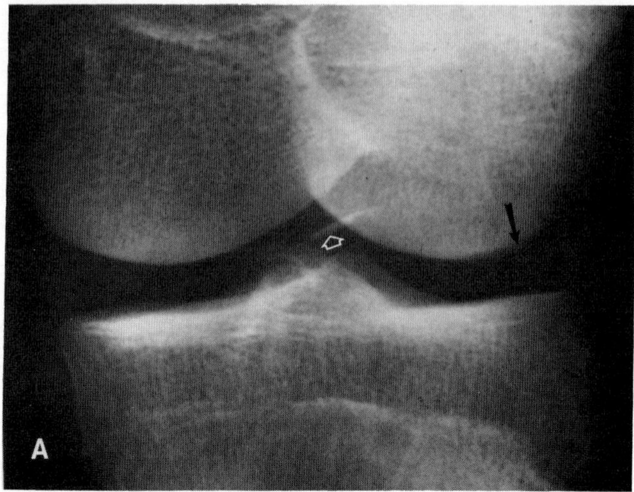

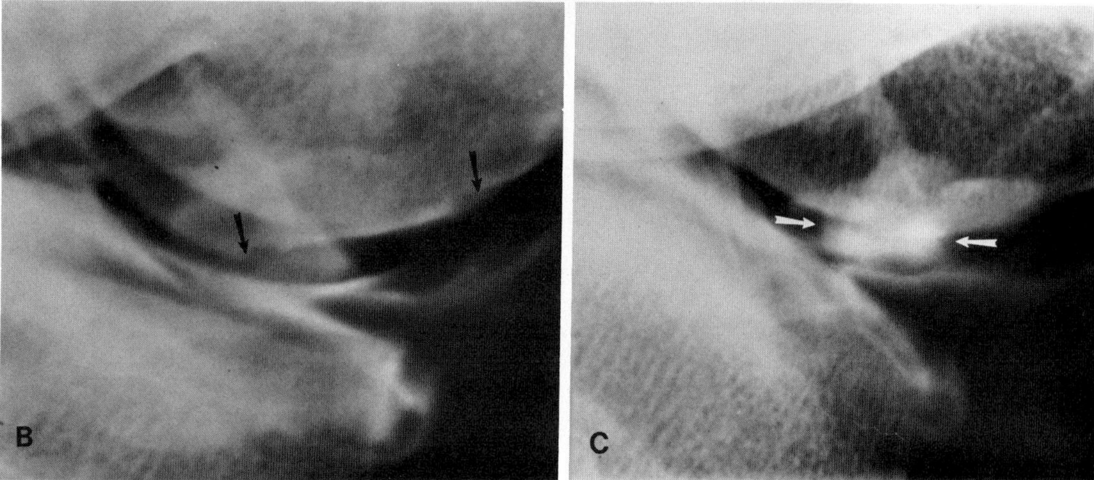

Figure 1.31. Osteochondral fracture. *A,* Preliminary film shows fracture defect of articular cortex (*arrow*) and loose bone fragment in joint (*open arrow*). *B,* Double contrast arthrogram demonstrates the cartilage defect (*arrows*). *C,* Different view of the anterolateral joint space demonstrates better the large cartilagenous loose body (*arrows*).

detached. *Hemangioma* of the synovium of the knee may be localized or diffuse. Smillie found skin involvement in each of his cases of diffuse synovial hemangioma.

The above mentioned synovial proliferative diseases can be demonstrated by arthrography. The synovial thickening in chronic inflammatory synovitis, pigmented villonodular synovitis (Fig. 1.34), villous synovitis, synovial chondromatosis and osteochondromatosis (see Prager and Mall), rheumatoid arthritis (Fig. 1.35), synovial hemangioma, other tumors, and hemophilic arthritis produce filling defects arising from the synovial surfaces of the joint and bursae. Bubbles of contrast agent may simulate filling defects on the double contrast arthrogram. Synovial inflammation, including rheumatoid arthritis, can produce lymphatic opacification during arthrography (Fig. 1.36).

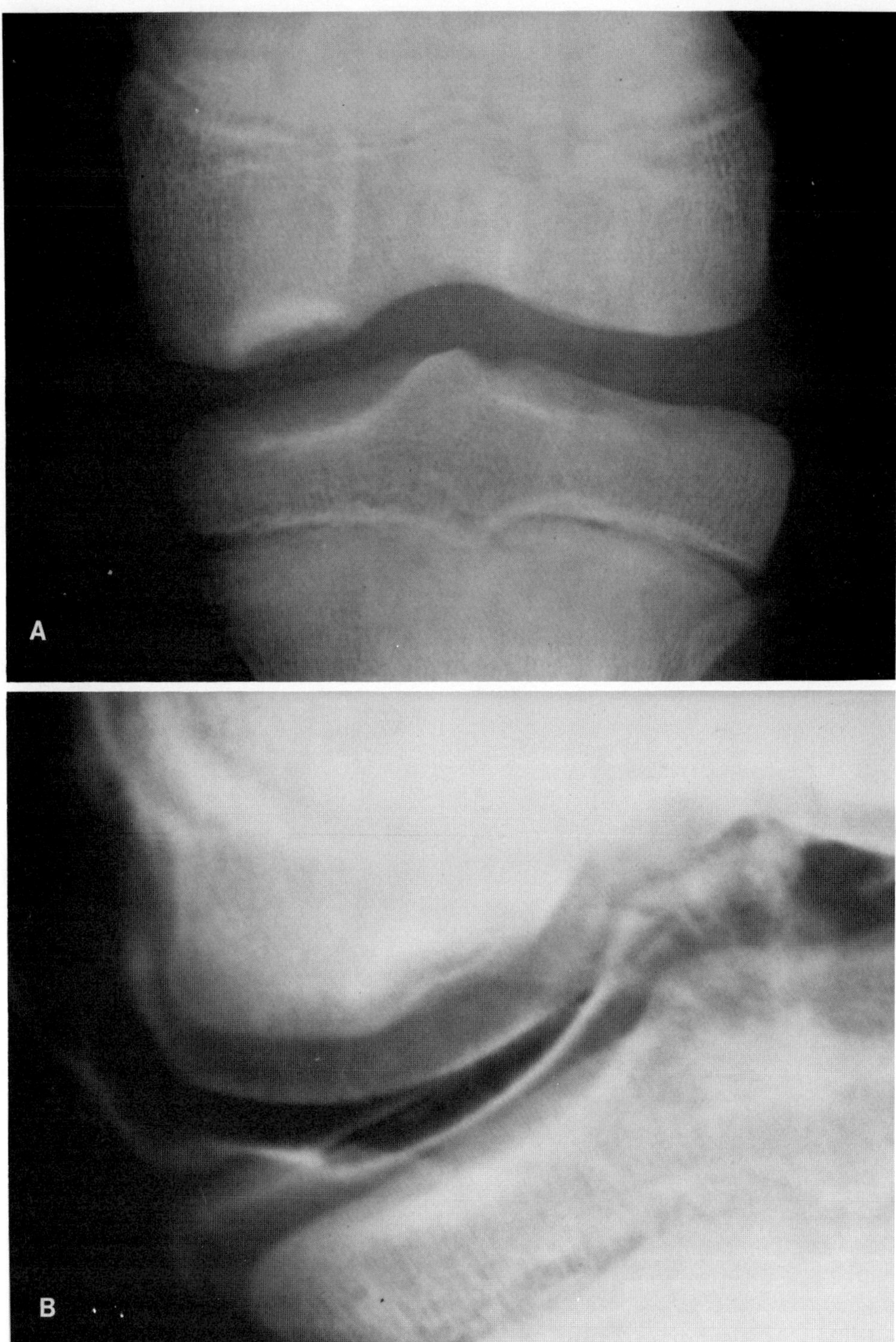

Figure 1.32. Osteochondritis with either uninvolved or completely healed articular cartilage. *A,* Preliminary film shows typical defect in the medial femoral condyle. *B,* Normal surface of cartilage seen on arthrogram.

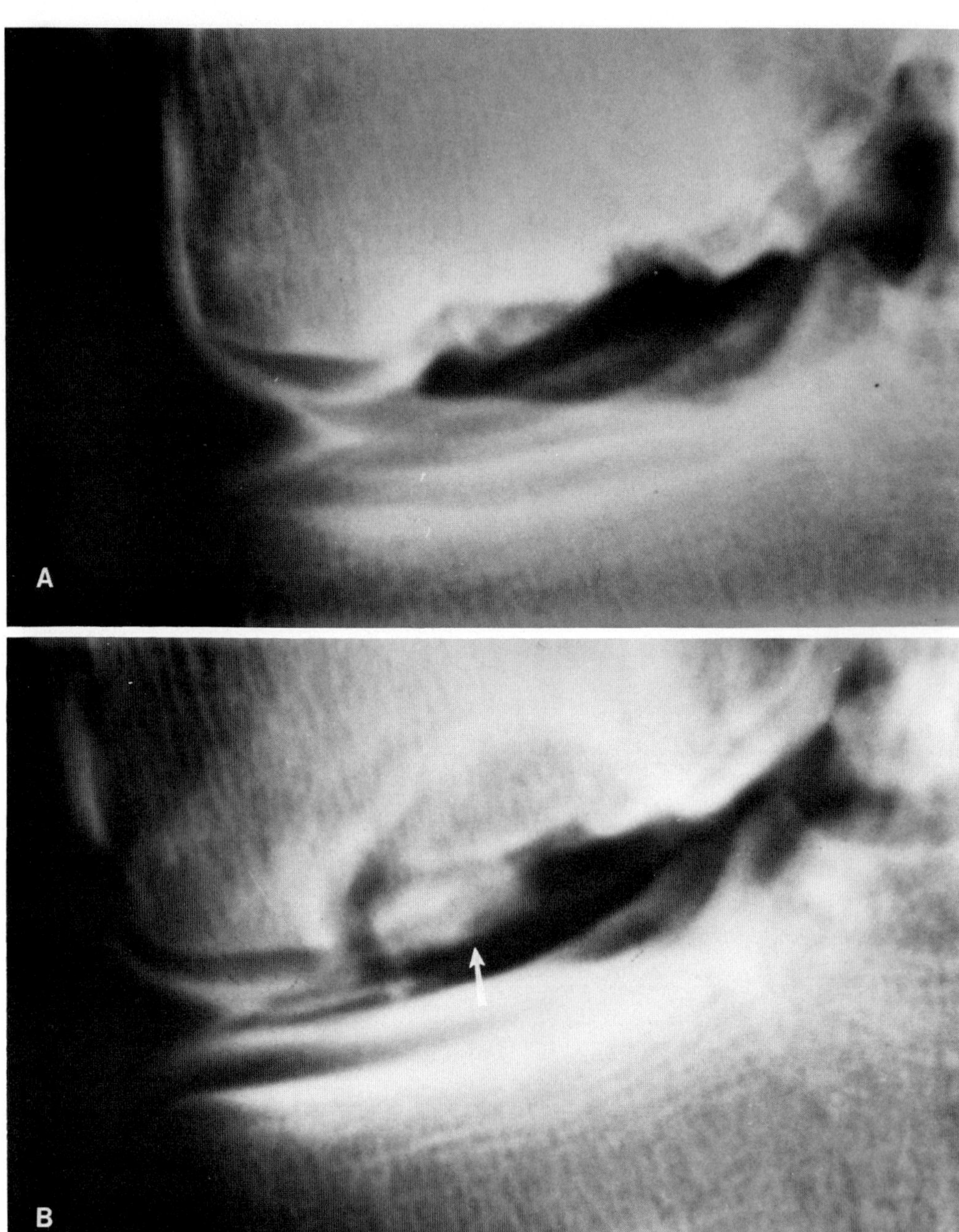

Figure 1.33. Osteochondritis, long standing case. *A,* Large crater in articular surface. *B,* Different view shows partially separated bone plug in the crater (*arrow*).

Popliteal Cyst (Baker's Cyst)

A cystic mass in the popliteal region which communicates with the joint is commonly called a Baker's cyst. Baker's description of this condition in 1885 was preceded by several reports of the same entity. Various mechanisms have

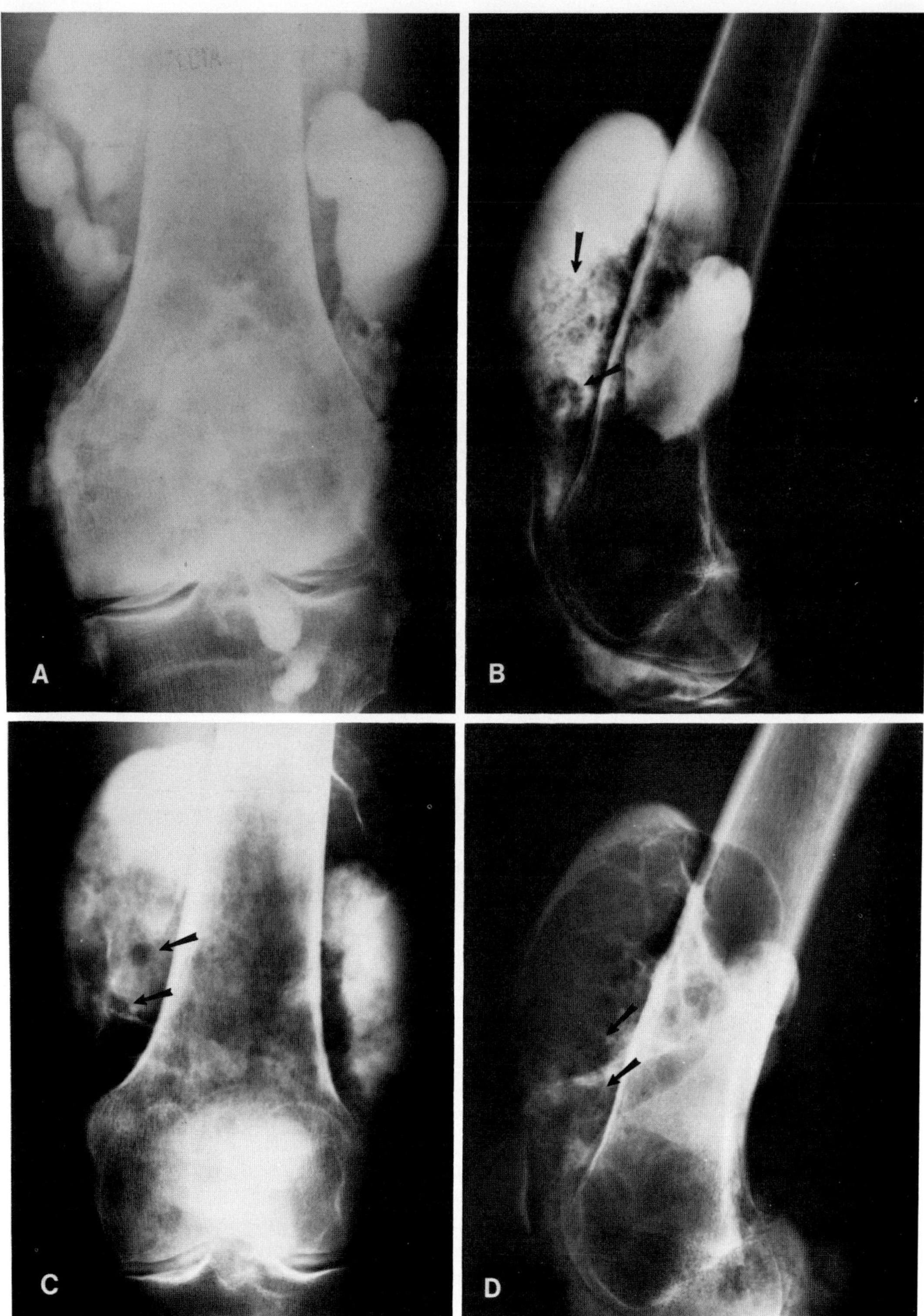

Figure 1.34. Villonodular synovitis. Enlargement of the synovial sac and filling defects due to synovial thickenings (*arrows*). *A* and *B*, Single contrast. *C* and *D*, Double contrast.

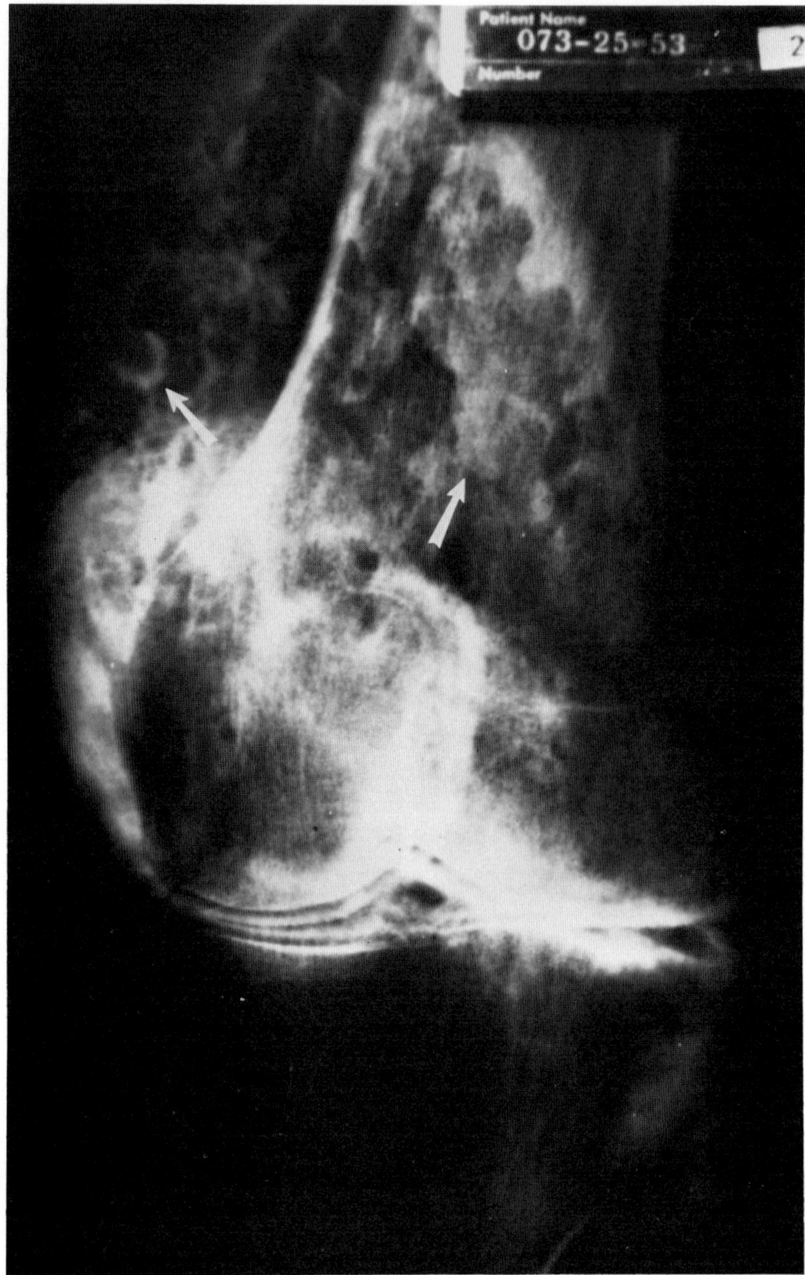

Figure 1.35. Rheumatoid arthritis. Note marked irregular thickening of the synovium in the suprapatellar bursa (*arrows*). Double contrast.

been theorized to explain the formation of these popliteal cysts, including (1) developmental anomaly, (2) synovial herniation through a posterior capsular defect, (3) rupture of the posterior capsule allowing leakage of joint fluid which becomes encapsulated, and (4) a communication through the capsule between the joint space and the normally occurring semimembranosus bursa located in

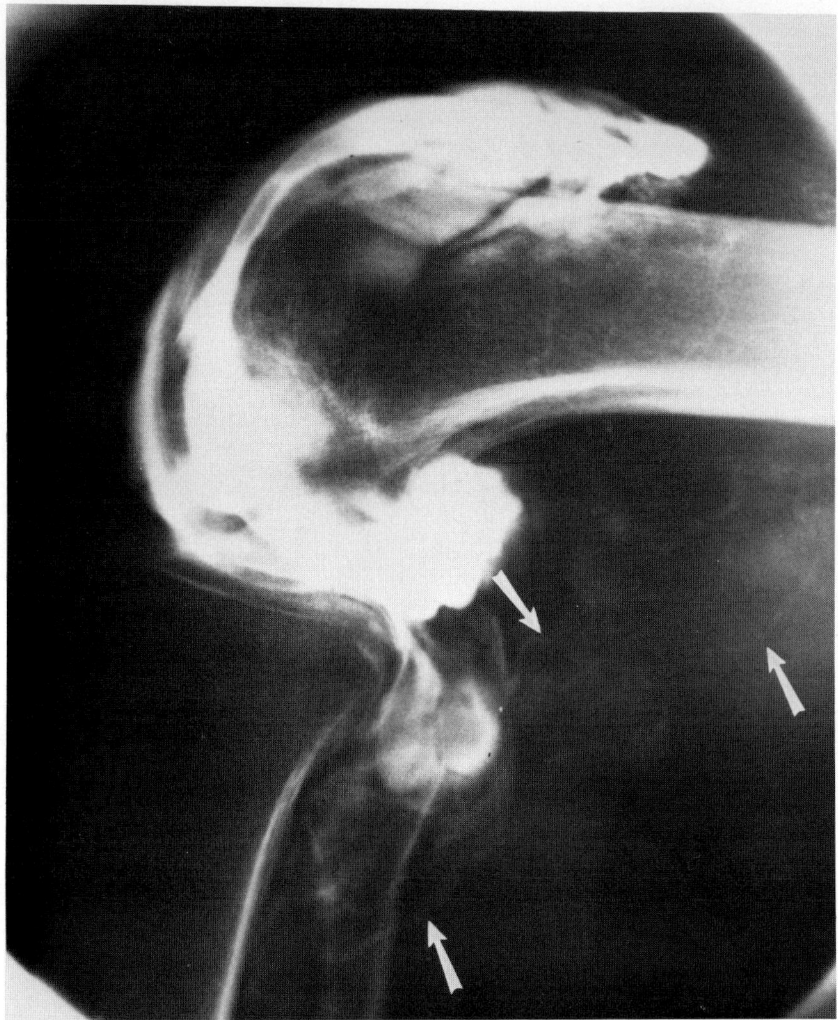

Figure 1.36. Rheumatoid arthritis. The lymphatic vessels opacify by arthrography in some cases of this disease (*arrows*). Single contrast.

the medial popliteal space, the more deeply situated medial gastrocnemius bursa, or the lateral gastrocnemius bursa. The bursae could be distended by an effusion resulting from an irritated synovium, which explains why popliteal cysts are frequently found concomitantly with intraarticular lesions. Lindgren and Willen resolved the controversy about the origin of the cysts by a correlative investigation of a large number of postmortem arthrograms and knee dissections. In no case did they find a herniation of synovium through a capsular defect or a cyst that was separate from the normally occurring bursae. They discovered instead "slit-shaped" communications between the joint space and the gastrocnemius and semimembranosus bursae in over half of the study population over age 50, a lower incidence below age 50, and no communication in 31 specimens under age 10. They concluded that the communication was

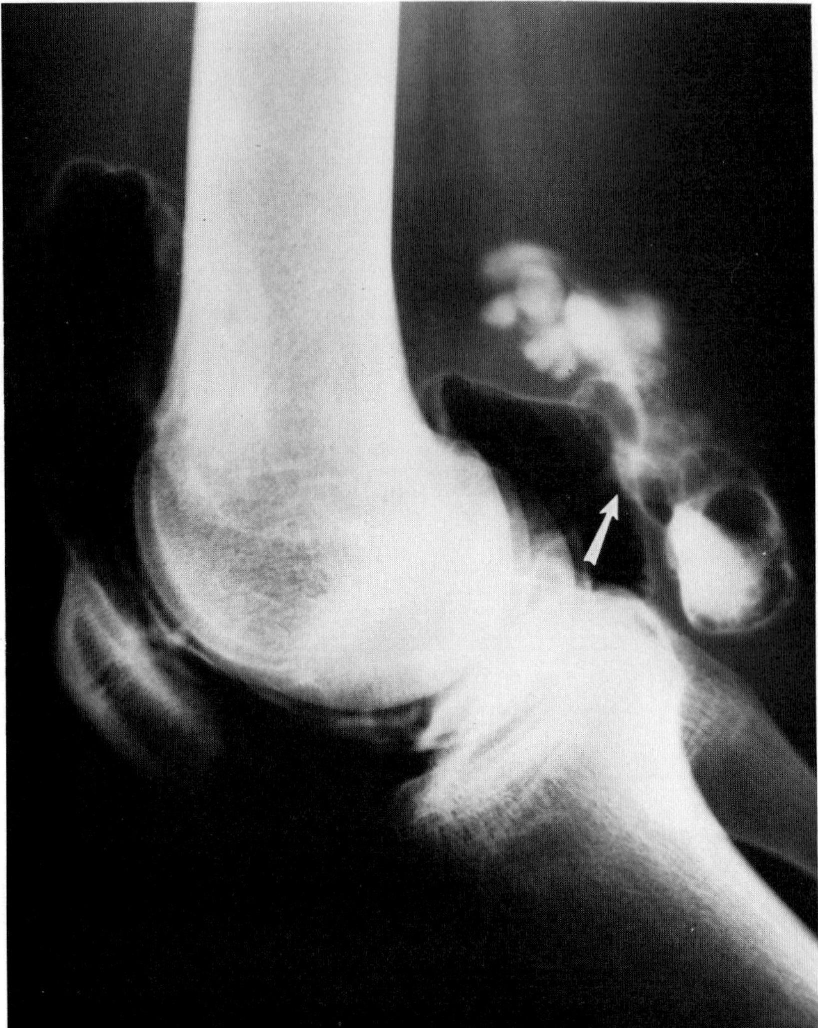

Figure 1.37. Popliteal cyst. Air and contrast material have entered distended gastrocnemius-semimembranosus bursa through communication with joint (*arrow*). Double contrast.

usually acquired. The rare congenital Baker's cyst would result from a developmental bursal communication.

Arthrography establishes the diagnosis of the popliteal cyst by the opacification of the involved gastrocnemio-semimembranosus bursa (Fig. 1.37). Since clinically palpable Baker's cysts in adults usually accompany intraarticular lesions, these lesions should be searched for on the arthrogram.

Rheumatoid arthritis or chronic effusion from other cause, can result in a huge popliteal cyst which dissects downward into the muscles of the calf, causing calf pain and swelling suggestive of venous obstruction (Fig. 1.38). These cysts sometimes rupture which may produce acute calf pain and a hot "ropy" swelling mimicking thrombophlebitis (Fig. 1.39). In the appropriate clinical situation, arthrography is indicated to differentiate between thrombo-

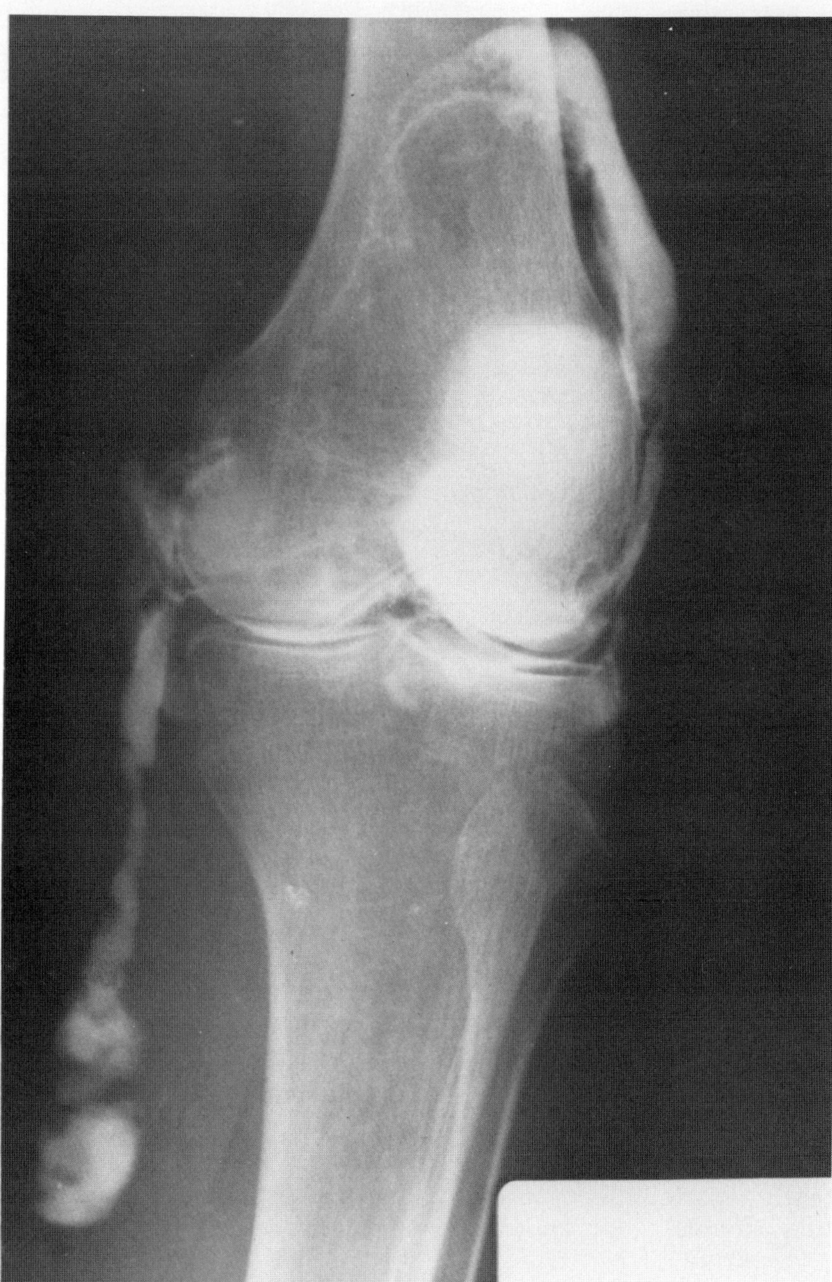

Figure 1.38. Dissecting calf cyst in rheumatoid arthritis. Single contrast arthrogram shows enlarged intact cyst extending into the calf.

phlebitis and dissecting calf cyst or ruptured cyst. A venogram might be avoided if the arthrogram is positive. However, the physician must realize that a dissecting cyst and thrombophlebitis may co-exist. Two instances of this in rheumatoid arthritis patients were recently revealed by Gordon et al. It has

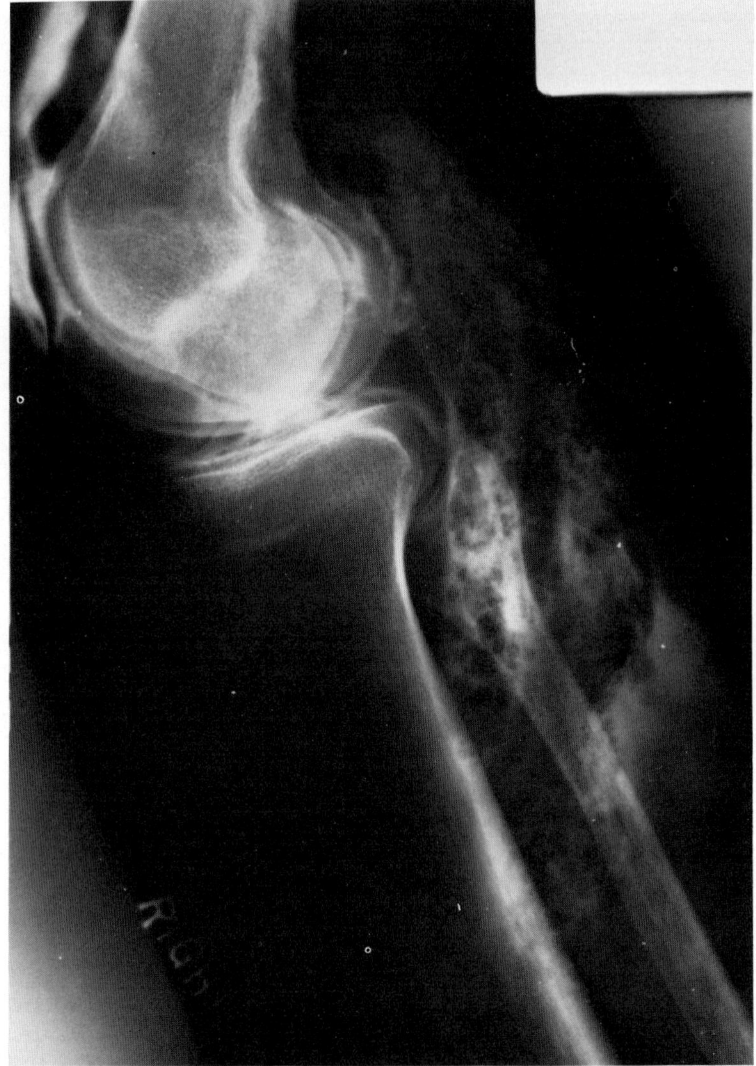

Figure 1.39. Ruptured popliteal cyst in rheumatoid arthritis. Double contrast arthrogram shows extravasation of contrast agent and air into the calf.

been recently reported that cysts of the knee also occur anterior to the femur in rheumatoid patients.

Synovial (Medial Plica) Shelf Syndrome

The medial patellar fold (plica) is often larger than the lateral fold (plica). The frequency with which a prominent medial plica occurs is reported to be in the range of 20 to 55%. A broad medial patellar plica can be a normal variant of no significance. However, some orthopedists feel that a large thick medial plica can produce symptoms because it impinges on the anteromedial portion of the medial femoral condyle and on the medial facet of the patella. They find that during flexion of the knee the plica becomes taut and transmits pressure to the condyle and patella that may be damaging. Names given to this condition include: synovial shelf, medial plica shelf, suprapatellar plica, Lino's band. and Pseudochondromalacia patellae. Other orthopedists feel that this is an area of controversy and a large medial patellar plica is rarely or never a cause of knee symptoms.

Most of the attention this structure has received has been from arthroscopists. Some arthroscopists cut large medial plica through the arthroscope and others advise open operation with division of the band.

Irregardless of the debate about this condition, it is possible to demonstrate a large medial patellar plica on an axial view of the patella at arthrography (Fig. 1.27A). The possible significance of this arthrographic finding has not been established.

ARTHROGRAPHY FOLLOWING MENISECTOMY

Most patients have a satisfactory return of normal joint function without troublesome symptoms following menisectomy. The clinical results following

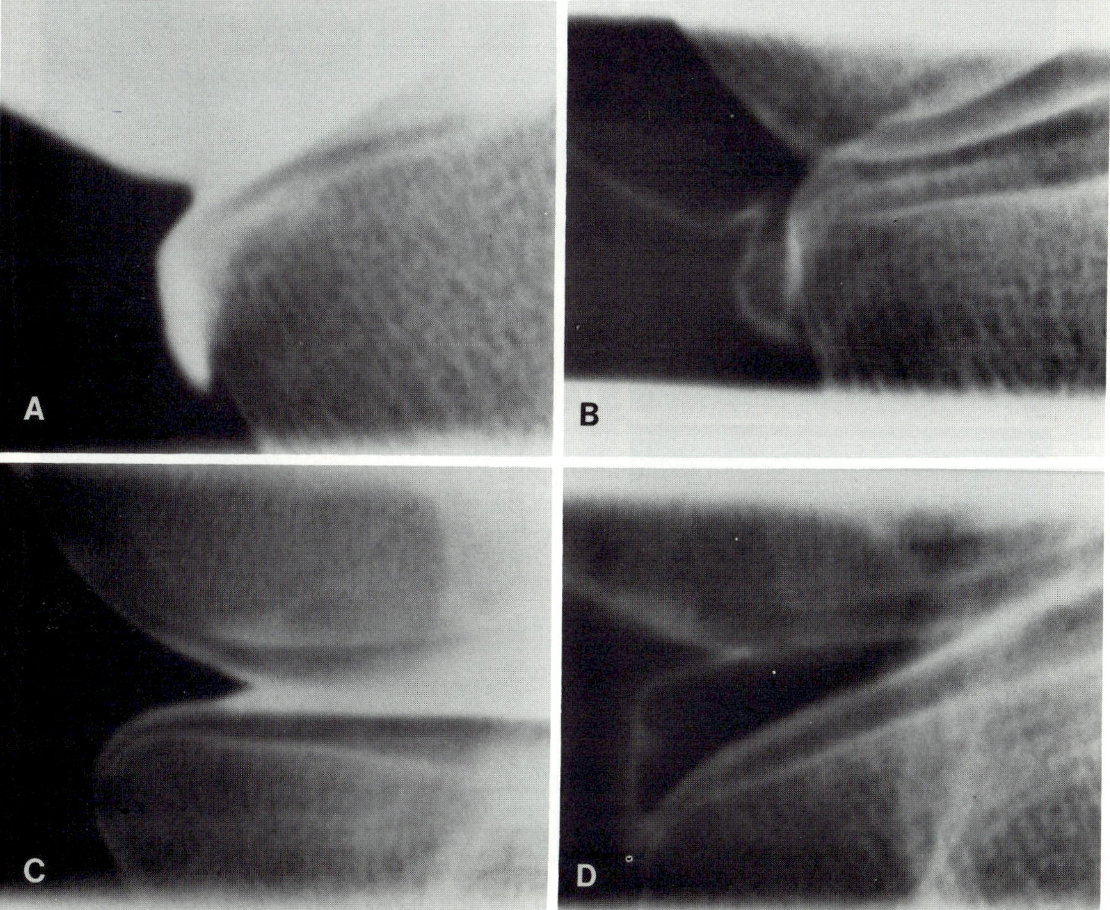

Figure 1.40. Medial menisectomy. Small residual rim of anterior portion on meniscus shown by positive contrast (*A*) and double contrast (*B*). Posteriorly there is a larger residual meniscus shown by positive contrast (*C*) and double contrast (*D*).

2

Arthrography of the Shoulder

R. D. Arndt, M.D.

Indications for shoulder arthrography include virtually any shoulder disability. The most common indications are suspicion of rotator cuff tear, and anterior capsular derangement resulting in recurrent glenohumeral dislocation. Occasionally, arthrography is helpful to diagnose adhesive capsulitis. Clinical symptoms associated with these conditions are similar, consisting of weakness during abduction and elevation, pain, diminished range of motion, and recurrent dislocation. Clinical diagnosis, although fairly certain, is not definite, and arthrography is indicated if surgical treatment is planned.

FUNCTIONAL ANATOMY

The shoulder is a multiaxial or ball-and-socket joint. Its main support consists of muscles and tendons. The joint is encased in a fibrous capsule with an inner synovial lining. The capsule has two extensions: a short extension below the coracoid process where it becomes the subscapularis bursa that contains the subscapularis tendon as it passes anterior to the glenoid rim; and the other, a longer extension, forming a synovial-lined sheath for the tendon of the long head of the biceps muscle as it courses within the bicipital groove of the humerus. The latter extension usually stops at the surgical neck of the humerus and is secured to the bone by the transverse humeral (bicipital) ligament which spans the bicipital groove transversely at its most proximal aspect (Fig. 2.1).

The upper portion of the joint capsule covering the humeral head is supported by a broad, tendinous aponeurosis originating from and consisting of the fused tendons of the rotator cuff muscles which insert on the greater tuberosity. This musculotendinous rotator cuff is comprised of the tendons of the supraspinatus muscle superiorly, the subscapularis muscle anteriorly, and the infraspinatus and teres minor muscle posteriorly. All unite into a broad aponeurosis which is in intimate contact with the shoulder joint capsule, particularly along its superior aspect where the supraspinatus tendon separates the glenohumeral joint from the subacromial-subdeltoid bursa complex superiorly. The latter is sometimes connected to the subcoracoid bursa anteriorly. These bursae, in turn, separate the rotator cuff from the deltoid muscle superolaterally, and coracoid process and acromion superiorly. Severe degeneration or rupture of the supra-

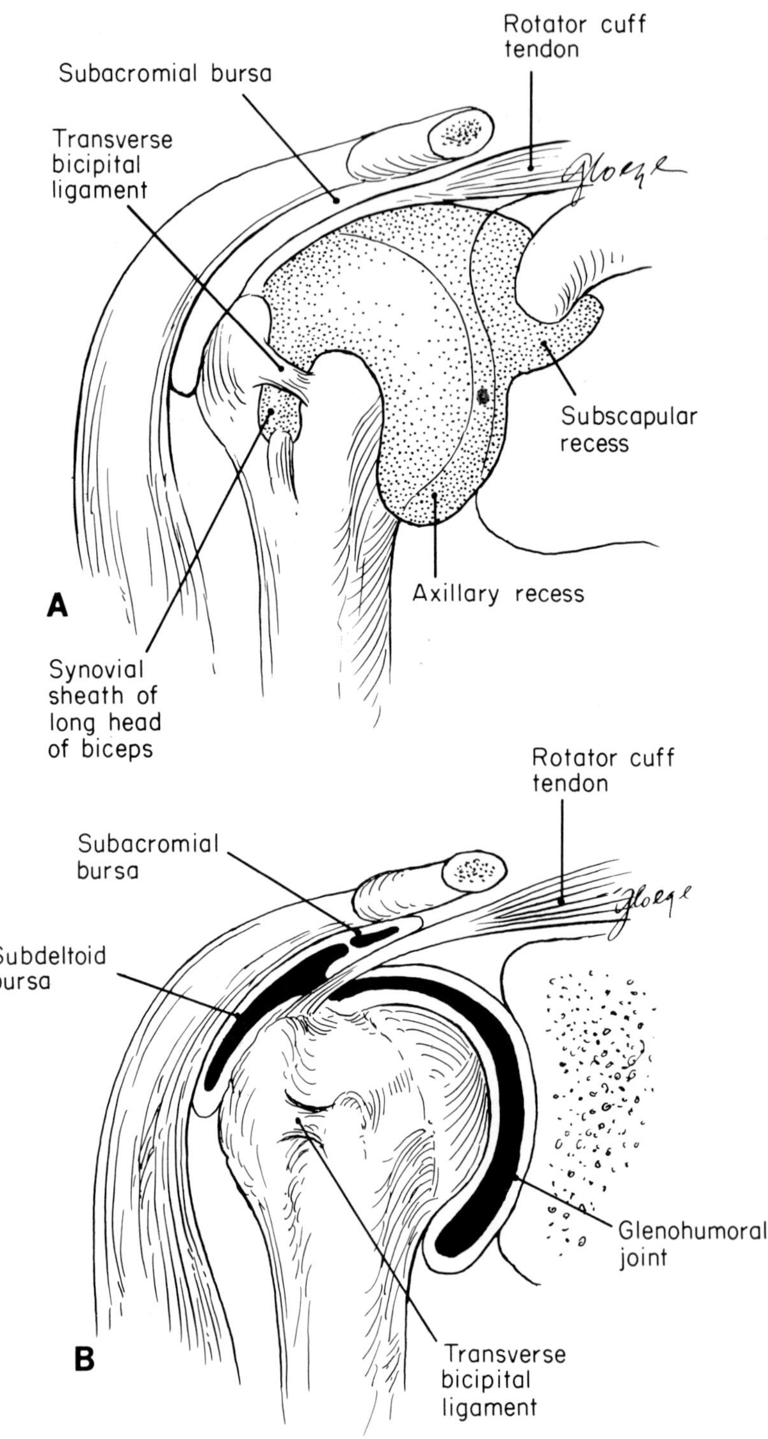

Figure 2.1. *A,* Distended synovial bursa of the glenohumeral joint. *B,* Coronal section of same. (Modified from Grant, J.C.B., *An Atlas of Anatomy,* Ed. 5. Williams & Wilkins, Baltimore, 1962.)

spinatus tendon will allow communication of the glenohumeral joint with the subacromial bursa. Rotator cuff degeneration, if prolonged, leads to sclerotic eburnation and irregularity of the contact surfaces of the humerus, particularly near the greater tuberosity, and the acromion which may be detected on plain radiographs. Degeneration of the supraspinatus portion of the rotator cuff is common in individuals over 60 and usually occurs bilaterally. In younger persons it may result from injury. A complete tear through the supraspinatus tendon just proximal to its insertion on the greater tuberosity is required before an abnormal communication can occur between the subacromial bursa and the glenohumeral joint. It is this communication and the ensuing filling with contrast material of the subacromial bursa which allows the arthrographic diagnosis of complete rotator cuff tear.

METHOD

Preliminary anteroposterior radiographs in internal and external rotation and a view of the bicipital groove are obtained. The patient lies supine with the arm in the anatomical position, palm-up. It may be helpful to elevate the contralateral shoulder on a pillow or sponge, so that the injured shoulder is rotated into a slightly oblique position permitting a tangential fluoroscopic view of the glenohumeral joint.

A site one finger breadth inferior and lateral to the coracoid process is chosen as the point of entry (Fig. 2.2). After sterile cleaning and draping, local anesthesia vith 1% lidocaine is performed. A 20- or 22-gauge spinal needle is inserted at this point and advanced under fluoroscopic guidance into the glenohumeral

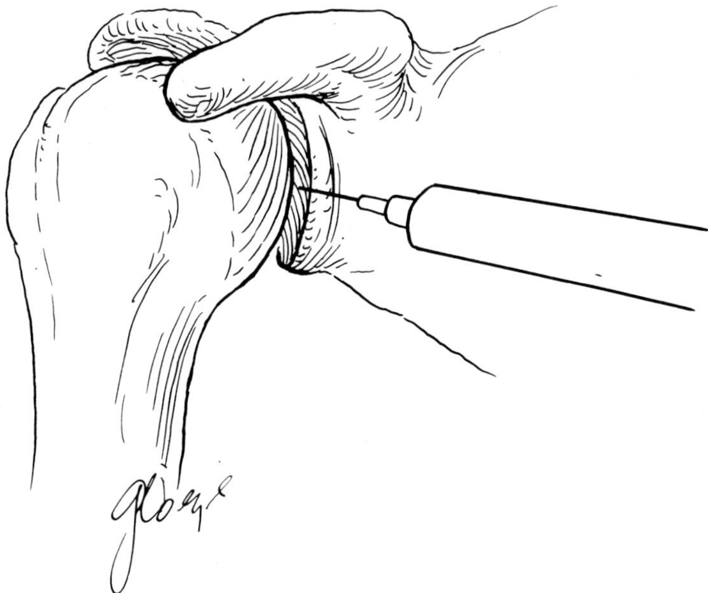

Figure 2.2. Site of arthrocentesis for shoulder arthrography.

space, with the needle remaining perpendicular to the tabletop. The glenohumeral joint is deeper than usually anticipated, and only a spinal needle provides adequate length. Periodic testing for ease of flow from a lidocaine or saline-filled syringe will help in identifying the intraarticular position of the needle. When the pressure necessary for injection becomes less, and especially if some of the injected fluid can be aspirated, the needle tip is certain to be in the joint space. Alternatively, if the needle tip has pierced the articular cartilage of the humerus or glenoid, the flow will be blocked. By continuing the pressure on the syringe plunger, while at the same time withdrawing the needle tip 1 or 2 mm, the tip usually finds its way into the space, and fluid flows freely from the syringe. Contrast material is then instilled under fluoroscopic guidance (Fig. 2.3). The axillary recess is usually the first to fill, then the subscapularis recess, with simultaneous outlining of the articular cartilage of the humerus (Fig. 2.4). The synovial sac of the glenohumeral joint communicates normally with the subscapularis bursa which lies below the coracoid process and contains the subscapularis tendon. An additional communication exists between the glenohumeral joint and the synovial-lined sheath covering the proximal portion of the long head of the biceps. The subacromial bursa which is immediately beneath the acromion does not normally communicate with the glenohumeral joint but may communicate with a potential space, the subcoracoid bursa. One must be cautious when injecting contrast in a patient with a history of recurrent glenohumeral dislocation, for that condition may lead to enlargement of the subacromial bursa which may communicate with and thus also enlarge the subcoracoid bursa. If these abnormally large bursae are punctured, contrast may appear as if it were flowing into the shoulder joint. Close inspection, however, fails to disclose contrast outlining the articular cartilage of the humerus or glenoid, proving that a bursagram rather than an arthrogram has been obtained.

We prefer to use dilute diatrizoate meglumine (Renografin 60 mixed with an equal amount of injectable saline or water). The usual capacity of the shoulder joint is 20 cc. When the joint and synovial recesses are filled, a few drops of contrast are allowed to flow out through the needle hub under its own hydrostatic pressure to reduce any excess intraarticular contrast fluid, thus preventing leakage into the soft tissue during subsequent exercise prior to filming. The needle is then removed and the patient is asked to briefly exercise the joint after which overhead Bucky grid film exposures are made. The importance of exercising the joint prior to radiography cannot be overemphasized because without it a rotator cuff may go undetected. Exercise evenly distributes the pressure of intraarticular fluid and forces contrast material into the subacromial bursa if a rotator cuff tear has created an abnormal communication between this bursa and the glenohumeral joint.

Supine anteroposterior neutral, internal, and external rotation views, a bicipital groove view, an axillary and a tangential film of the glenoid fossa should be obtained. After these have been inspected for quality, the study can be terminated. We usually advise our patients to avoid vigorous exercise for the remainder of the day, and prescribe salicylates for pain which is usually minor. The source of the pain is a chemical synovitis induced by the hyperosmolar contrast medium.

Although single contrast arthrography is the usual method of examination

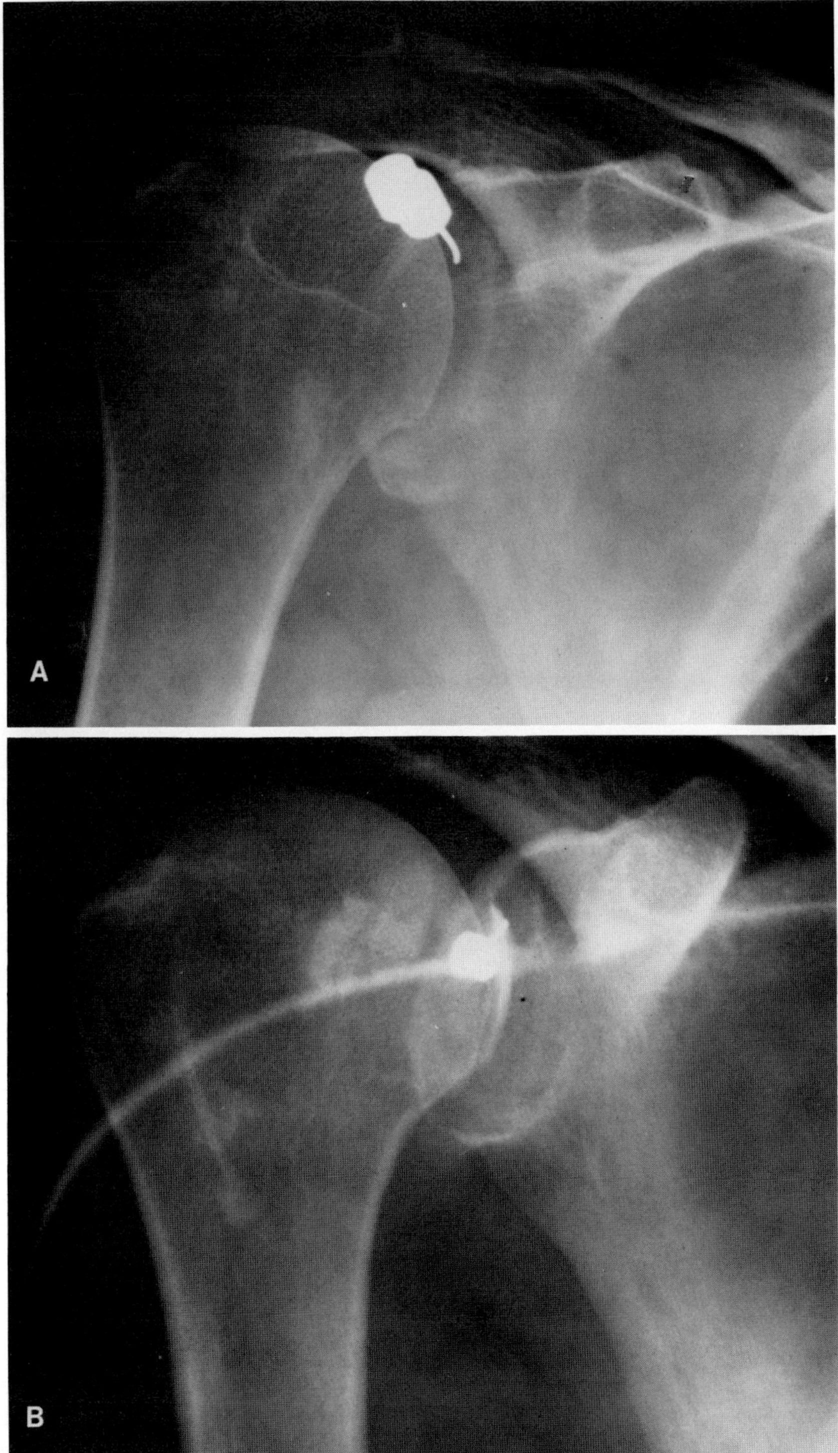

Figure 2.3. *A,* Needle position for injection of shoulder arthrogram. *B,* Early injection phase; contrast flows away from needle tip outlining articular cartilage.

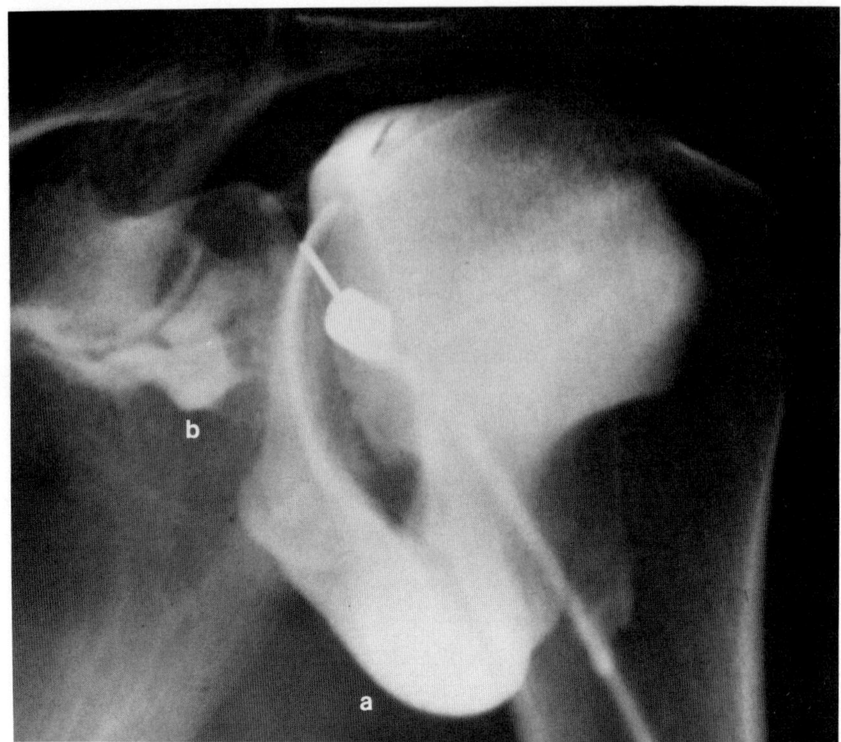

Figure 2.4. Shoulder arthrogram: Late injection phase showing axillary recess (*a*), and subscapularis recess (*b*).

for the shoulder, double-contrast technique is very valuable in demonstrating the true extent of incomplete tears and for showing the actual width of a complete tear. Most importantly, the double-contrast method can show the size and quality of the rotator cuff tendon, which is helpful to the orthopedic surgeon in deciding on the feasibility of surgical repair.

After single contrast film exposures have been completed, the needle is reinserted according to the method described. This is now much easier since the synovial sac is distended with contrast medium. Approximately 5 to 10 cc of contrast agent is aspirated and an equal volume of filtered room air (drawn into a syringe through several layers of sterile gauze sponges) is injected. The needle is withdrawn and, following exercise, the same series of films as for the single contrast arthrogram are repeated, but now with the patient upright and turned slightly posterior-oblique to the affected side, and the x-ray tube angled 15° caudad. The technical factors are decreased to a range around 65 mA and 65 kVP. If double contrast is preferred as the primary technique of arthrography, 10 cc of dilute diatrizoate meglumine and 10 to 15 cc of filtered room air are injected by the method outlined above and films obtained accordingly (Fig. 2.5). It is our custom to perform single contrast shoulder arthrography first. If the rotator cuff tendon is intact, the arthrogram is completed. In the event the films reveal a tear, we proceed immediately to the double contrast examination for assessment of the tendon itself.

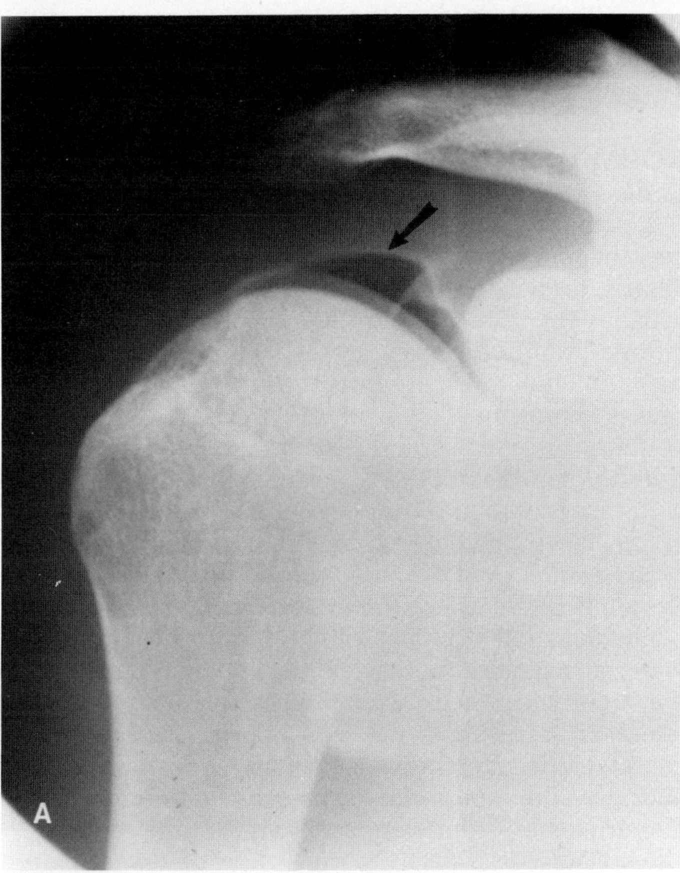

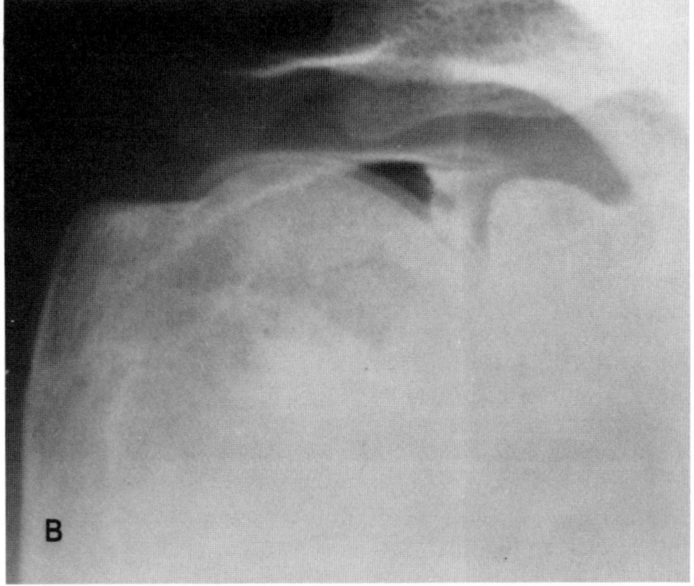

Figure 2.5. Normal double contrast shoulder arthrogram. *A*, Internal rotation. *B*, External rotation. Note intact inferior surface of rotator cuff aponeurosis (*arrow*) and articular cartilage of humerus. Film exposure for double contrast study is deliberately lower than single contrast.

Complications are few and consist primarily of allergic reactions to the contrast agent and local anesthetic. A remote possibility of infection is slightly increased in a previously infected or postsurgical shoulder. Our experience indicates a rate of postarthrographic infection of less than 0.5%.

NORMAL SHOULDER ARTHROGRAM

A smooth, rounded axillary recess is seen at the medial edge of the surgical neck of the humerus. The slender subscapularis recess containing the subscapularis tendon extends medially from the glenohumeral joint to the region beneath the coracoid process (Fig. 2.1). This recess is most distended on the internal rotation view and becomes less capacious during external rotation when the taut subscapularis muscle lying anteriorly compresses the recess and causes expulsion of some of its contrast material (Fig. 2.6). Similarly, the contrast agent in the axillary recess is expressed during abduction of the arm by pressure from the taut pectoralis major muscle against the humeral head. It follows that both recesses should best be seen on the internal rotation view. The long tendon of the biceps muscle is visible as a linear filling defect within its opacified synovial sheath and extends to its insertion on the supraglenoid tubercle. The tendon is best seen on the external rotation and bicipital groove views (Fig. 2.7).

The articular cartilage of the humerus is outlined by a thin line of contrast material which tapers to end on the medial margin of the greater tuberosity at the anatomical neck. No contrast should normally be present superior and lateral to this line. A few words of caution: In the external rotation view, the contrast-filled synovial sheath of the long head of the biceps tendon may project laterally and superiorly to the greater tuberosity and articular cartilage of the humerus; the tendon can usually be identified within the sheath and this should allow differentiation from the abnormal opacification of the subacromial bursa resulting from a rotator cuff tear (Fig. 2.8). This tendon and its sheath will rotate medially and anteriorly in the internal rotation view; if contrast material remains superior and lateral to the greater tuberosity in that projection, it indicates opacification of the subacromial-subdeltoid complex and, hence, a rotator cuff tear.

ABNORMAL SHOULDER ARTHROGRAM

Rotator Cuff Tear

In a rotator cuff tear with complete severance of the tendinous aponeurosis, an abnormal communication is established between the glenohumeral joint and the subacromial bursa (Fig. 2.9). Thus, contrast material injected into the glenohumeral joint will enter the subacromial bursa and will be recognized as a collection superior to the greater tuberosity of the humerus, as well as superior to the line of contrast-outlined articular cartilage where it thins out just medial to the greater tuberosity. This abnormality is most dramatically demonstrated in the internal rotation projection (Figs. 2.10 to 2.12). The size of the subacromial bursa is variable, particularly along the lateral aspect of the humeral head. It is, however, always closely apposed to the inferior edge of the acromion. If a

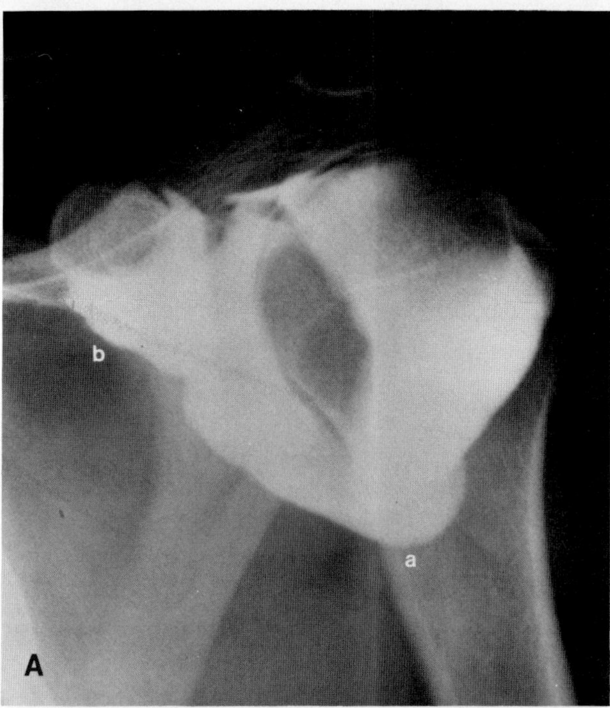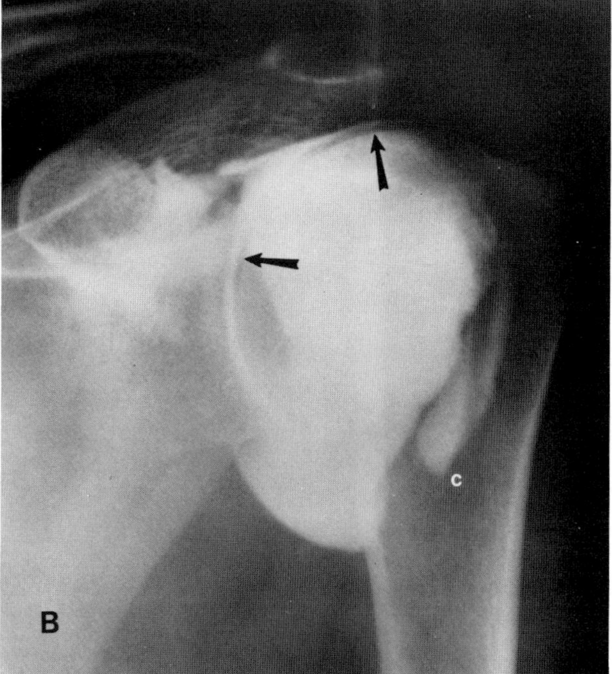

Figure 2.6. Normal single contrast shoulder arthrogram. *A,* Internal rotation. *B,* External rotation. Note axillary recess (*a*), subscapularis recess (*b*), long head of biceps tendon in its synovial sheath (*c*), and articular cartilage of humerus outlined by contrast material (*arrows*). In external rotation (*B*) taut subscapularis muscle flattens subscapularis bursa anteriorly expressing contrast media; with internal rotation this recess fills again (*A*).

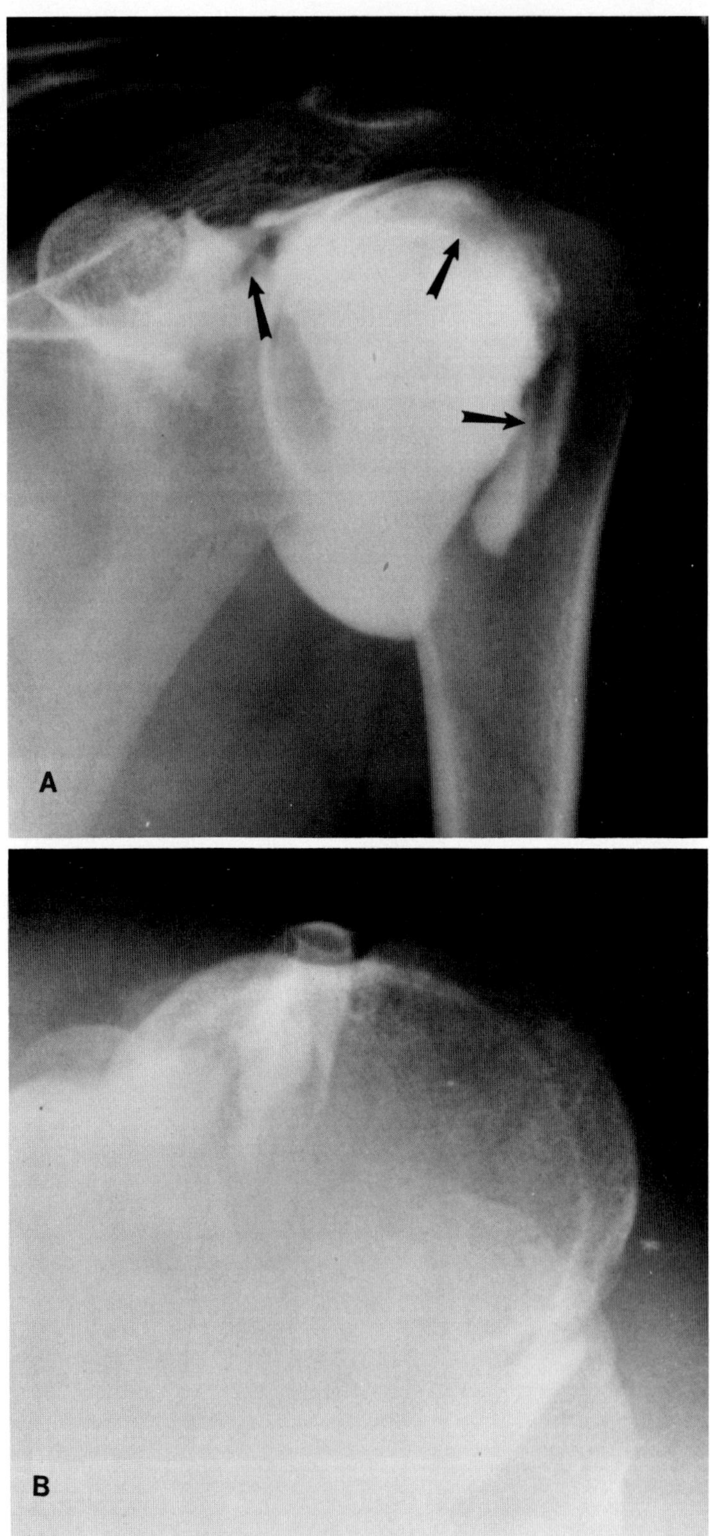

Figure 2.7. Normal single contrast shoulder arthrogram. *A*, External rotation view shows course of long head of biceps tendon within its synovial sleeve and insertion on supraglenoid tubercle (*arrows*). *B*, Tangential view of bicipital groove clearly outlines the tendon within its contrast-filled sleeve, which is within the bony groove on the anterior aspect of the proximal humeral shaft and head.

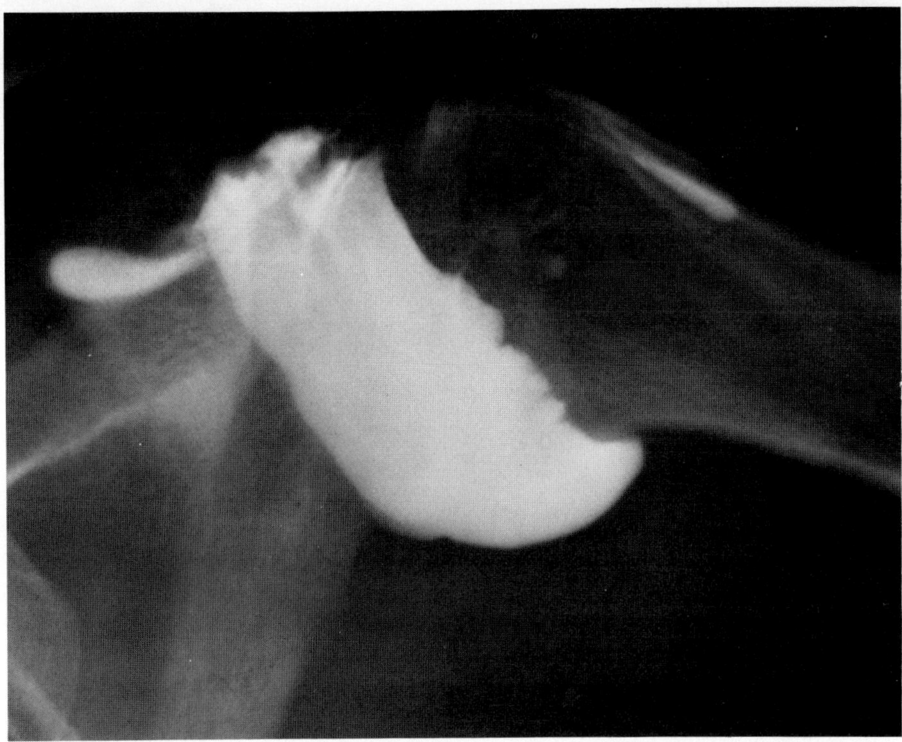

Figure 2.8. Normal single contrast shoulder arthrogram. Anteroposterior view in extreme external rotation. The superolateral position of the long head biceps tendon in this projection can simulate contrast in the subacromial bursa and hence a rotator cuff tear. Identification of the outline of the tendon within the contrast-filled sleeve differentiates.

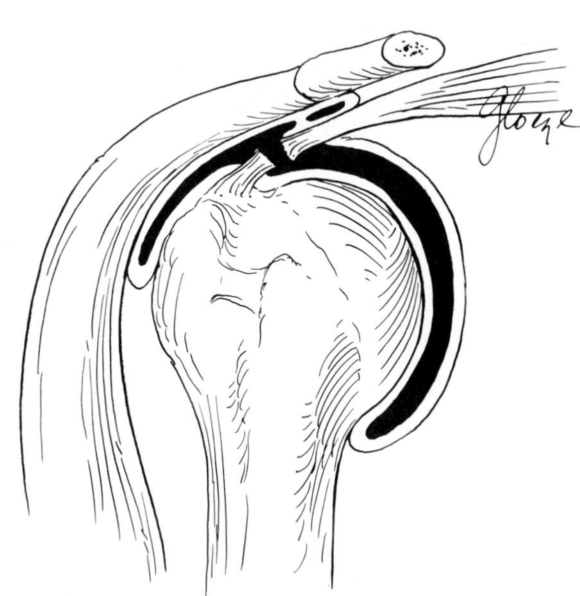

Figure 2.9. Torn rotator cuff tendon allowing communication of glenohumeral joint and subacromial bursa.

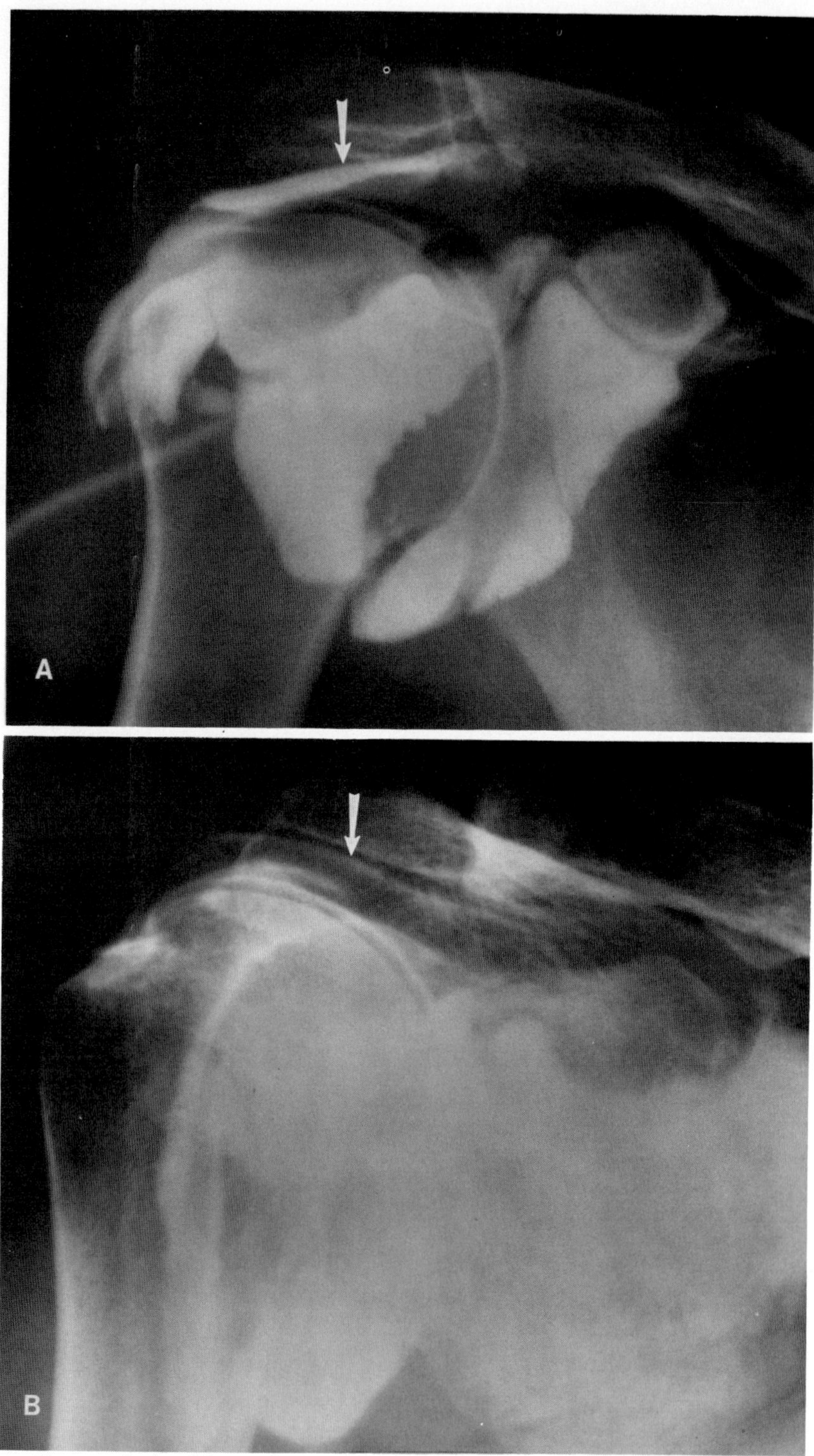

Figure 2.10. Abnormal shoulder arthrograms, single contrast. *A,* Contrast within subacromial bursa (*arrow*) indicates communication with glenohumeral joint and hence a rotator cuff tear. *B,* Inferior and superior surface of rotator cuff tendon is opacified (*arrow*), implying a leak into the subacromial bursa due to a rotator cuff tear.

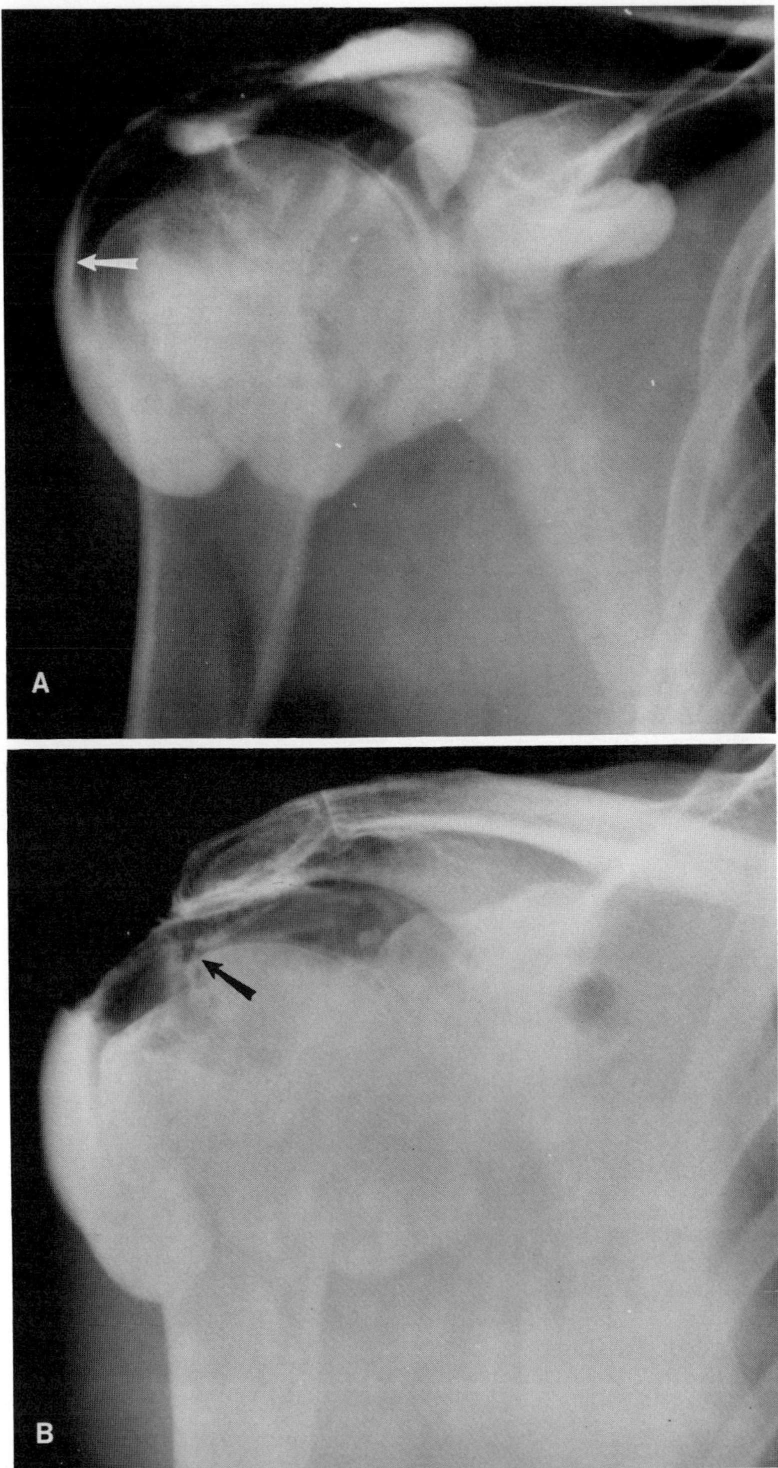

Figure 2.11. Abnormal shoulder arthrogram. *A,* Single contrast study with contrast in subacromial bursa, indicating a complete rotator cuff tear (*arrow*). *B,* Double contrast study, same patient. The actual rent in the rotator cuff tendon is well seen (*arrow*), and the condition of the tendon is easily assessed.

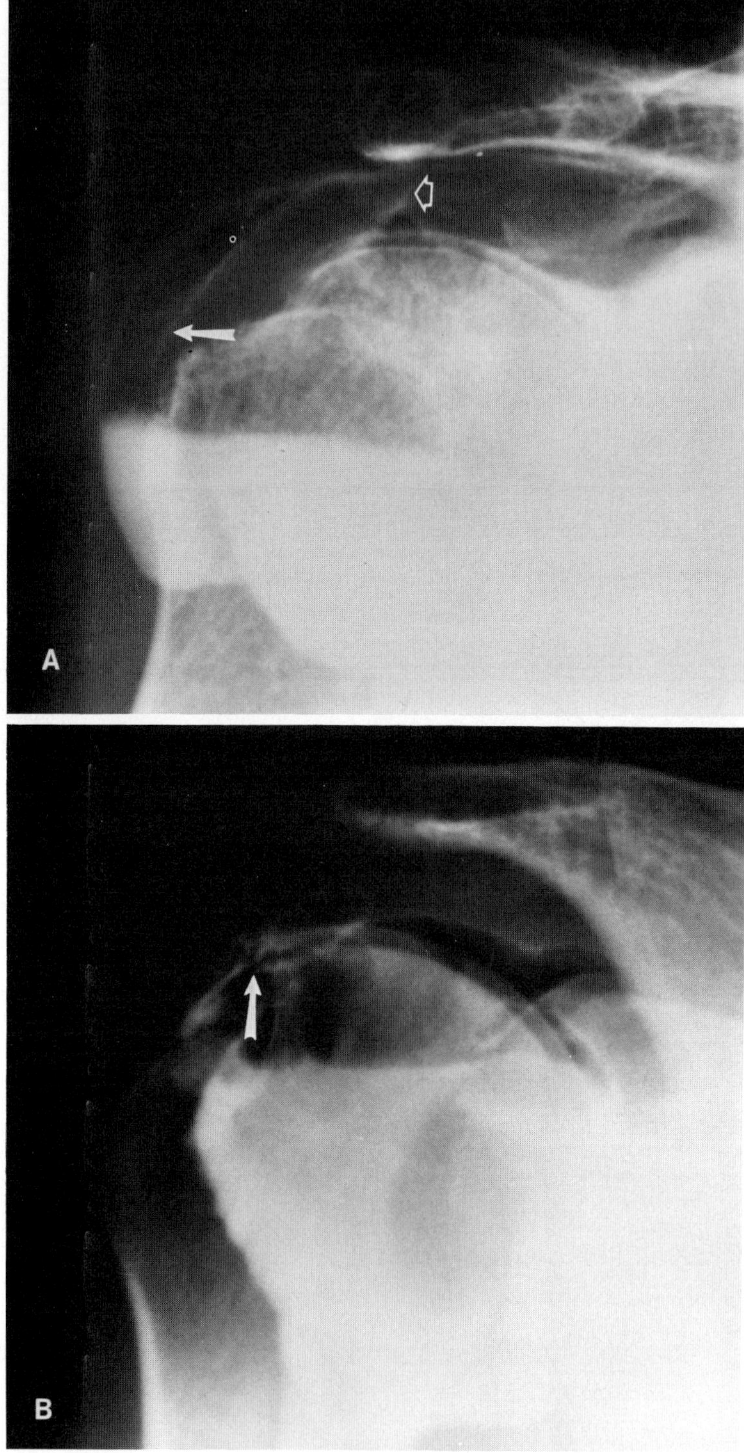

Figure 2.12. Abnormal shoulder arthrogram, double contrast. *A,* Note contrast and air within subacromial bursa (*arrow*), indicating a rotator cuff tear. The entirety of the tendon, including the tear (*open arrow*), is clearly seen. *B,* Another case. The rotator cuff tendon is torn in its distal aspect, near its insertion on the greater tuberosity of the humerus (*arrow*).

communication exists between the subacromial and subcoracoid bursae, a large collection of contrast will form a broad, dense perimeter around the superior and lateral aspect of the humeral head (Fig. 2.13). In a normal arthrogram, both of these spaces are free of contrast material. It is our judgment that the size of the subacromial bursa may be greater in those patients whose shoulder injury is of long duration, suggesting that long-term communication with the glenohumeral space enlarges this bursa (Fig. 2.14). According to other authors, however, severity of injury has no bearing on the size of the bursa in that its volume and extent is normally variable. Occasionally, when a tear is incomplete, careful observation may reveal an ulceration outlined by contrast on the undersurface of the tendon just medial to the greater tuberosity above the anatomical neck of the humerus (Fig. 2.15).

The importance of exercising the joint following injection of contrast material prior to filming cannot be overemphasized. We have frequently demonstrated a communication only on postexercise films, whereas films made during or immediately after contrast injection were normal.

In addition to lack of adequate exercise following contrast injection, there are three other possible sources of error, according to Killoran et al. The first is an error in technique: not injecting enough contrast media. At least 20 cc is the capacity of the normal joint, and up to 30 cc or more is required if the rotator

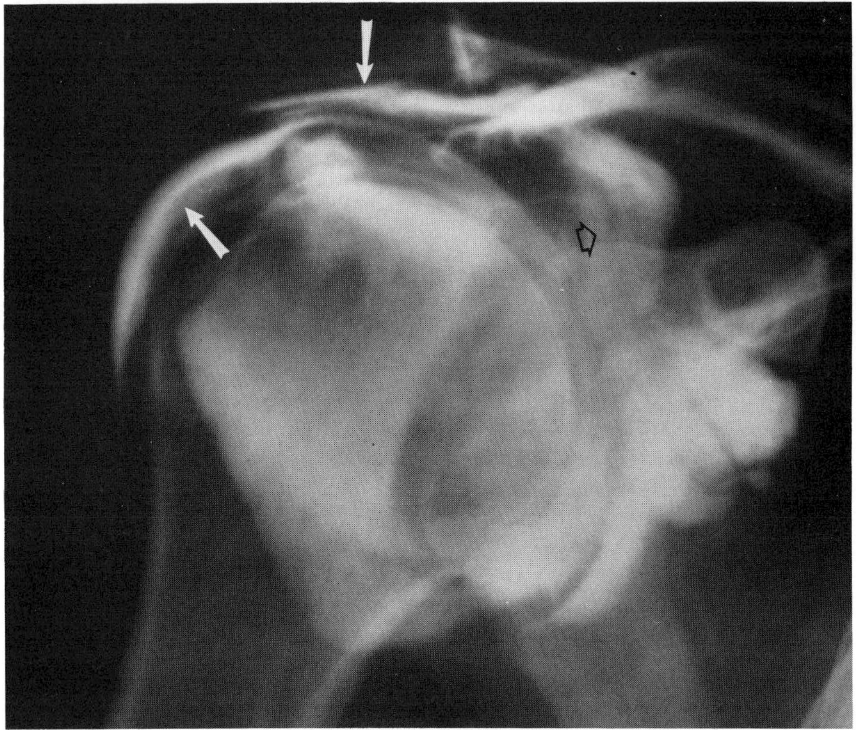

Figure 2.13. Abnormal shoulder arthrogram, single contrast. A rotator cuff tear has allowed contrast medium to enter the subacromial-subdeltoid bursa complex (*arrows*) which in turn communicates with and has enlarged the subcoracoid bursa (*open arrow*), suggesting the tear is of long standing.

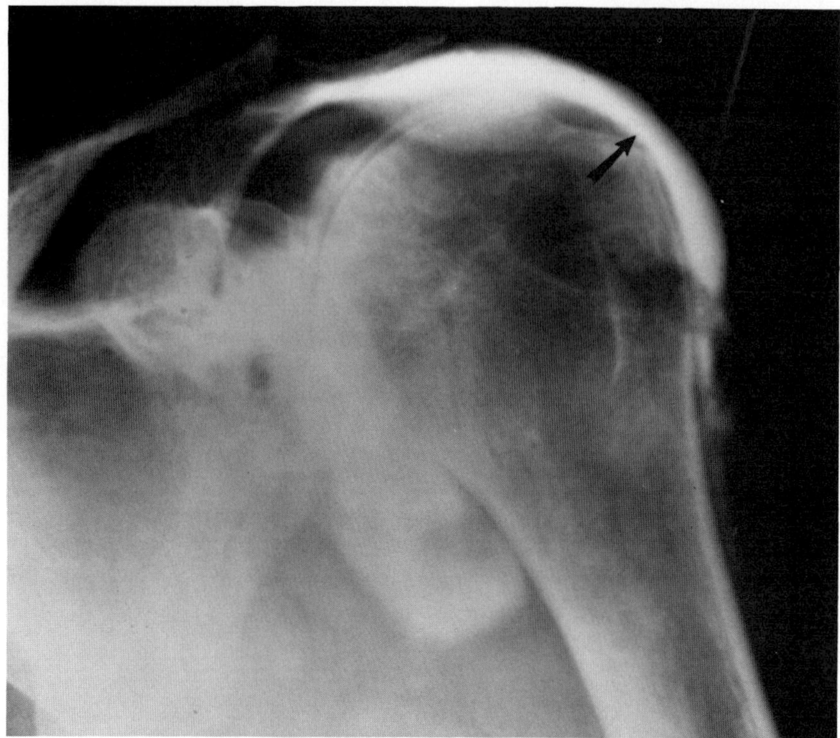

Figure 2.14. Abnormal shoulder arthrogram. Rotator cuff tear has allowed passage of contrast medium into the subacromial bursa (*arrow*). Large size of this bursa suggests a chronic communication with the glenohumeral joint and probably a tear of long duration.

cuff is torn. The contrast agent should be injected until the patient indicates a definite sensation of pressure within the joint and contrast material flows freely back from the needle hub when the syringe or extension tubing is disconnected. The second error is one of interpretation which occurs on the external rotation film. In this projection, the contrast agent-filled sheath of the long head of the biceps, an anterior structure, moves outward and projects slightly laterally to the greater tuberosity and humeral head, simulating a collection of contrast medium in the subacromial bursa (Fig. 2.8). The differentiation is made by identifying the linear filling defect of the tendon within the sheath and by noting that the opacified tendon sheath moves medially on the internal rotation film. In contradistinction, an opacified subacromial bursa remains superior and lateral to the greater tuberosity in both projections, is usually broader, and does not contain the filling defect of the tendon (Fig. 2.16).

The third source of error, as described earlier, is the inadvertent injection of the subcoracoid bursa. This is only a potential space in most persons but if this bursa is enlarged and also communicates with the subacromial bursa, injection of contrast will result in a bursagram simulating a rotator cuff tear (Fig. 2.17). Careful inspection, however, will show no contrast material outlining the articular cartilage of the humerus, indicating that a bursagram rather than a glenohumeral arthrogram has been performed. If contrast medium does enter the glenohumeral joint from the subcoracoid injection by way of the subacro-

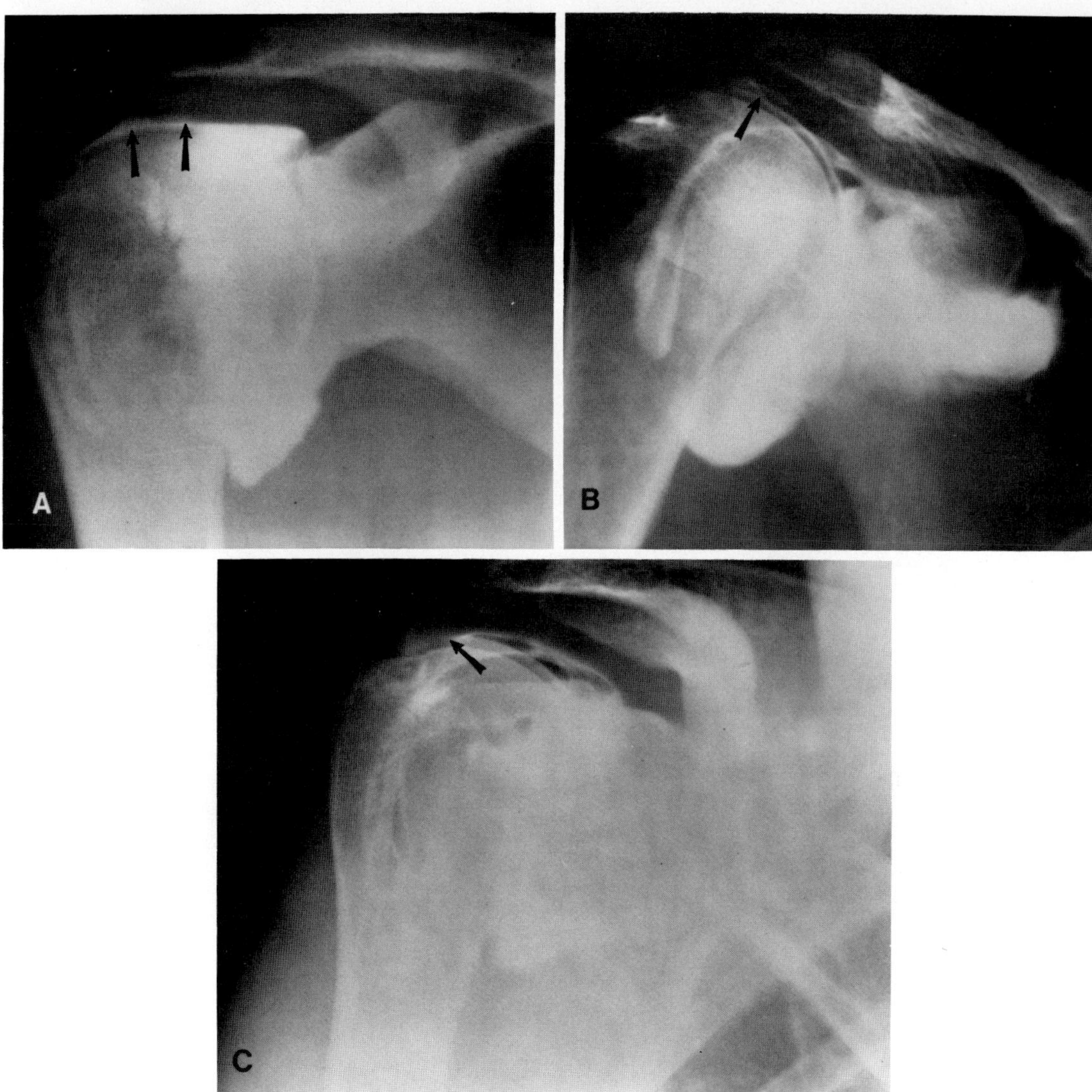

Figure 2.15. Abnormal shoulder arthrograms. *A,* Note irregularity of undersurface of rotator cuff tendon indicating ulceration (*arrows*). This represents an incomplete tear of the tendon—there is no opacification of the subacromial bursa. The scalloped margins and small volume of the joint recesses indicate associated adhesive capsulitis. *B,* Note opacified fissure in distal portion of rotator cuff tendon (*arrow*). This represents an incomplete tear of the tendon since no contrast enters the subacromial bursa. *C,* Double contrast study shows large opacified cavity on undersurface of distal portion of rotator cuff tendon (*arrow*). No contrast is visible in the subacromial bursa indicating an incomplete tear.

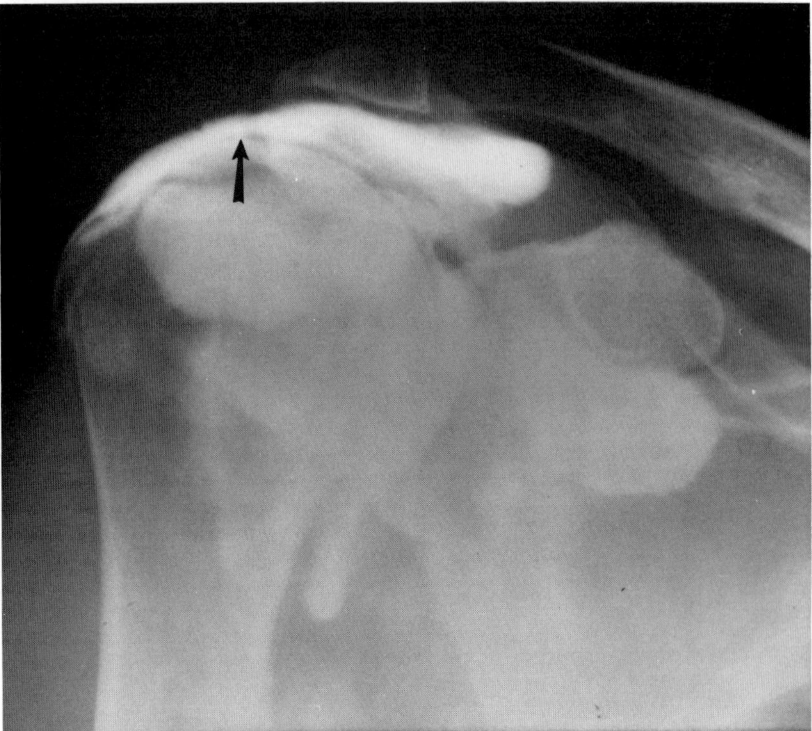

Figure 2.16. Abnormal shoulder arthrogram, single contrast. A majority of the contrast medium injected into the glenohumeral joint has passed into the subacromial bursa (*arrow*) verifying the clinically suspected complete tear of the rotator cuff tendon.

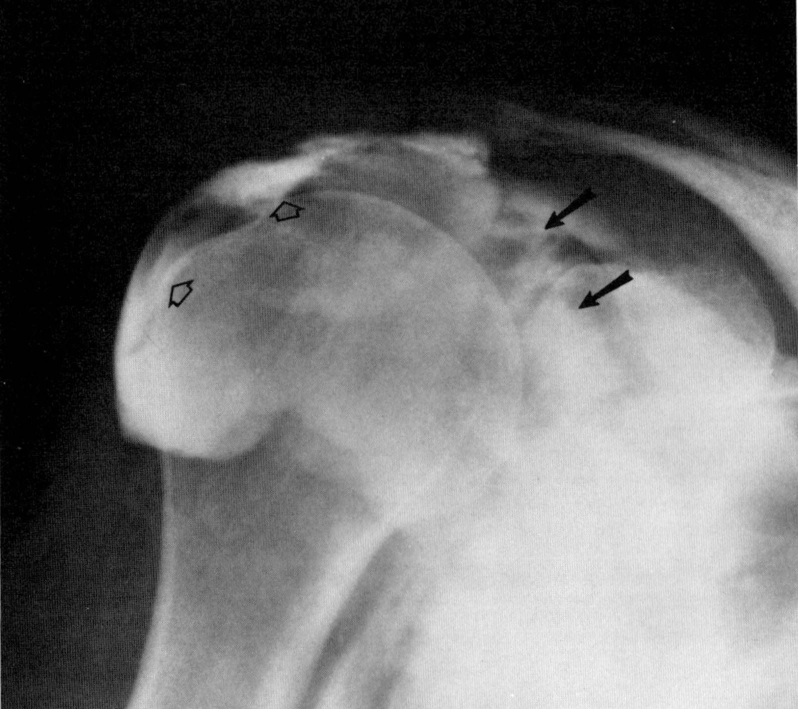

Figure 2.17. Shoulder bursagram. Inadvertent contrast injection of the subcoracoid bursa (*arrows*), and the communicating subacromial bursa (*open arrows*). No contrast outlines the articular cartilage of the humerus, indicating failure to inject the glenohumeral joint. The examination is nondiagnostic and must be repeated.

mial bursa, an abnormal communication exists and a rotator cuff tear is implied. This represents a "retrograde" positive shoulder arthrogram (Fig. 2.18).

Anterior Capsular Derangements

The anterior support of the shoulder consists of the joint capsule, subscapularis tendon, anterior glenohumeral ligaments, and the fibrocartilaginous glenoid labrum (Fig. 2.19). Anterior glenohumeral dislocation usually results in injury of these structures and may include rupture of the capsule, tears of the glenohumeral ligaments which anchor the capsule to the glenoid labrum, and labrum

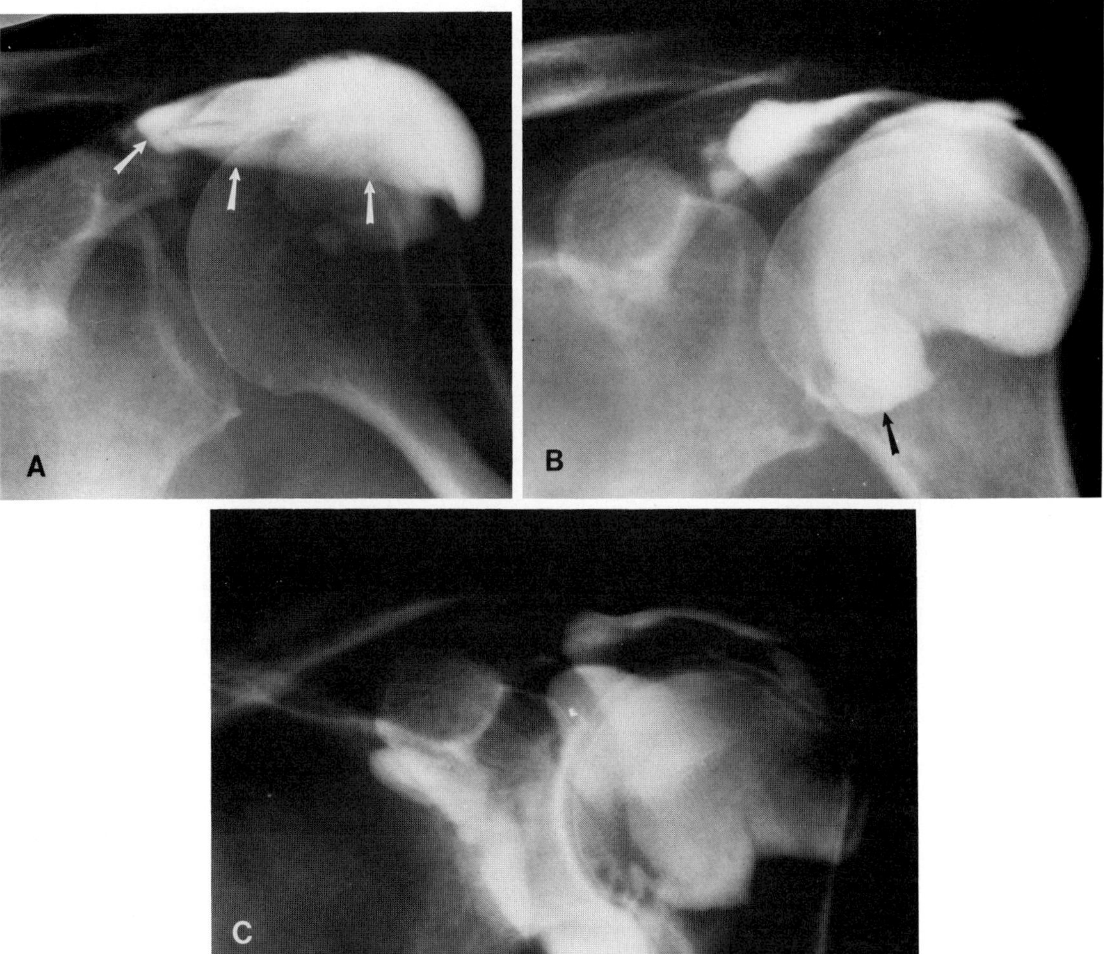

Figure 2.18. Single contrast shoulder arthrogram. A, Bursagram, due to inadvertent injection of an enlarged subcoracoid bursa communicating with a very large subacromial bursa (*arrows*). B, After exercise some of the contrast medium seeps into the recesses of the glenohumeral joint including the axillary recess (*arrow*). C, After further vigorous exercise there is complete filling of the glenohumeral joint (note contrast outlining articular cartilage of humerus), indicating a complete rotator cuff tear. This represents a positive "retrograde" shoulder arthrogram!

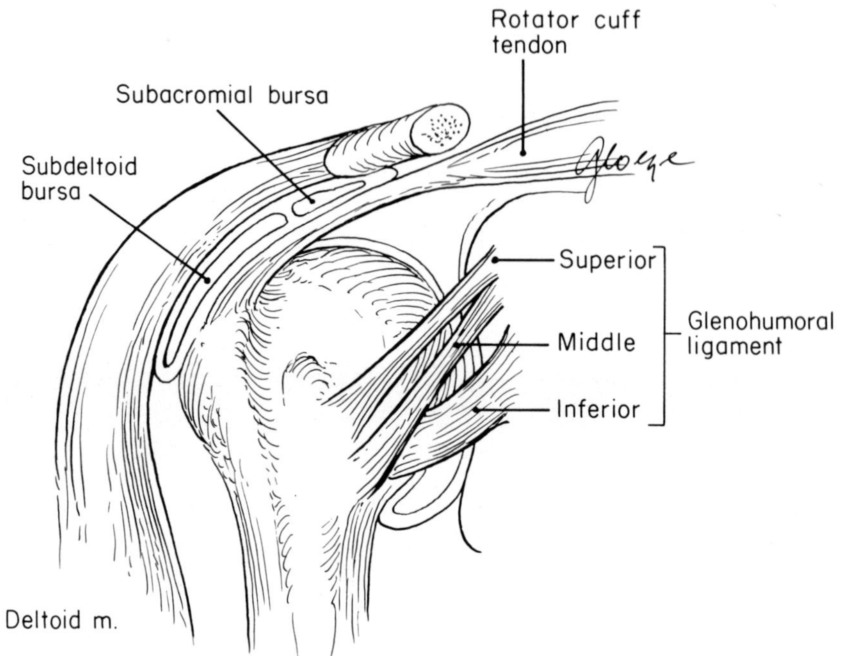

Figure 2.19. The anterior glenohumeral ligaments of the shoulder joint.

detachment. If the glenohumeral ligament tears are severe or heal incompletely, recurrent dislocation may result.

Arthrographic findings are best demonstrated in the internal rotation view and, as described by Kummel (1972), consist of the following: (1) free extravasation of contrast agent from the shoulder joint down the musculature of the arm or beneath the subscapularis muscle into the axilla (Fig. 2.20), indicating an acute tear of the capsule, anterior glenohumeral ligaments, or subscapularis tendon; and (2) enlargement of the subscapularis recess and obliteration of the normal indentation between it and the axillary recess, resulting in a large anteromedial pouch. This is caused by avulsion, incomplete healing and stretching of one or more anterior glenohumeral ligaments which may be accompanied by detachment of the glenoid labrum. An enlarged anterior pouch assuming a teardrop shape indicates a chronic or recurrent injury. The volume of the shoulder joint may exceed two or three times the normal (Fig. 2.21). This has been referred to as the balloon shoulder joint and is best appreciated on the internal rotation film when the anterior muscles are relaxed. External rotation tenses the subscapularis muscle which will obliterate this sac and express all contrast from it. Such anterior capsular derangements may be accompanied by a rotator cuff tear (Fig. 2.22). It is to rule out this tear and to evaluate the degree of detachment of the joint capsule from the labrum or the labrum from the glenoid that shoulder arthrography is performed. The larger the anteromedial ballooned pouch, the greater the detachment or derangement of the anterior ligaments. A comparison arthrogram of the opposite normal shoulder may be helpful to clarify the synovial sac alteration of the abnormal shoulder.

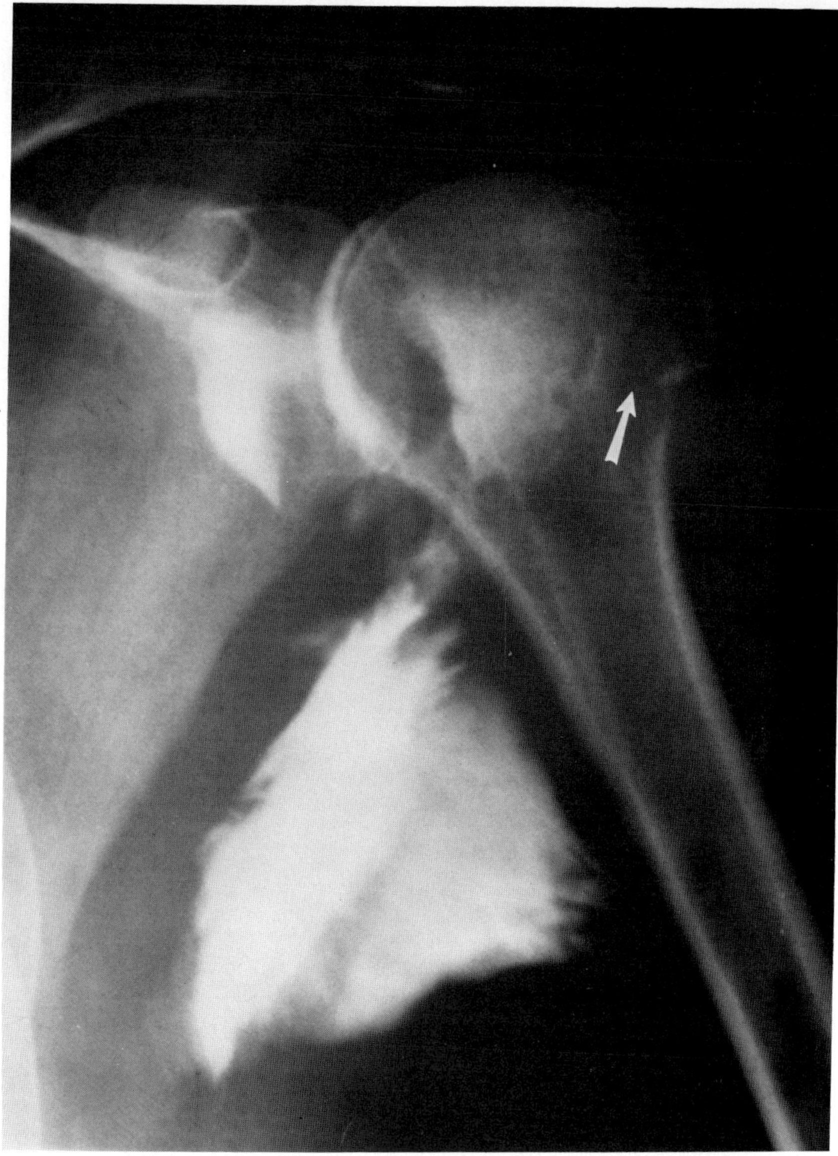

Figure 2.20. Abnormal shoulder arthrogram. Contrast leakage beneath subscapularis muscle into axilla was evident immediately upon injection of the shoulder joint. At surgery this proved to be an acute capsular-glenoid detachment and tear of an anterior glenohumeral ligament, following dislocation. Note also an avulsion fracture of the greater tuberosity (*arrow*).

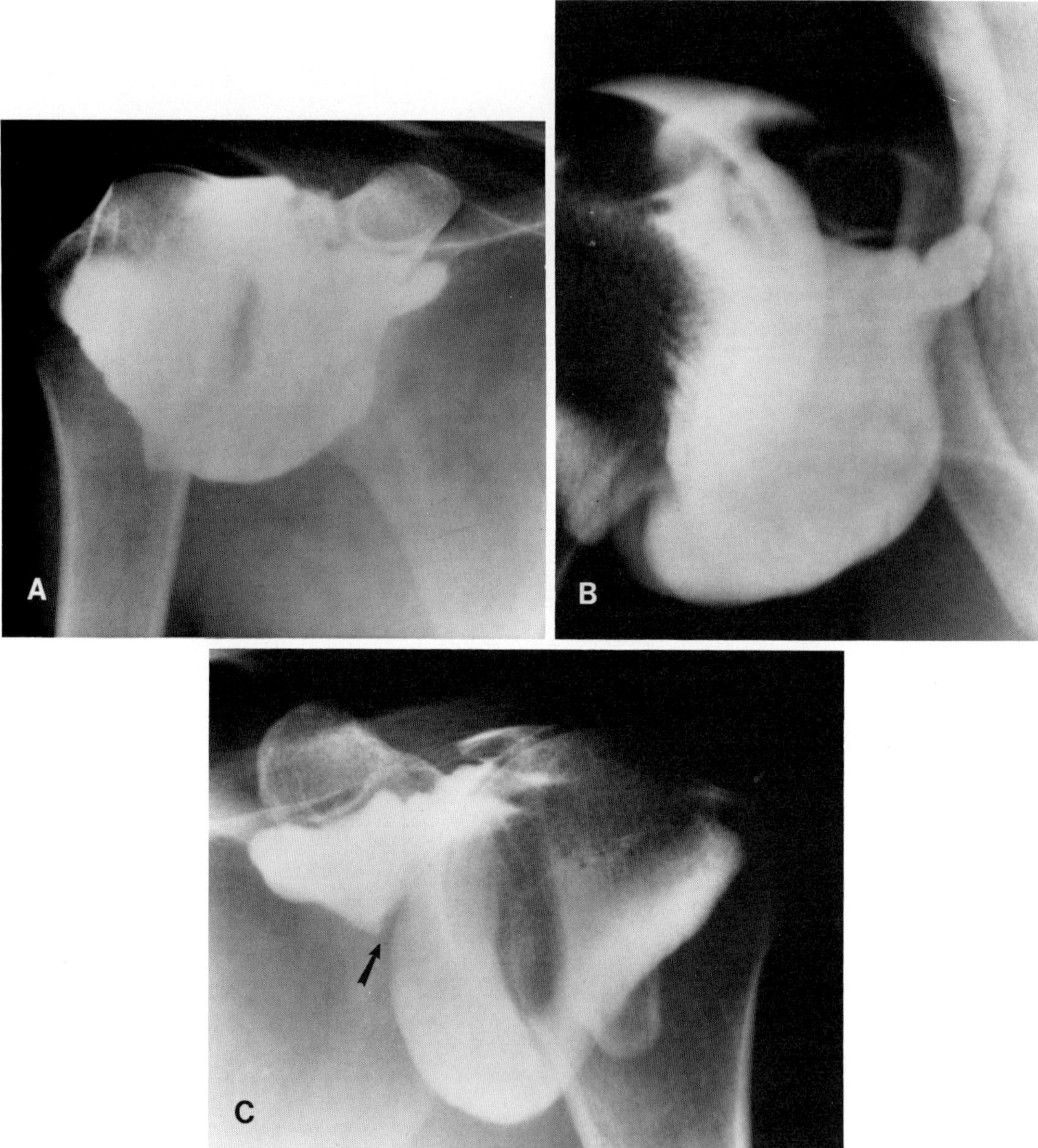

Figure 2.21. Abnormal shoulder arthrogram: recurrent dislocation. *A,* and *B,* Two patients with recurrent dislocation. Arthrogram shows large inferomedial pouch, absence of incisura between axillary and subscapularis recesses, and increased volume of the shoulder joint. *C,* Normal shoulder arthrogram for comparison. *Arrow* indicates the incisura.

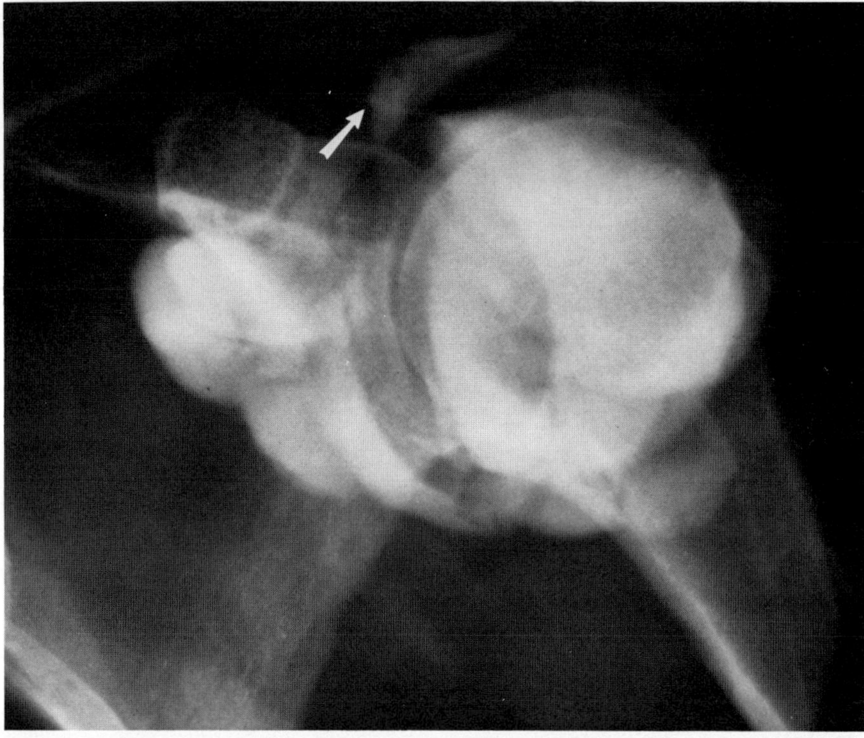

Figure 2.22. Abnormal shoulder arthrogram. "Balloon shoulder joint" in patient with recurrent dislocation showing multiple bulging sacs, increased volume (more than 30 ml of contrast media injected), and an associated rotator cuff tear (*arrow*).

The cartilaginous labrum may be injured with recurrent anterior shoulder dislocation. Detachment and tears of the labrum, most frequently the anterior lip, was first described by Bankart. Single and especially double contrast arthrography can be highly effective in examining for injuries of the labrum. The supine and prone axillary and upright external rotation films are the most informative (Fig. 2.23). The typical bony Bankart deformity, a healed impacted fracture of the anterior-inferior glenoid rim (Fig. 2.24), and the impacted fracture of the Hill-Sachs notch deformity on the posterolateral aspect of the humeral head should be sought on plain films as additional evidence of acute or recurrent glenohumeral dislocation. Absence of these bony lesions, however, does not rule out damage to anterior ligaments or the glenoid labrum.

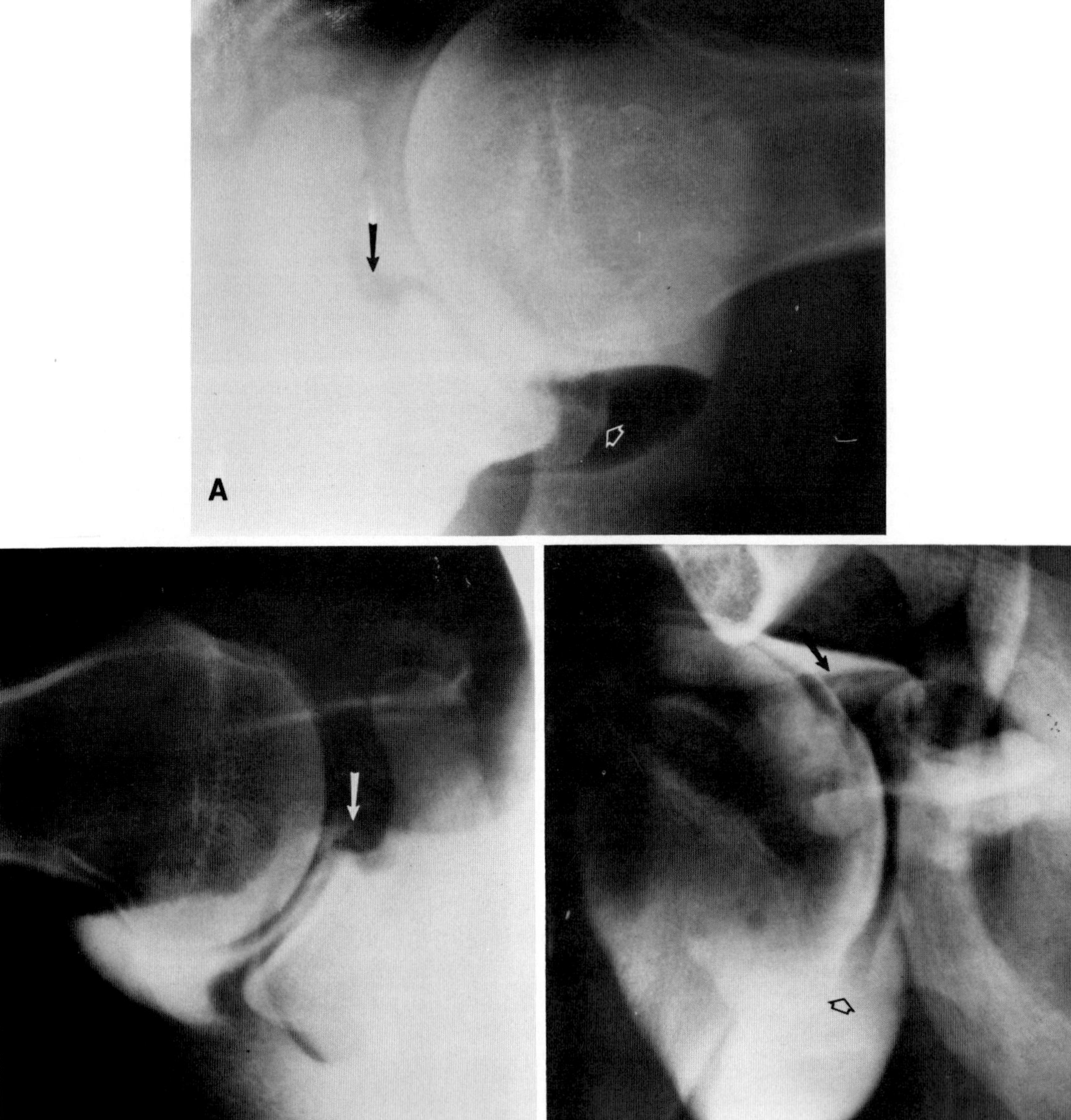

Figure 2.23. Abnormal shoulder arthrogram, double contrast. *A,* Recurrent dislocation. Prone axillary view shows irregular small anterior lip of cartilaginous glenoid labrum (*arrow*). Posterior lip is also deformed (*open arrow*) (courtesy of Jerrold H. Mink, M.D.). *B,* Another patient, supine axillary view, reveals normal rounded posterior glenoid lip, but anterior lip of glenoid labrum is small, irregular, and partially amputated (*arrow*). This patient also suffered recurrent shoulder dislocation. *C,* Normal glenoid labrum. Anterior lip (*arrow*) and posterior lip (*open arrow*).

Bicipital Lesions

In most shoulder arthrograms injected with sufficient volumes of contrast, the synovial reflection of the long head of the biceps anterior to the humerus will be opacified. Nonfilling may be normal or mean an insufficient volume of contrast. It may occasionally indicate adhesions, subluxation, or rupture of the tendon. Leakage of contrast from the synovial sheath into the musculature of the upper arm is commonly observed in asymptomatic persons, and there is disagreement about its significance. In most cases, it probably reflects high

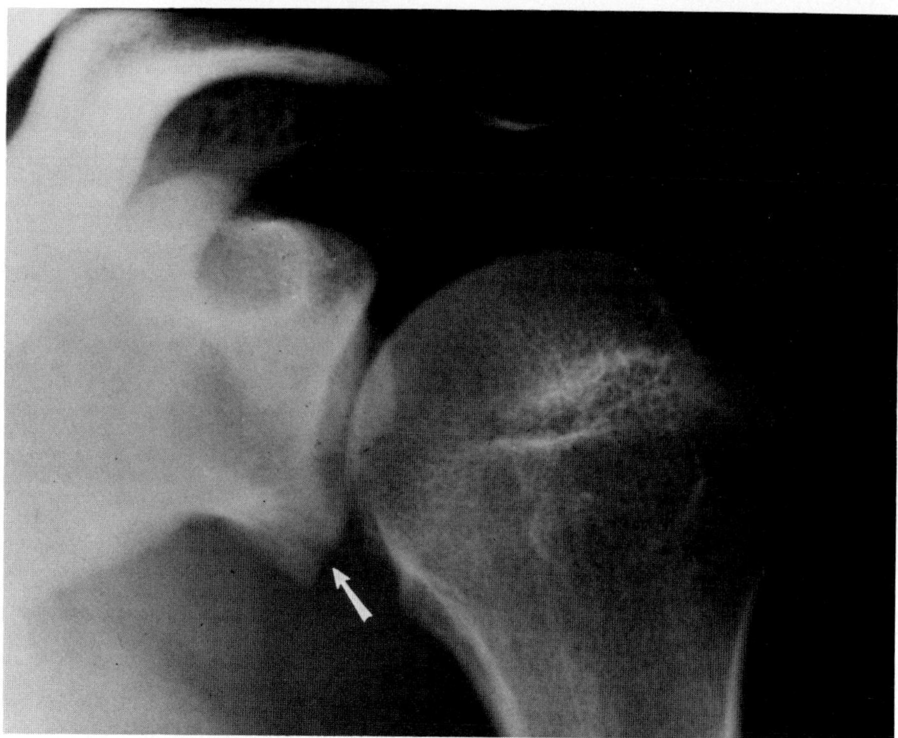

Figure 2.24. Plain film showing a healed, impacted fracture of the anterior inferior glenoid rim in a patient with a history of recurrent shoulder dislocation: bony Bankart type deformity (*arrow*).

injection pressure or vigorous exercise prior to filming. In a few patients, however, this finding indicates direct injury to the biceps tendon such as a complete tear or, more commonly, rupture of the transverse bicipital ligament (Fig. 2.1A) which usually results from medial subluxation of the long head of the biceps tendon from the bicipital groove (Fig. 2.25). Surgical correlation for the latter is difficult to obtain. In general, however, when contrast leakage from the bicipital sleeve is observed, the diagnosis of a bicipital lesion should be made with caution unless there is strong clinical correlation, recalling that, in most instances, it is a nonspecific finding.

Adhesive Capsulitis

The hallmark of this condition is diminished volume of the shoulder joint. The volume of contast that can be injected is usually only 5 to 10 cc and considerable resistance to injection is felt. The anatomical recesses are small

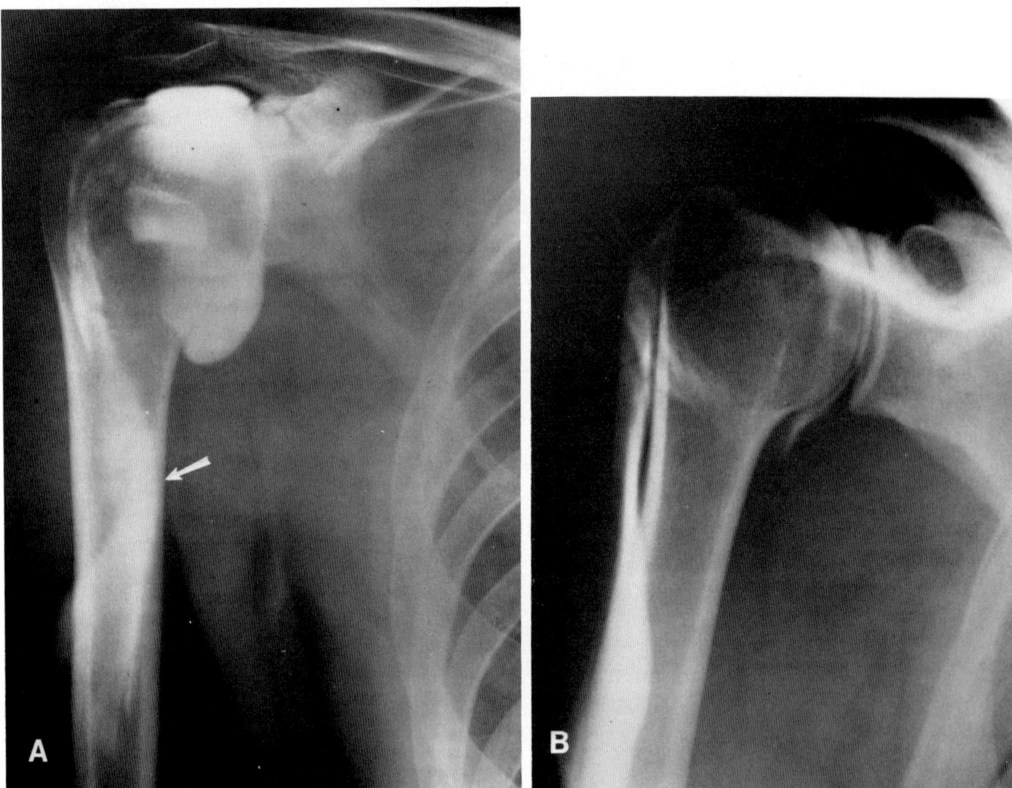

Figure 2.25. Abnormal shoulder arthrograms: bicipital lesions. *A,* Contrast medium passes freely from synovial sleeve of biceps tendon into musculature of arm (*arrow*). Torn transverse bicipital ligament. *B,* Complete rupture long head of biceps tendon. External rotation view shows massive leak from synovial sleeve and absence of outline of the tendon within it. *C,* Tangential view of bicipital groove shows empty bicipital canal indicating dislocation or rupture of biceps tendon. *D,* Tangential view of bicipital groove shows an empty groove. Clinical signs indicated complete rupture of the tendon. Contrast within the subacromial bursa (*arrow*) indicates an associated rotator cuff tear.

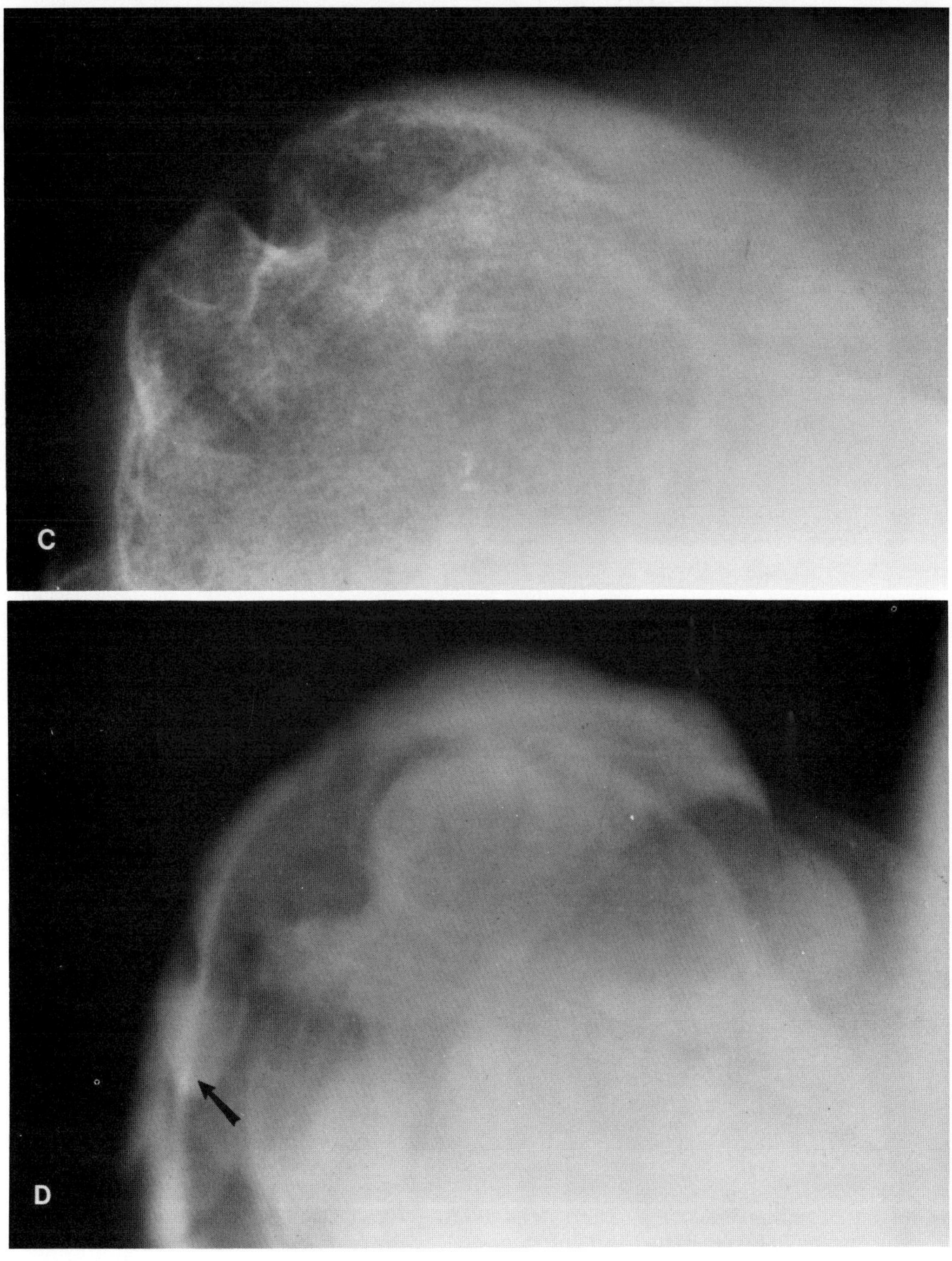

Figure 2.25 (*C* and *D*)

with irregular, retracted margins, and the biceps tendon sheath fills poorly or not at all (Fig. 2.26). In severe cases, contrast may not even outline all the articular cartilage of the humerus because of the reduced volume of the gleno-humeral joint. The causes of adhesive capsulitis may be traumatic, inflammatory, or prolonged disuse of the joint due to pain or immobilization. The value of arthrography is to verify the condition and its severity. At the time of arthrography, a specimen of joint fluid or contrast agent should be aspirated and sent for bacteriologic studies (Fig. 2.27). Additionally, depot corticosteroid preparations may be injected. Occasionally, distention by arthrography may at least temporarily improve the mobility of the joint and allow exercise maneuvers to improve the condition.

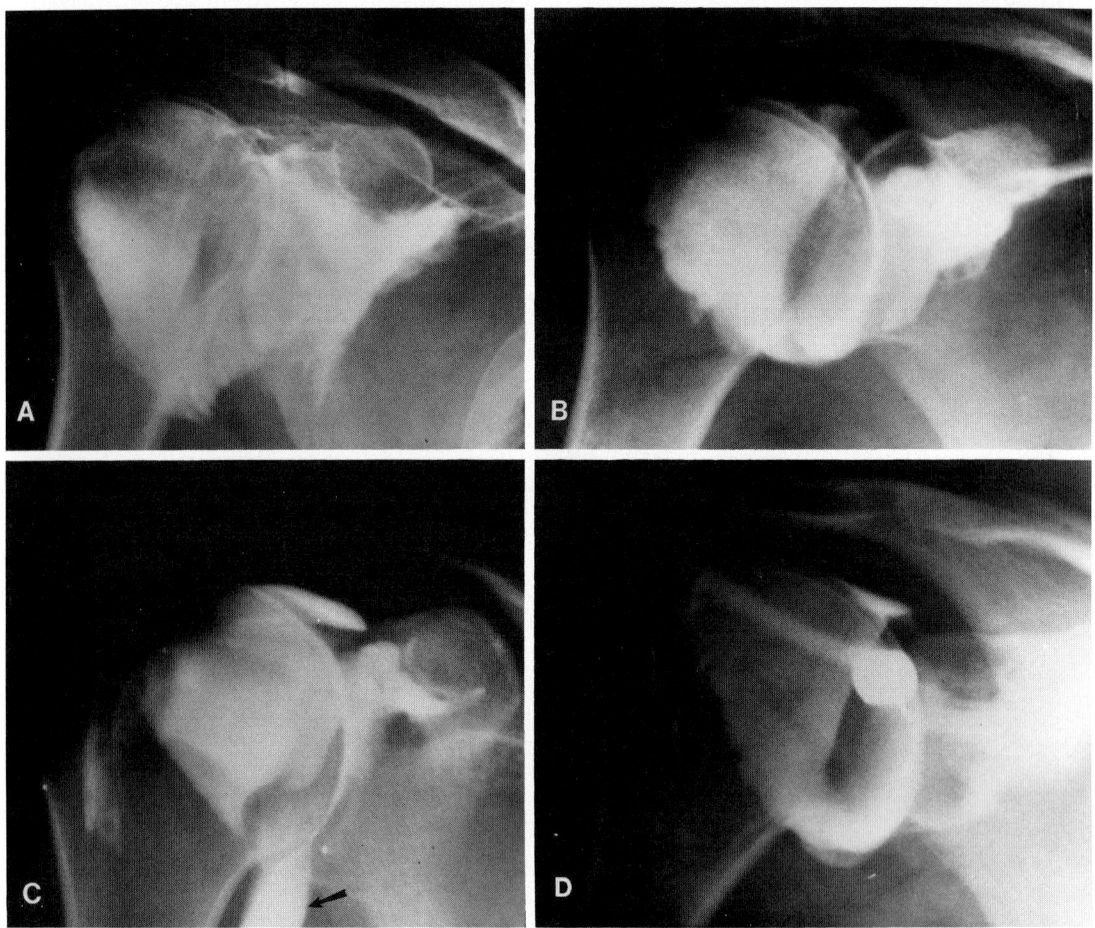

Figure 2.26. Abnormal shoulder arthrograms. *A,* Adhesive capsulitis. Note retracted, serrated margins of synovial recesses in a patient with reduced range of motion. *B,* Adhesive capsulitis. The synovial recesses are small. Joint capacity was only 10 ml. Note nonfilling of the biceps tendon sleeve. *C,* Adhesive capsulitis with severe retraction of synovial recesses, diminished joint volume (8 cc), and formation of pseudodiverticulum (*arrow*). *D,* Adhesive capsulitis. Joint volume, 6 cc. There was improvement in range of motion after the arthrogram.

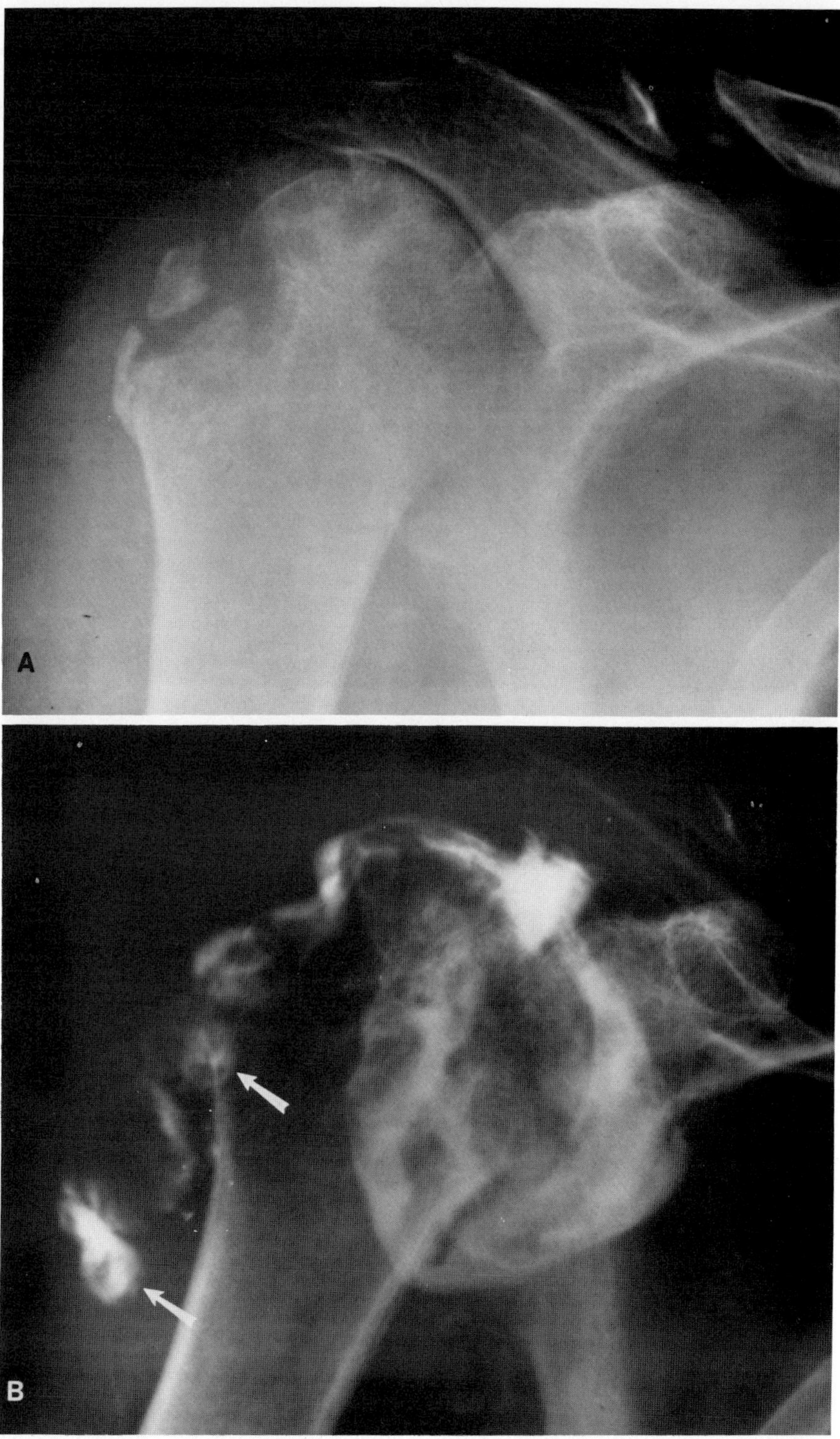

Figure 2.27. Abnormal shoulder arthrogram: pyogenic arthritis in a rheumatoid shoulder. *A,* Preliminary film reveals destruction and fragmentation of the humeral head and marked narrowing of the glenohumeral joint. *B,* Arthrogram verifies total destruction of articular cartilage, retracted synovial recesses, synovial hypertrophy, and dissecting synovial inflammatory cyst superolaterally (*arrows*). Joint aspirate at time of arthrography yielded *Staphylococcus aureus* on bacterial culture.

Inflammatory Arthritis and Other Conditions

Shoulder arthrography is occasionally useful in established diseases of the shoulder when a superimposed rotator cuff tear needs to be excluded before treatment for joint disability can begin. This is particularly true in rheumatoid arthritis when corticosteroid therapy is being considered. The arthrographic findings in this condition consist of multiple, nodular filling defects due to nodular hypertrophy of the synovial lining of the capsule (Fig. 2.28). Other findings include adhesive capsulitis, lymphatic filling during arthrography, enlargement of the synovial sac, dilatation of the biceps tendon sheath and,

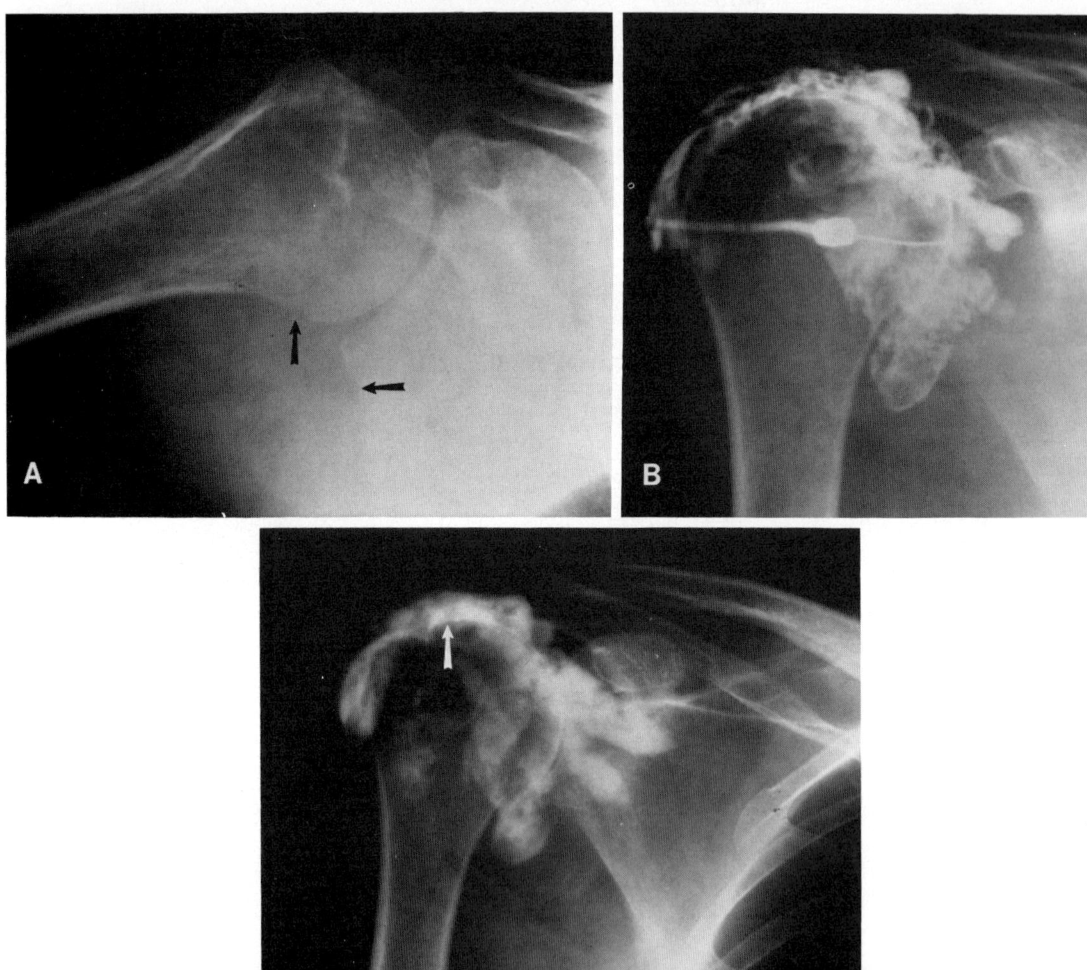

Figure 2.28. Abnormal shoulder arthrogram: rheumatoid arthritis. *A,* Preliminary film reveals subcortical erosions of humerus and glenoid (*arrows*). *B,* Arthrogram, early injection phase, reveals numerous, nodular filling defects within synovial recesses of the joint indicating synovial hypertrophy. *C,* Final film of arthrogram shows synovial hypertrophy, retraction of joint recesses, and a rotator cuff tear (*arrow*).

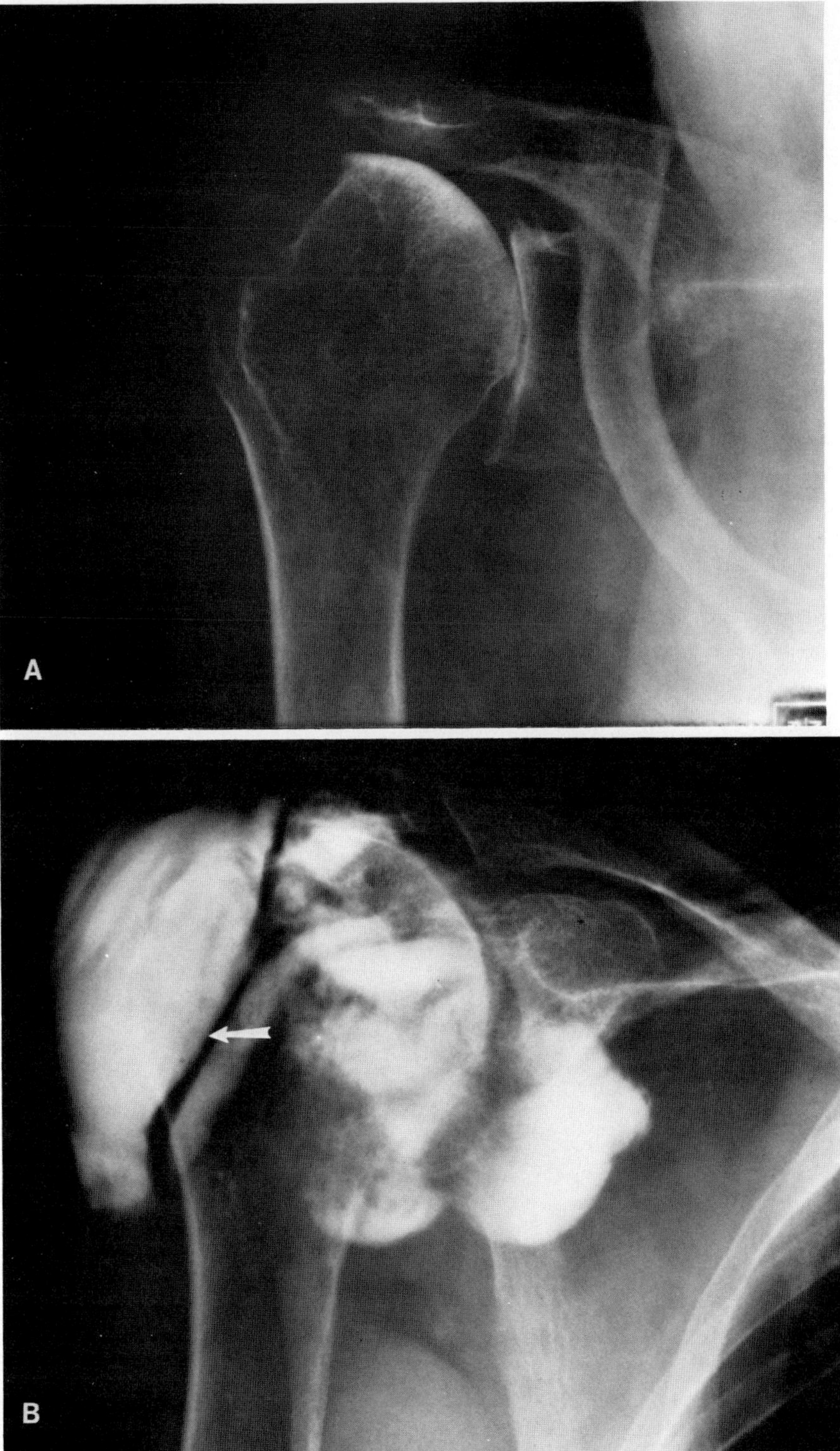

Figure 2.29. Abnormal shoulder arthrogram: rheumatoid arthritis: *A,* Preliminary film shows advanced narrowing of the joint space, eburnation of superior aspect of humeral head, and generalized osteoporosis. *B,* Arthrogram reveals nodular synovial hypertrophy, enlarged anterior recesses from chronic joint effusion and/or glenohumeral ligament relaxation, and large contrast-filled subacromial bursa secondary to a chronic rotator cuff tear (*arrow*).

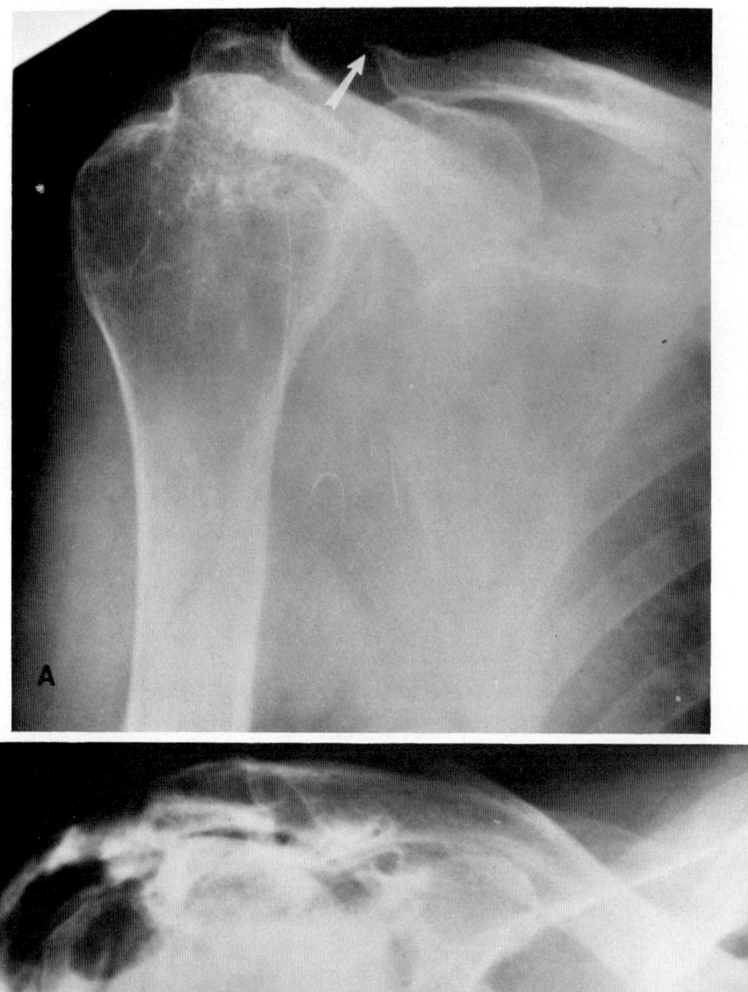

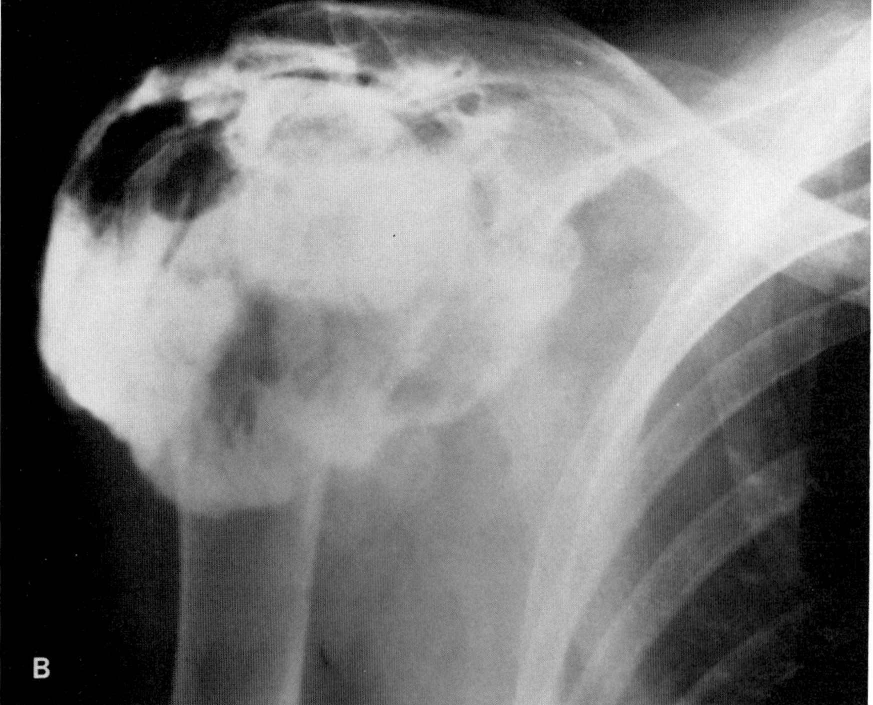

Figure 2.30. Abnormal shoulder arthrogram: rheumatoid arthritis: *A,* Preliminary film shows osteoporosis, narrowing of the glenohumeral joint, and "pencil point" erosion of lateral head of clavicle (*arrow*). *B,* Arthrogram reveals enlarged joint sac due to chronic effusion, with irregular margins and synovial hypertrophy, and a rotator cuff tear.

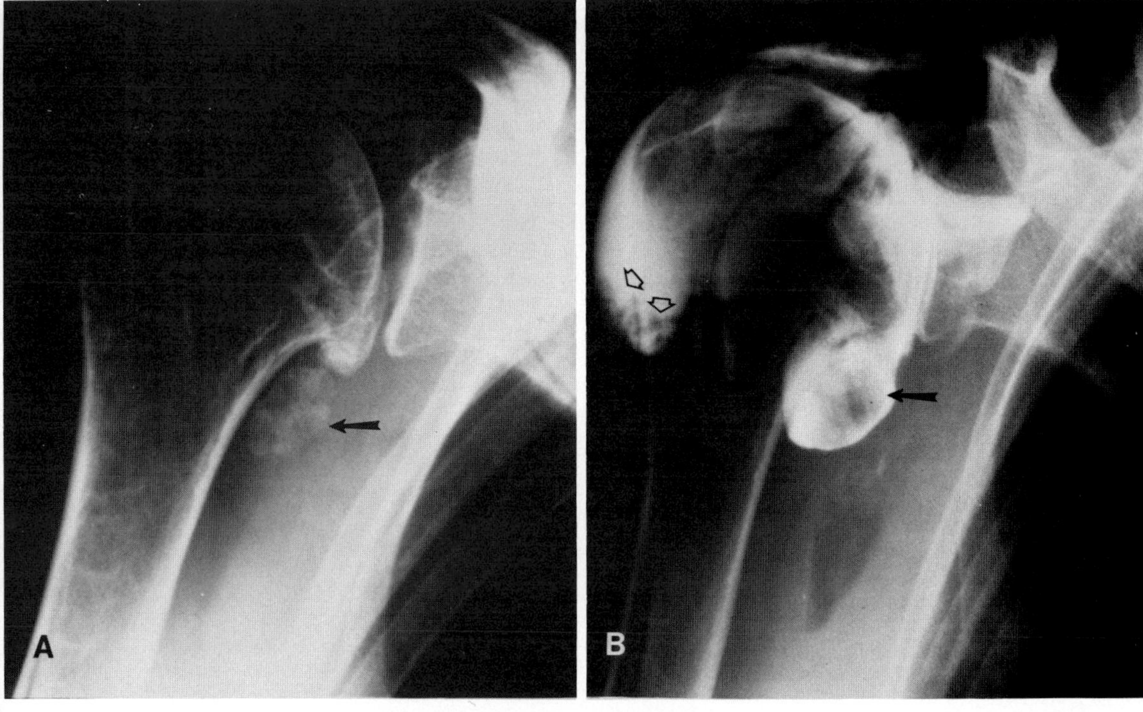

Figure 2.31. Abnormal shoulder arthrogram: synovial osteochondromatosis. *A*, Preliminary film indicates a calcified body within the glenohumeral joint (*arrow*). *B*, Arthrogram verifies the loose body within the axillary recess (*arrow*) and shows multiple, smaller "stones" in a contrast-filled subacromial bursa (*open arrows*), the latter indicating a rotator cuff tear.

occasionally, a dissecting synovial cyst along the anterolateral aspect of the shoulder joint. Since the incidence of associated rotator cuff tear in shoulders involved with rheumatoid arthritis is high, probably caused by inflamed synovium eroding the inferior surface of the tendon, as well as trauma, there is some value in confirming this diagnosis rather than assuming that shoulder pain in a rheumatoid patient is an exacerbation of the basic disease (Figs. 2.29 and 2.30).

Rarely, arthrography may be of use in identifying other conditions such as pigmented villonodular synovitis, and synovial osteochondromatosis (Fig. 2.31).

References

Andren, L., Lundberg, B.J., Treatment of rigid shoulders by joint distention during arthrography. Acta Orthop Scand, *36*:45–53, 1965.

Bankart, A.B., The Pathology and treatment of recurrent dislocation of the shoulder joint. Br J Surg, *26*: 23–29, 1938.

De Smet, A.A., Ting, Y.M., Weiss, J.J., Shoulder arthrography in rheumatoid arthritis. Radiology, *116*: 601–605, 1975.

El-Khoury, G.Y., Albright, J.P., Abu Yousef, M.M., et al. Arthrotomography of the glenoid labrum. Radiology, *131*:333–337, 1979.

Ennevaara, K., Painful shoulder joint in rheumatoid arthritis: Clinical and radiologic study of 200 cases with special reference to arthrography of the glenohumeral joint. Acta Rheumatol Scand, Suppl. II, 11–116, 1967.

Ghelman, B., Goldman, A.B., The double contrast shoulder arthrogram: Evaluation of rotator cuff tears. Radiology, *124*:251–254, 1977.

Goldman, A.B., Ghelman, B., The double contrast shoulder arthrogram. Radiology, *127*:655–663, 1978.

Grant, J.C.B., *A Method of Anatomy*, Ed. 6, pp. 180–188. Williams & Wilkins, Baltimore, 1958.

Grant, J.C.B., *An Atlas of Anatomy,* Ed. 5, Figs. 35–43. Williams & Wilkins, Baltimore, 1962.

Killoran, P.J., Marcove, R.C., Freiberger, R.H., Shoulder arthrography. AJR, 103:658–668, 1968.

Kummel, B.M., Arthrography of anterior capsular derangements of the shoulder. Clin Orthop, 83:170–176, 1972.

Kummel, B.M., When shoulder complaints limit athletic performance. Physician Sports Med, pp.46–51, Aug. 1974.

Lindblom, K., Arthrography and roentgenography in ruptures of the tendons of the shoulder joint. Acta Radiol, 20:548–562, 1939.

Meschan, I., *An Atlas of Normal Radiographic Anatomy,* Ed. 2, pp. 66–88. W.B. Saunders, Philadelphia, 1968.

Mink, J.H., Richardson, A., Grant, T.T., Evaluation of glenoid labrum by double-contrast shoulder arthrography. AJR, 133:883–887, 1979.

Nelson, C.L., Burton, R.I., Upper extremity arthrography. Clin Orthop., 197:62–72, 1975.

Nelson, C.L., Razzano, C.D., Arthrography of the shoulder, a review. Trauma, 13:136–141, 1973.

Neviaser, J.J., Arthrography of the shoulder joint. J Bone Joint Surg, [Am] 44:1321–1330, 1962.

Neviaser, J.J., *Arthrography of the Shoulder,* pp. 179–190, Charles C Thomas, Springfield, Illinois, 1975.

Samilson, R.L., Raphael, R.L., Post, L., et al. Arthrography of the shoulder joint. Clin Orthop, 20:21–31, 1961.

Schinz, H.R., et al., *Roentgen Diagnosis,* edited by L.G. Rigler, Ed. 2, Vol. I, pp. 352–355. Grune and Stratton, New York, 1968.

Weiss, J.J., Thompson, G.R., Doust, V., et al., Rotator cuff tears in rheumatoid arthritis. Arch Intern Med, 135:521–525, 1975.

3

Arthrography of the Hip

R. D. Arndt, M.D.

INDICATIONS FOR HIP ARTHROGRAPHY

Prior to the advent of total hip replacement in adults, hip arthrography found its primary application in infants for the evaluation of congenital malformations, especially dislocation, where the objective was the detection of an infolded acetabular labrum which prohibited reduction by conservative means. Less frequent indications in children are evaluation of the articular cartilage in Legg-Perthes disease and, occasionally, neonatal septic hip.

In adults, hip arthrography is performed to examine the painful joint in infectious, posttraumatic and sometimes inflammatory arthritis, but most importantly to confirm the presence of loosening or infection of a total hip prosthesis. The latter now constitutes the major indication for all hip arthrography performed in radiological practice.

FUNCTIONAL ANATOMY

The hip joint is a ball-and-socket joint comprised of the three segments of the innominate bone which form the acetabulum—ischium, ilium, and pubis—and the femoral head which completes the joint. The acetabulum is a hollow half-sphere with a ventral notch, or acetabulae incisura bridged by the transverse ligament. The perimeter of the acetabular cuff is lined by a thick border of fibrocartilage, the acetabular labrum (limbus), attached to the rim of the acetabulum and ventral transverse ligament. This labrum grasps the head of the femur just beyond its articular surface. In the base of the acetabular fossa, there is a fat pad which serves as a shock absorber. Imbedded in this fat pad is the ligamentum teres which originates from the transverse ligament of the acetabular notch and extends to the fovea centralis, a flattened portion of the femoral head which is not covered by articular cartilage. This ligament connects the head to the transverse ligament, and is surrounded by its own synovial sheath within which arteries and veins course between the acetabulum and the head of the femur. The sheath is not opacified during arthrography (Fig. 3.1).

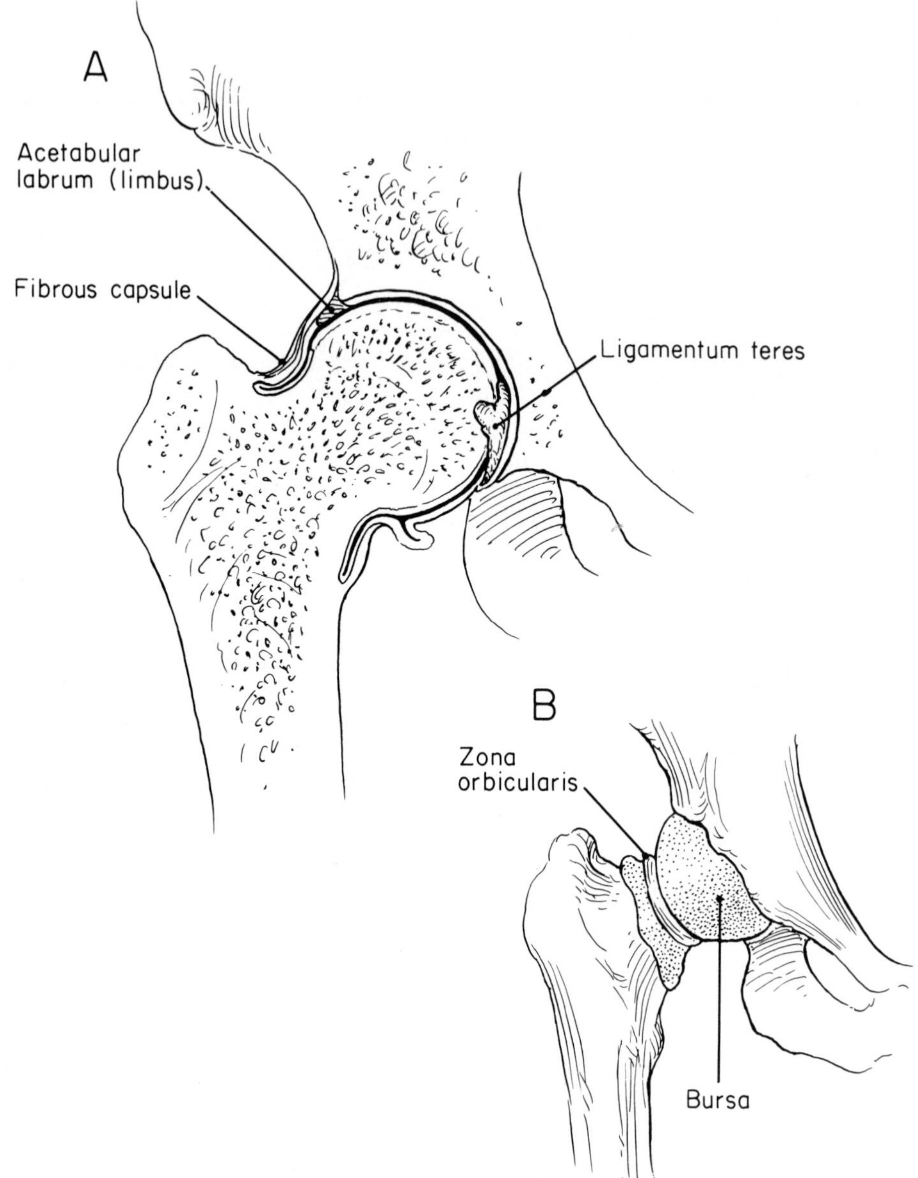

Figure 3.1. Synovial bursa of the hip joint. *A,* Coronal section. *B,* Distended synovial bursa.

The hip joint is contained within a strong fibrous capsule that is lined by synovium. The joint capsule is comprised of several ligamentous contributions from each bony compartment of the acetabulum—the ileofemoral, pubofemoral, and ischiofemoral ligaments. The capsule is attached to the rim of the acetabulum as well as the labrum and transverse ligament. Distally, it inserts on the femur anteriorly along the intertrochanteric line just proximal to the lesser trochanter. Although the fibers of the capsule cross the femur posteriorly, there are no posterior or superior attachments.

The synovial sac frequently bulges below and beyond the fibrous capsule for 1 or 2 cm along the posterior aspect of the femoral neck, acting as a bursa for the obturator externus tendon. Several deep circular fibers of the capsule at the level of the femoral neck constrict the synovial sac of the joint and are recognized as the zona orbicularis at arthrography.

NORMAL HIP ARTHROGRAM

The synovium lines the joint capsule over the entire joint, except for the bare surfaces of the articular cartilage. The synovial recesses consist of the supra- and infraarticular recesses, the acetabular recess, and the recess colli. The latter is actually an outpouching of the synovial sac beneath the fibrous joint capsule at a point where it is not attached directly to the femoral neck. Several circular fibers of the capsule at the midpoint of the femoral neck constrict the synovial sac in a ring-like fashion, resulting in an extrinsic impression on the contrast material—the zona orbicularis (Fig. 3.2). The labrum of the articular cartilage of the acetabulum is readily identifiable. The sheath of synovium enveloping the ligamentum teres and vessels entering the fovea centralis of the femur is not visible. The articular cartilage of femur and acetabulum can be easily assessed.

METHOD OF HIP ARTHROGRAPHY IN CHILDREN

General anesthesia is usually required in children under 5 years of age. The method of arthrocentesis is the same as in adults, although the preferred point of entry is along the medial aspect of the femoral neck below the growth plate of the capital femoral epiphysis (Fig. 3.3). This avoids puncture of the growth plate itself, the epiphysis, and femoral vessels.

With the leg in the anatomical position, a 22-gauge spinal needle with stylet in place is advanced perpendicular to the tabletop down to the periosteum. A syringe containing saline or lidocaine is attached, and the needle bevel is rotated slightly and withdrawn 1 or 2 mm until fluid can be freely injected. Extension tubing is then attached to a syringe containing iodinated contrast material (diatrizoate meglumine), and contrast is slowly infused under fluoroscopic guidance. If a bone stain is observed, the needle tip is rotated or withdrawn further until contrast medium flows freely into the joint space, usually filling first the medial recesses and the joint reflection beneath the zona orbicularis, and thereafter outlining the cartilaginous head. The capacity of the joint varies according to age and is usually about 2 cc in newborns, 3 or 4 cc in toddlers, and 5 to 7 cc in 10-year-old children. Slight traction on the leg aids in filling the joint. Before removing the needle, a few drops of contrast are allowed to flow out, reducing the intraarticular pressure and preventing extravasation of contrast material through the needle hole in the capsule. A slight amount of contrast or joint fluid should be aspirated and sent for bacterial culture. Immediately after needle withdrawal, overhead films are taken, including anteroposterior films in neutral position, adduction, abduction, with internal and external ("frog-leg") rotation, and lateral projections. These films must be taken promptly insofar as contrast absorption is rapid and considerable detail may be lost even

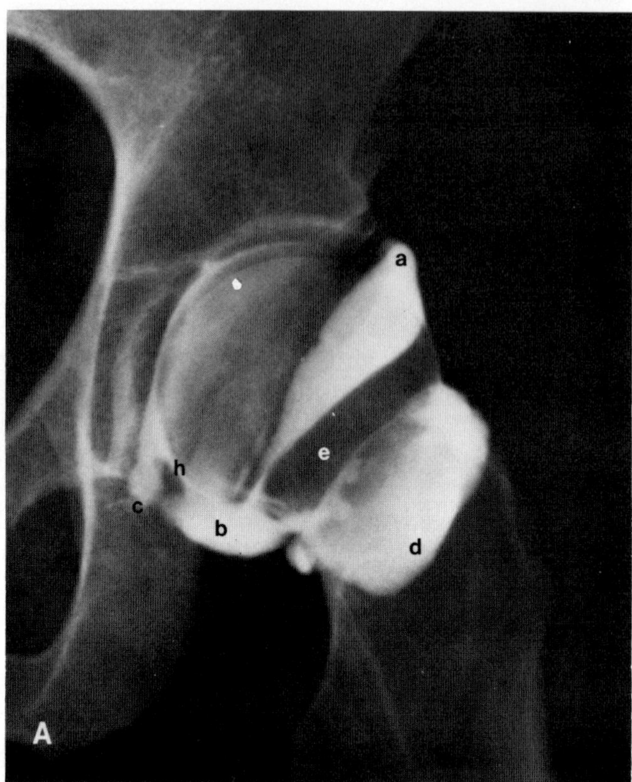

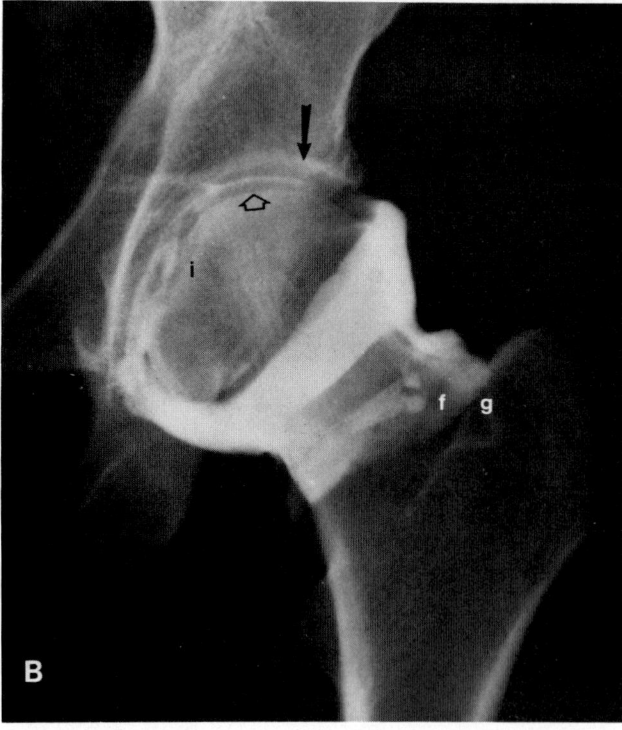

Figure 3.2. Normal adult hip arthrogram. *A* and *B* antero-posterior views show articular cartilage of the acetabulum (*arrow*) and femoral head (*open arrow*), as well as (*a*) supraarticular recess, (*b*) infraarticular recess, (*c*) acetabular recess, (*d*) recess coli, (*e*) zona orbicularis, (*f*) distal border of capsule anteriorly, (*g*) distal border of capsule posteriorly, (*h*) outline of transverse acetabular ligament, (*i*) fovea centralis.

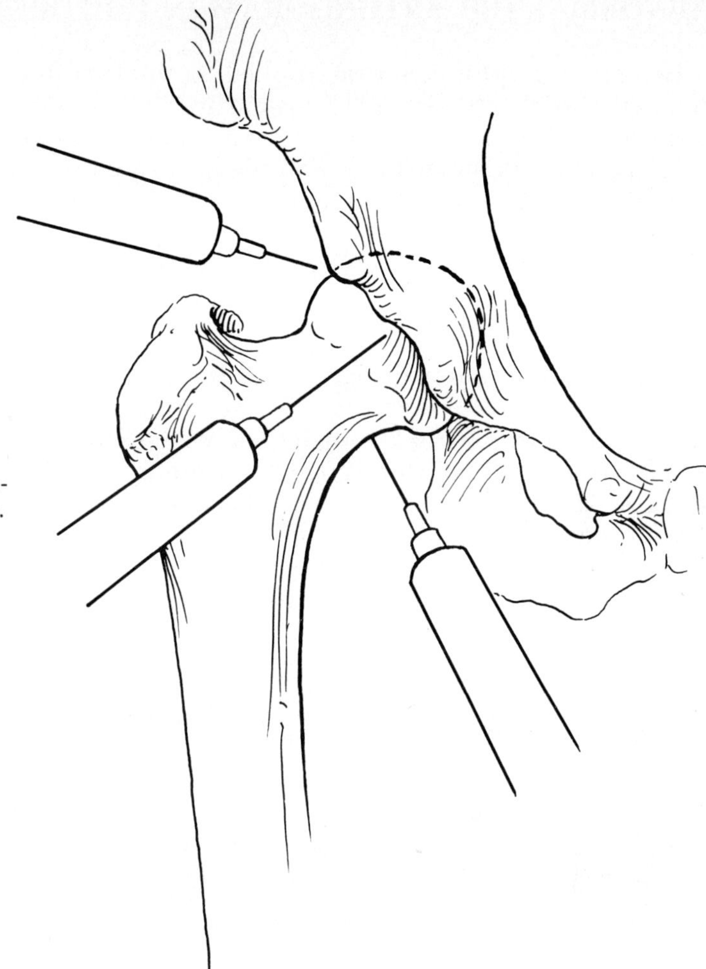

Figure 3.3. Sites for arthrocentesis in hip arthrography.

after only 10 minutes. In a dislocated hip, joint puncture is often easiest using
the medial approach because the joint capsule is often pulled medially in this
condition.

In children, as well as adults, the radiologist is occasionally requested to
perform a hip aspiration without contrast arthrography. When no fluid is
obtained during aspiration, a dilemma arises. Is the joint dry? Is the needle
intraarticular? This can only be resolved by injecting contrast media and
verifying the intraarticular location of the needle tip with a roentgenogram.
Saline, sterile water, or more contrast agent can then be injected and reaspirated
for bacteriological culture, assuring both the radiologist and clinician that the
aspirate and culture results are reliable. If the joint is distended with contrast
agent, films should be obtained to maximize the diagnostic yield of the joint
aspiration.

ABNORMAL HIP ARTHROGRAM IN CHILDREN

Hip arthrography was first applied to children during the early part of this century and continues today primarily for the evaluation of congenital hip dislocation, particularly to detect the presence of an interposed, infolded labrum between the acetabular fossa and the dislocated femoral head. Such deformity of the labrum is a barrier to conservative management of dislocation. The hip arthrogram is also useful in evaluation of the articular cartilage and sphericity of the femoral head in Legg-Perthes disease.

Congenital Hip Dislocation

The normal infant arthrogram has been described by Severin (Fig. 3.4). The cartilaginous labrum comprises the superolateral border of the opacified joint space and resembles a nonopacified wedge with contrast medium lining its undersurface and the lateral edge of the innominate bone attached to its superior surface. The cartilaginous femoral head should be spherical and the cartilaginous acetabulum should cover no less than the medial half of the femoral head. Excessive pooling of contrast medium in the inferomedial portion of the acetabulum, in association with superolateral displacement of the cartilaginous femoral head, indicates subluxation.

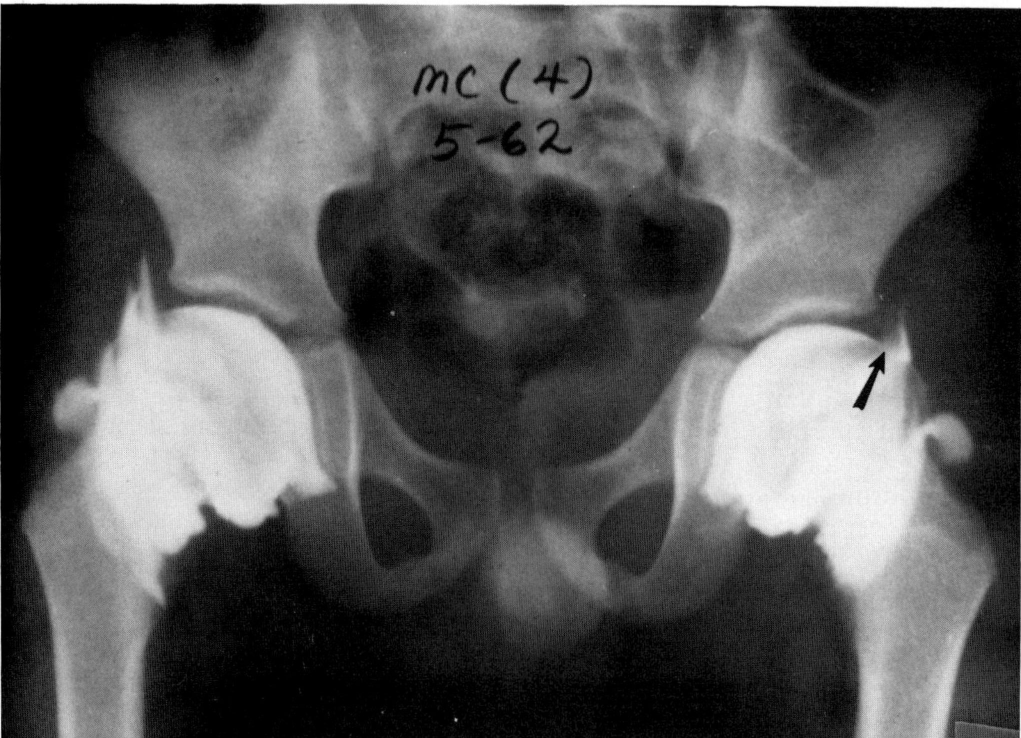

Figure 3.4. Normal bilateral hip arthrogram in a child. Note the cartilagenous acetabular labrum or limbus (*arrow*). (Courtesy of Robert Watanabe, M.D.)

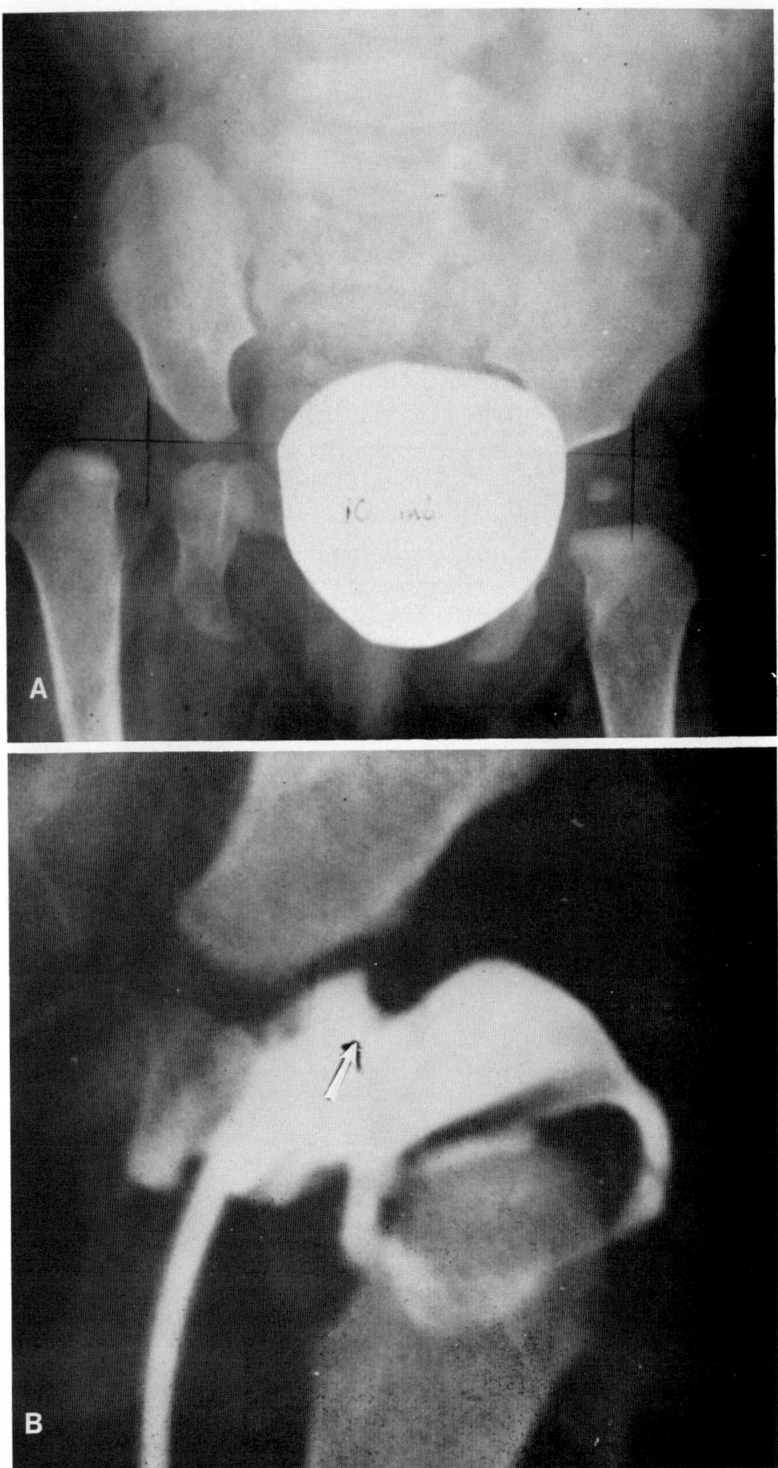

Figure 3.5. Congenital hip dislocation. *A,* Plain film: all signs are present on the right side, including: delayed ossification of the femoral head, increased acetabular angle, disruption of Shenton's line, and superolateral subluxation of the femoral head. *B,* Arthrogram in a congenital hip dislocation with infolded acetabular labrum. The filling defect of the labrum (*arrow*) is clearly seen interposed between the acetabulum and the dislocated femoral head.

With complete dislocation, the femoral head slips beneath and beyond the labrum. The latter, being an elastic structure, then moves back to its original position, coming to rest medial to the femoral head where it can be recognized as a wedge-shaped filling defect in the contrast-filled joint space (Fig. 3.5).

In the patient with a fully dislocated femoral head, according to Severin, four arthrographic signs are found: (1) a large amount of contrast material in the inferomedial aspect of the joint, since most of the capsule has now been retracted medially; (2) failure of the cartilaginous acetabulum to cover at least the medial half of the femoral head; (3) a filling defect caused by the labrum, located between the acetabulum and the femoral head; and (4) the femoral head displaced laterally and superiorly (Fig. 3.6).

Occasionally, in a complete dislocation, the arthrogram reveals an hourglass constriction of the capsule between the femoral head and acetabulum, indicating that a fold of capsule has become inverted, with the labrum lying anterior to it. This capsular fold may be an insurmountable obstruction to conservative relocation of the femoral head. Although prolapse of the femoral head lateral to the labrum often requires surgical reduction, this is not always the case and,

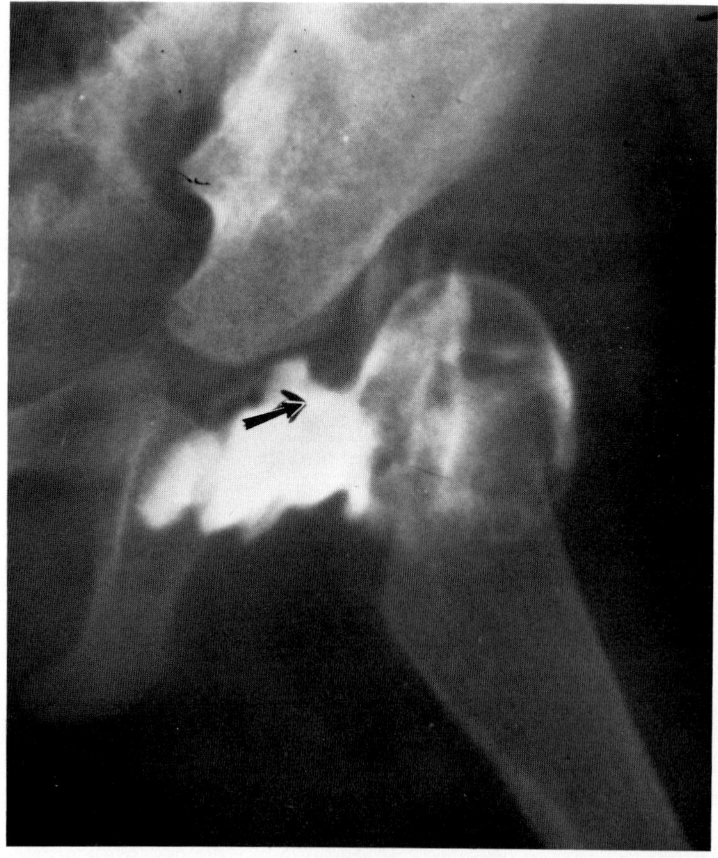

Figure 3.6. Abnormal hip arthrogram: congenital hip dislocation. The infolded acetabular labrum is obvious (*arrow*). Note the medially retracted joint capsule containing most of the injected contrast medium.

occasionally, gradually progressive and prolonged abduction will allow the head to return under the edge of the labrum to its normal position. Prolonged dislocation results in atrophy of the labrum which is undesirable since it results in a shallow acetabulum. Although the atrophic labrum allows the femoral head to be relocated, the shallow acetabulum predisposes to future subluxation and premature secondary osteoarthritis. Preservation of the cartilaginous labrum allows formation of a normal acetabulum, which is the final determinative factor in producing a normal hip joint.

Another arthrogram following reduction of the femoral head may be necessary to verify the reduction as complete by identifying the normal location of the limbus.

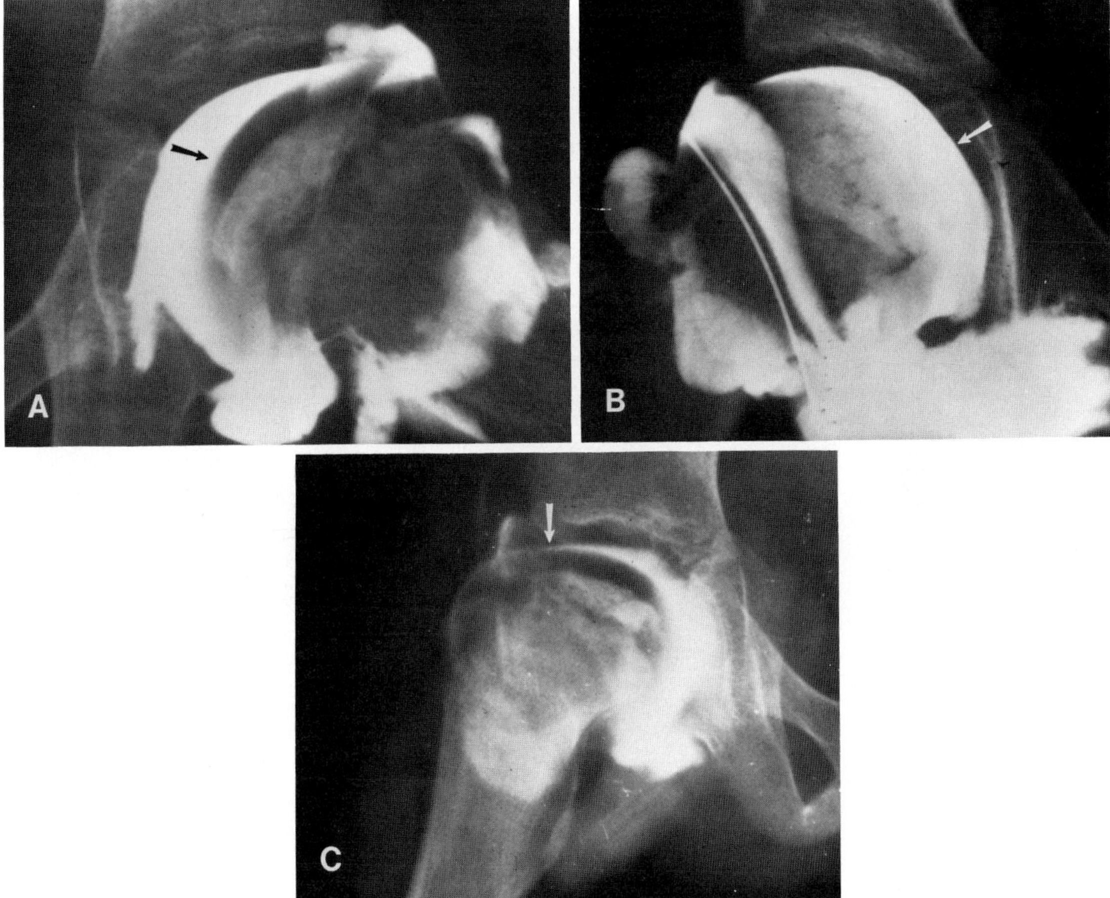

Figure 3.7. Abnormal hip arthrogram: Legg-Calvé-Perthes disease, fragmentation stage. *A*, Contrast pooling in the joint centrally over femoral head cartilage (*arrow*) indicates head-acetabular incongruity. *B*, Early coxa plana. The bony portion of the femoral capital epiphysis is still intact, but there is flattening of the central portion of the contrast-outlined femoral head articular cartilage (*arrow*) due to size incongruity between the femoral head and acetabulum. *C*, Flattening of the articular cartilage of the superolateral aspect of the femoral head (*arrow*) suggests pressure changes induced by the acetabular labrum on the swollen femoral head. There is head-acetabulum size incongruity. Note pooling of contrast in medial portion of joint.

Legg-Calvé-Perthes Disease

The role of hip arthrography in Legg-Perthes disease is limited. In the earliest stages of the disease, the examination adds no information because the cartilaginous portion of the femoral head and acetabular cartilage will be normal. According to Katz, it is in the fragmentation and healing stages that arthrography is of value in establishing the size and shape of the cartilaginous head. During the fragmentation stage, the femoral head may be normal in contour but enlarged, compressing the acetabular cartilage medially and laterally to varying degrees, resulting in size incongruity between the head and acetabulum. Contrast may pool between the incongruous cartilaginous surfaces (Fig. 3.7). If femoral head enlargement becomes extreme, compression of the lateral aspect of the enlarged head by the acetabular labrum produces an indentation and sometimes future deformity of the articulating surface of the head (Fig. 3.8). These changes need not be permanent, however, and may revert to normal in the reconstitution or healing phase of the disease. This is particularly true if the evolution of the disease is slow (Fig. 3.9). During the healing phase, an arthrogram is helpful to demonstrate the final outcome in terms of femoral head size and shape, thickness and uniformity of the acetabular cartilage, and overall size

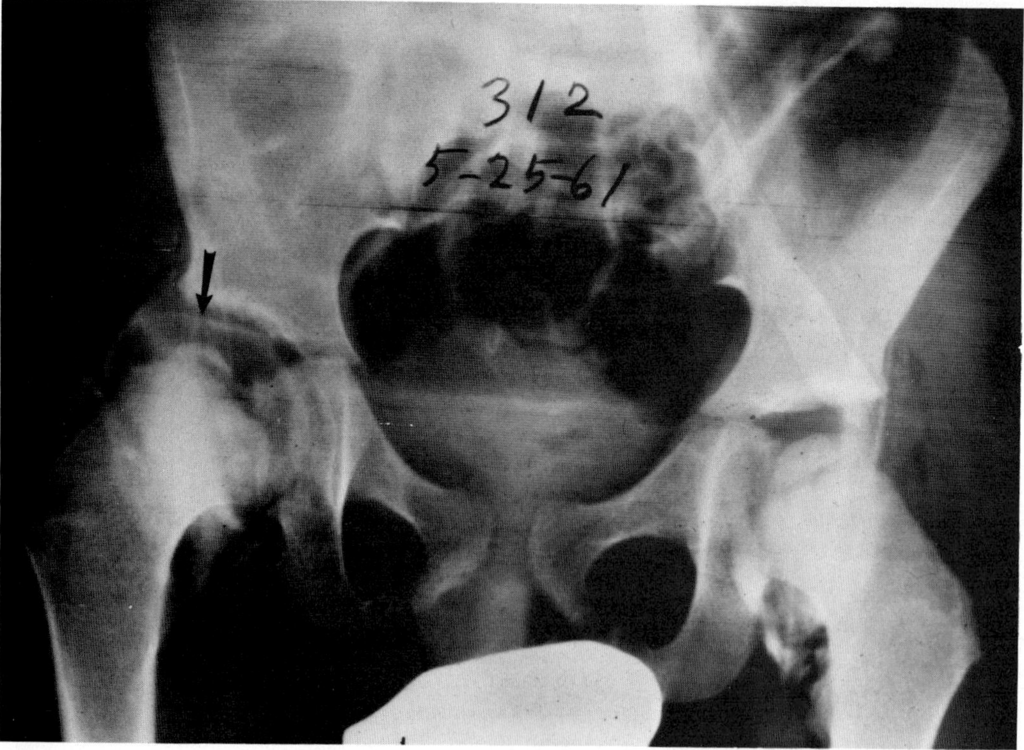

Figure 3.8. Abnormal hip arthrogram: Legg-Calvé-Perthes disease. Note contrast outlining a swollen cartilaginous femoral head with superolateral flattening (*arrow*). Femoral head circumference exceeds capacity of acetabulum indicating head-acetabulum size incongruity. (Courtesy of Robert Watanabe, M.D.)

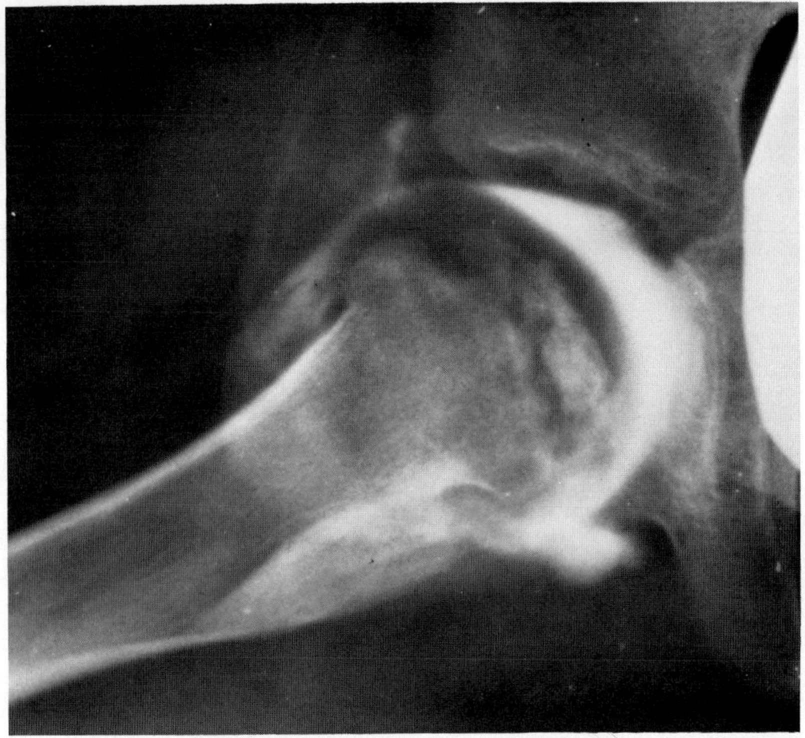

Figure 3.9. Abnormal hip arthrogram: Legg-Calvé-Perthes disease. There is central flattening of the femoral head articular cartilage. This results from pressure effects of the acetabulum on the swollen femoral head when size incongruity exists. The contour of the femoral head may revert to normal during the healing stage.

congruity of the head and acetabulum. A prediction regarding future degenerative arthritis and stability of the hip joint can thus be made and patient management directed accordingly.

ABNORMAL HIP ARTHROGRAM IN ADULTS—PAINFUL HIP JOINT

Method of Arthrography

Preliminary scout films include an anteroposterior and lateral radiograph of the hip joint. For arthrography of the adult hip, a 20-gauge spinal needle is ideal since it is flexible yet still wide enough in caliber to allow aspiration of joint fluid. The femoral artery is palpated and, following local anesthesia, the needle is inserted about 2 cm laterally from it and 2 cm beneath the inguinal crease, directing the needle perpendicular to the tabletop and toward the medial junction of the femoral head and neck (Fig. 3.3). This is performed under fluoroscopic guidance. The needle is advanced with stylet in place until it strikes or is just medial to the medial edge of the femoral neck (Fig. 3.10) (or the

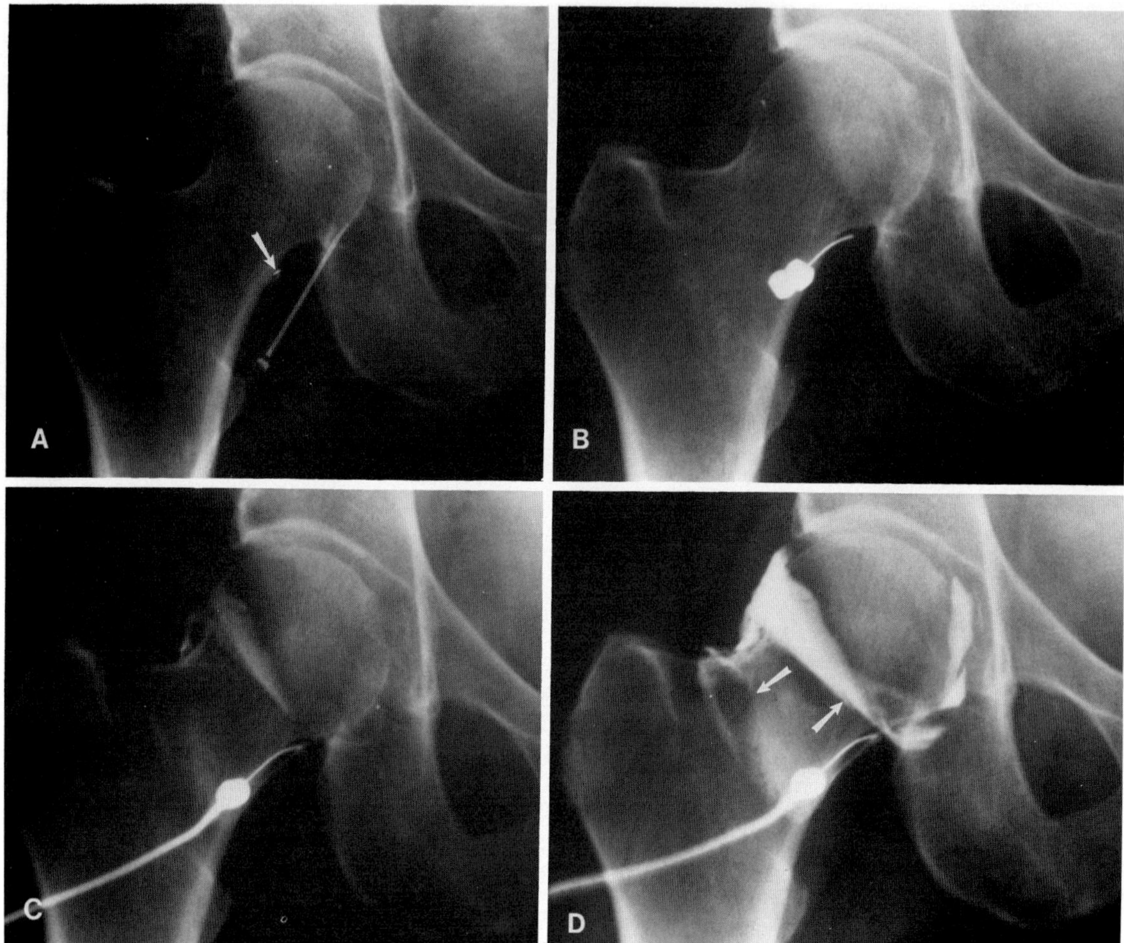

Figure 3.10. Normal adult hip arthrogram. *A,* Long needle indicates location of femoral artery. Short vertical needle indicates preferred site of arthrocentesis (*arrow*). *B,* Twenty-gauge spinal needle in place for joint injection. *C,* Early injection phase. *D,* Approximately 5 ml of contrast has been injected outlining synovial reflections above and below zona orbicularis (*arrows*). *E,* Nearly complete filling of the joint. *F,* Contrast-filled normal hip joint (20 ml) opacifying all synovial recesses and, finally, the articular cartilage (*arrow*).

prosthesis in the case of a total hip replacement). The bevel of the needle is then turned toward the femoral neck and the needle tip slides off into the joint capsule. Positive pressure on the barrel of a lidocaine- or saline-filled syringe is used to confirm the intraarticular location of the needle tip. When the liquid flows freely or joint fluid can be aspirated, the needle tip is certain to be within the joint space. In the event the medial approach is unsuccessful, the joint can be punctured laterally at the junction of the superolateral aspect of the femoral head with the acetabulum. Osteophytes projecting from the acetabulum may make this approach difficult. Finally, another method is to advance the needle directly into the central portion of the upper femoral neck until the needle

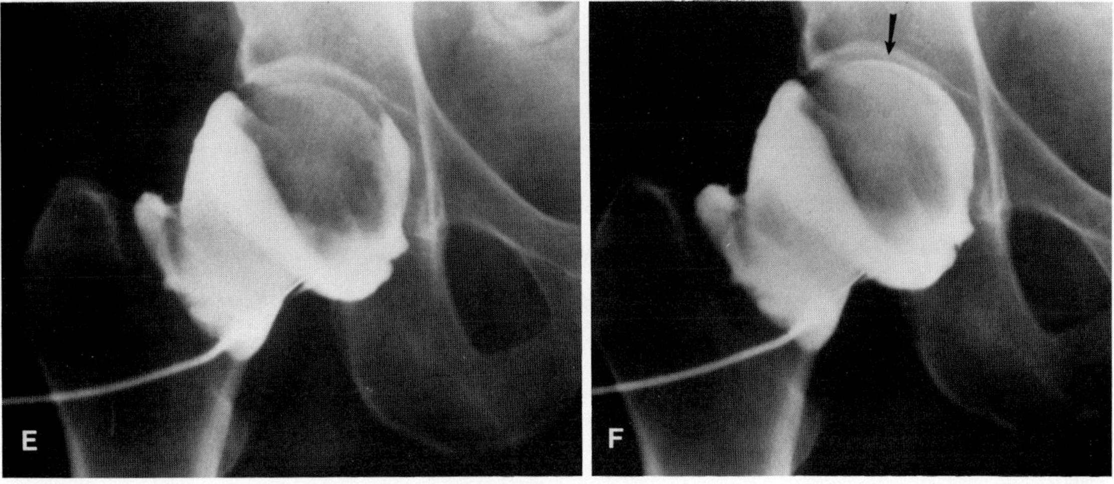

Figure 3.10 (*E* and *F*)

strikes bone. The fluid-filled syringe is attached to the hub of the needle and 1 cc of the fluid is injected as the needle tip is slowly withdrawn 1 or 2 mm. If the needle is within the periosteum or cortex, no fluid will flow, but upon minimal withdrawal of the needle tip, the pressure of injection should suddenly diminish, indicating the needle tip to be intraarticular. There may be temporary discomfort when the needle strikes the femoral periosteum.

After successful placement of the needle, aqueous contrast material is injected. If the injection is intraarticular, fluoroscopy reveals that the contrast flows readily within the confines of the joint. In the anatomical hip, contrast is first seen outlining the synovial sac below the zona orbicularis and thereafter the articular cartilage of the femoral head. The normal capacity is 15 to 20 cc. Before withdrawal of the needle, a sample of joint fluid or contrast medium may be aspirated for bacterial culture. Following active or passive exercise of the joint for several minutes, overhead radiographs consisting of at least antero-posterior films in internal and external rotation, neutral position, and a lateral radiograph are obtained.

Complications are those of arthrography in general. An occasional patient may have temporary difficulty walking after the arthrogram due to pain or because the local anesthetic may have transiently impaired function of the femoral nerve. Assistance in traveling home is usually advised for outpatients. Each patient is asked to refrain from heavy exercise for 24 hours after the arthrogram. Aspirin is recommended for relief of the mild discomfort of occasional chemical synovitis resulting from the hyperosmolar contrast material.

ARTHROGRAPHIC FINDINGS

The routine use of arthrography in the nonsurgical adult hip joint is limited. Pain or loss of mobility in the absence of plain film findings occasionally calls for an arthrogram. This is usually performed as part of arthrocentesis for bacterial culture of joint fluid. The arthrogram will demonstrate the condition of the articular cartilage, allow examination of the synovial membrane, and proves the intraarticular source of the aspirate.

Evaluation of the cartilage and demonstration of the synovium have been of value in determining the cause for the "frozen" or painful hip which is usually the result of infection, loose bodies, and rarely conditions such as synovial

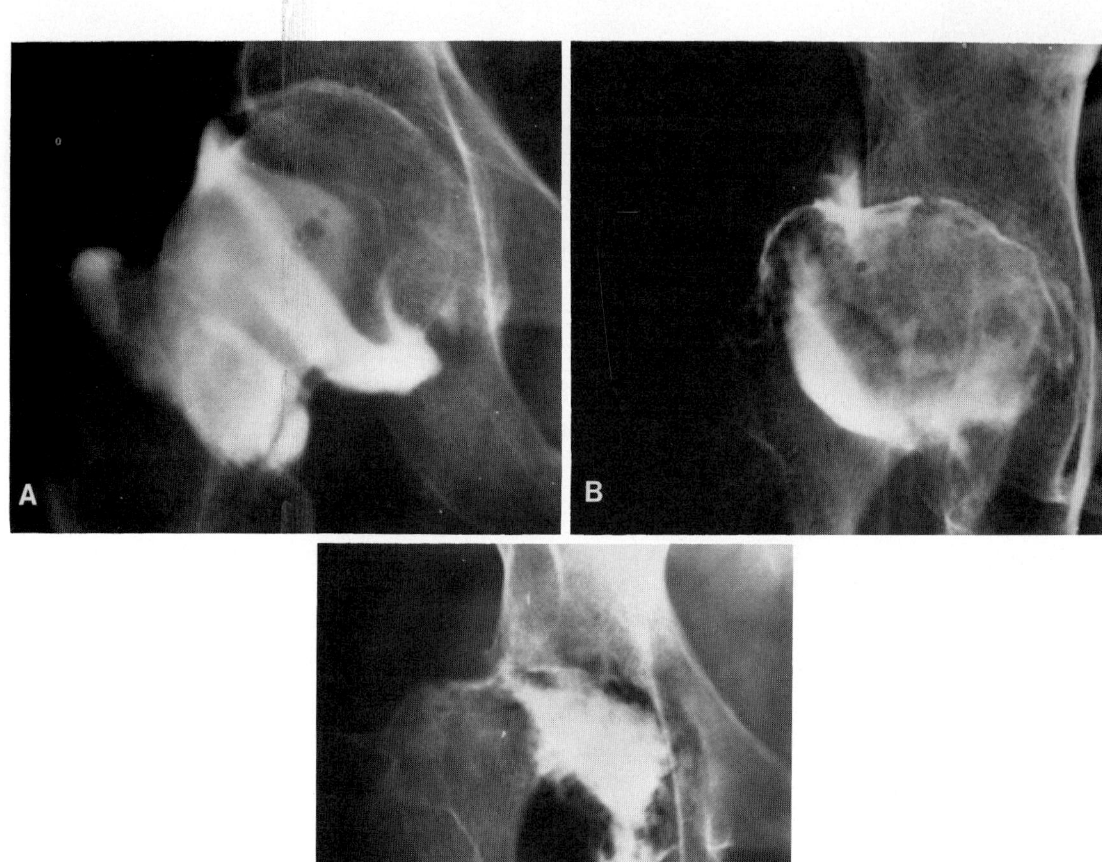

Figure 3.11. Abnormal hip arthrogram. *A,* Early infectious arthritis. Note marked narrowing of articular space due to destruction of articular cartilage. No contrast enters between cartilaginous surfaces. *B,* Infectious arthritis, late. Nearly all of the femoral articular cartilage has been destroyed. There is dissolution of the subchondral bone of the femoral head. The diminished joint volume and retracted synovial recesses indicate advanced adhesive capsulitis. *C,* Rheumatoid arthritis, secondarily infected. Note destroyed femoral head, retracted joint recesses, and rheumatoid synovial hypertrophy indicated by small nodular filling defects.

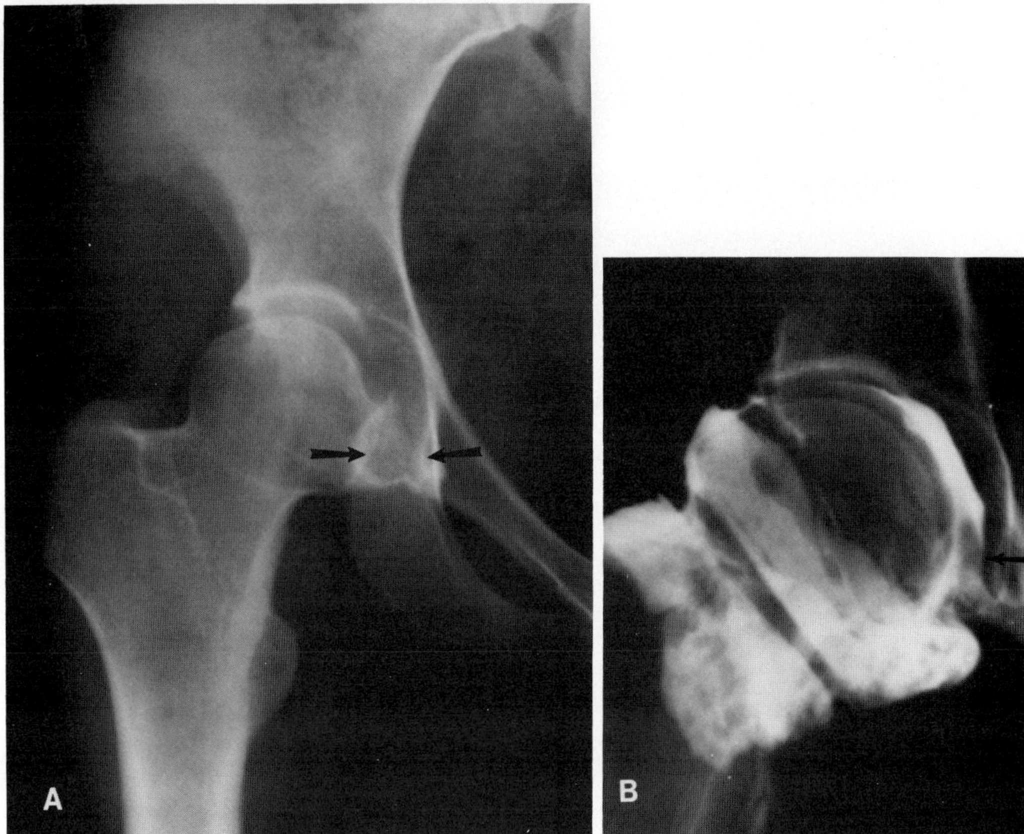

Figure 3.12. Abnormal hip arthrogram: synovial osteochondromatosis. *A,* Preliminary film shows an abnormally wide distance between the femoral head and inferomedial surface of the acetabulum (*arrows*). *B,* Arthrogram reveals radiolucent chondromatous body wedged between femoral head and acetabulum, medially (*arrow*). Note multiple synovial-filling defects of osteochondromatosis within joint recesses. (Reproduced with permission from L. W. Bassett: Hip Arthrography, Clinical Teachings, No. 1425. Westport, Conn., Medical Education Programs Ltd., 1979)

osteochondromatosis and pigmented villonodular synovitis. In infection the cartilage is destroyed, and retracted synovial margins indicate adhesive capsulitis (Fig. 3.11). Loose bodies are recognized as filling defects in the opacified joint recesses. Villonodular synovitis and synovial osteochondromatosis have a similar arthrographic appearance consisting of multiple nodules outlined as filling defects over the synovial surfaces (Figs. 3.12 and 3.13).

Relatively few arthrograms are ordered for aseptic necrosis of the femoral head in adults unless a femoral surface replacement is planned, in which case evaluation of the acetabular cartilage may require preoperative arthrography. Occasionally, there is an indication for arthrography in acute trauma of the hip joint when a torn capsule or a loose fragment of bone or cartilage is suspected (Fig. 3.14).

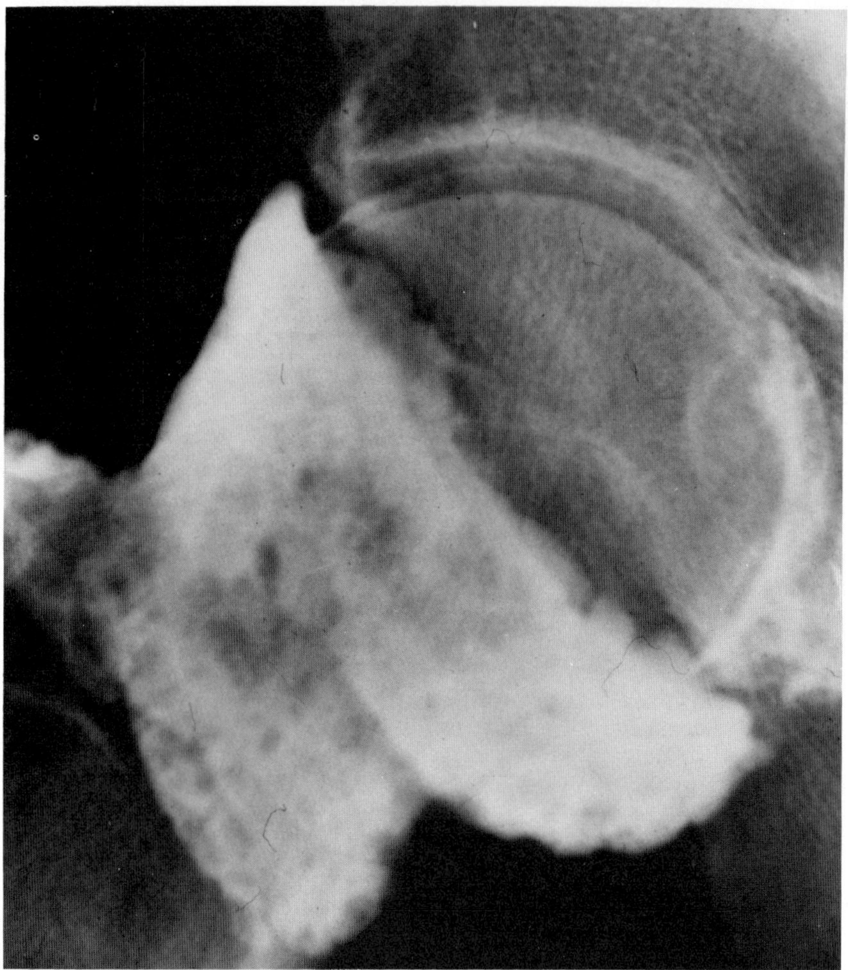

Figure 3.13. Abnormal hip arthrogram: synovial osteochondromatosis. Note retracted synovial margins and diminished joint capacity simulating inflammatory arthritis. The appearance at arthrography is often indistinguishable from the synovial proliferation of pigmented villonodular synovitis. (Reproduced with permission from L. W. Bassett: Hip Arthrography, Clinical Teachings, No. 1425. Westport, Conn., Medical Education Programs Ltd., 1979)

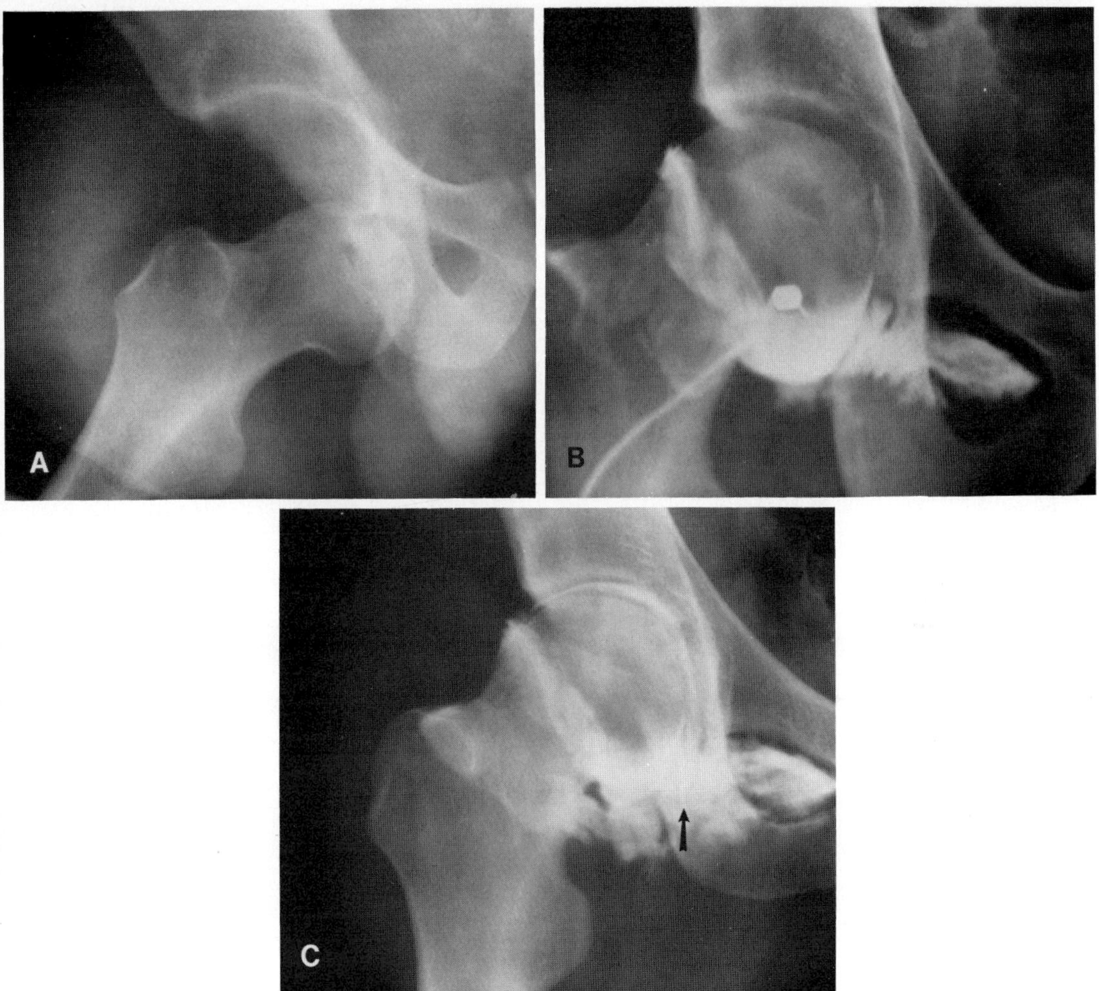

Figure 3.14. Abnormal hip arthrogram: capsular tear. *A*, Preliminary film shows anteroinferior dislocation of femoral head. *B*, Early filling phase of arthrogram after reduction of dislocation, reveals immediate extravasation of contrast medium from joint capsule anteromedially. *C*, Final film of arthrogram with joint and site of capsule tear opacified (*arrow*).

ABNORMAL HIP ARTHROGRAM IN ADULTS—LOOSE TOTAL HIP REPLACEMENT

Prior to the era of total hip replacement, there were few indications for hip arthrography in the adult. Now, however, a hip arthrogram is an important step in the workup of the patient with a painful total hip prosthesis. The arthrogram serves two primary functions: to establish the presence of loosening of the prosthesis and to aid in determining whether or not infection is present. For the latter, joint fluid or contrast material is aspirated and bacterial cultures of the aspirate are obtained. Prior to arthrography, plain roentgenograms of the symptomatic total hip prosthesis must be obtained and carefully examined for signs of prosthesis failure.

Plain Film Analysis

Dislocation usually occurs in the immediate postoperative period or when ambulation has occurred too early and a neocapsule has not fully formed around the joint. The early roentgen signs include loss of symmetry of the distance laterally and medially between the femoral head and the edge of the wire ring within the base of the acetabular component in the case of a Charnley-Mueller prosthesis. In true profile, the wire ring of a Charnley-Mueller acetabular cup appears as a straight line. However, because of slight anteversion

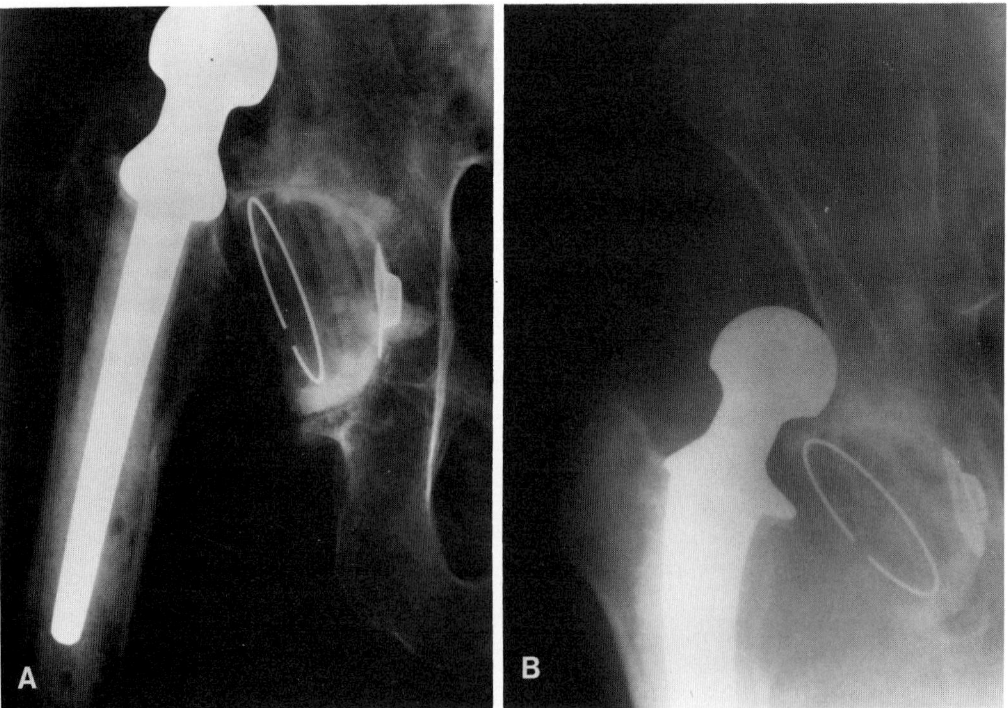

Figure 3.15. Total hip replacement with complete dislocation. *A* and *B*, Note that in both cases the angulation of the acetabular cup is greater than 45° from the horizontal.

during correct surgical positioning of the cup, the ring becomes an oval on the anteroposterior radiograph. The distance between the lateral and medial edges of the femoral head and the edge of the ring, however, remains constant and symmetrical in the normally seated prosthesis.

Dislocation and loosening are more likely to occur in the total hip replacement with suboptimal alignment or seating of the prosthesis such as excessive vertical orientation (45° from the horizontal plane of the acetabulum is ideal), or excessive anteversion of the cup (Fig. 3.15), and eccentric location of the metal stem within the femur. In the anteroposterior view of the commonly used Charnley-Mueller prosthesis, the normal oval profile of the acetabular cup metallic ring may become circular with extreme anteversion. A small degree of anteversion is the desired position of the cup. However, it is important for the radiologist to realize that anteversion and undesirable retroversion are indistinguishable on frontal radiographs, and a lateral view is necessary. Retroversion usually results in dislocation of the femoral head in any position of the joint other than neutral. This can be verified by obtaining views in adduction, abduction, and internal and external rotation.

Foreshortening of the metallic femoral stem on the anteroposterior film usually indicates anterior or posterior perforation of the surrounding femoral cortex. A lateral film will verify this complication.

In patients who have had an accompanying trochanteric osteotomy, disruption of the wire attachment of the greater trochanter due to fatigue fractures of the retaining wire sutures is common, but is unimportant if it occurs later than the immediate postoperative stage. Within 2 to 3 months following surgery, fibrous union of the greater trochanter to the femoral shaft is strong enough to allow abduction without being secured by intact wire sutures. If disruption of the wire sutures should occur early after surgery, it may result in upward migration of the trochanter, requiring reattachment.

Heterotopic bone formation is commonly seen, especially in the patient with multiple surgical procedures on the same hip. It is more likely to diminish range of motion than to cause pain. If excessive, it may require excision.

Extravasation of acrylic cement into the pelvis occurs frequently and is usually of no clinical significance. A small hat-shaped wire mesh retainer may be placed in the central portion of a thin refashioned acetabulum to prevent this.

Loosening of the acetabular component is more likely to occur than loosening of the stem because the cup is the most difficult component of the total hip replacement to secure. The onset of pain resulting from loosening tends to occur at a longer interval following surgery than pain from infection, but this observation is not certain to exclude the latter since some infections may not become overt for months to years after surgery. Loosening and infection are usually subtle, both clinically and radiologically. The usual sign of these conditions on roentgenograms is a progressively widening radiolucent zone between the acrylic cement and the adjacent bone (Fig. 3.16). It is important to understand, however, that a thin zone of radiolucency may be present normally and probably results from bone necrosis, secondary to the heat of polymerization as the acrylic cement solidifies (Fig. 3.17), and subsequent fibrous connective tissue response. Identification of a progressively widening radiolucent zone on serial

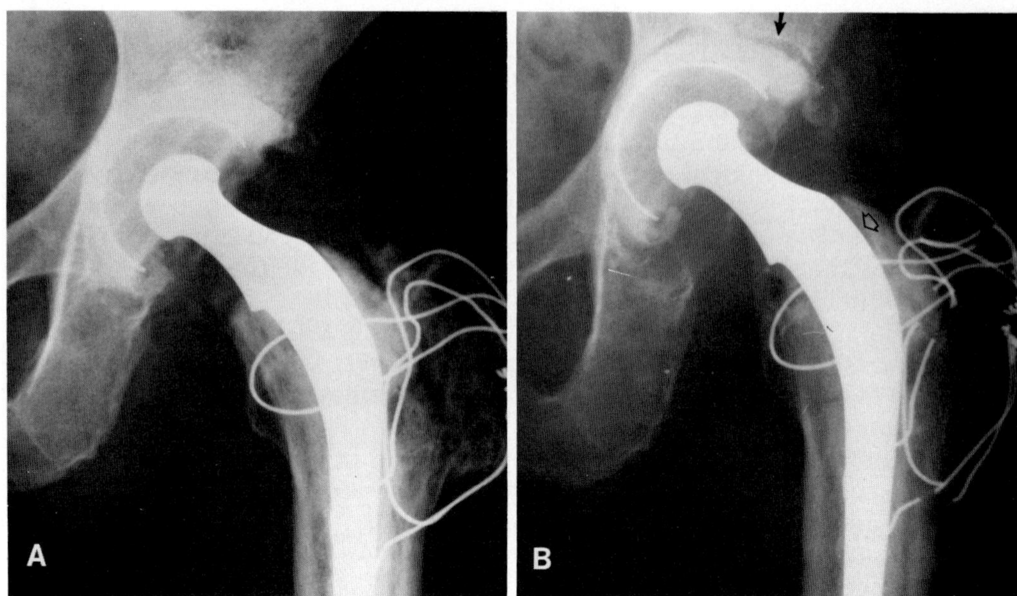

Figure 3.16. Loose total hip replacement. *A,* Early postoperative film reveals total hip replacement satisfactorily seated and aligned. *B,* Same patient, 6 years later, shows progressive widening of radiolucent zone between acrylic cement of cup and acetabulum (*arrow*) and along superlateral aspect of stem and femur (*open arrow*).

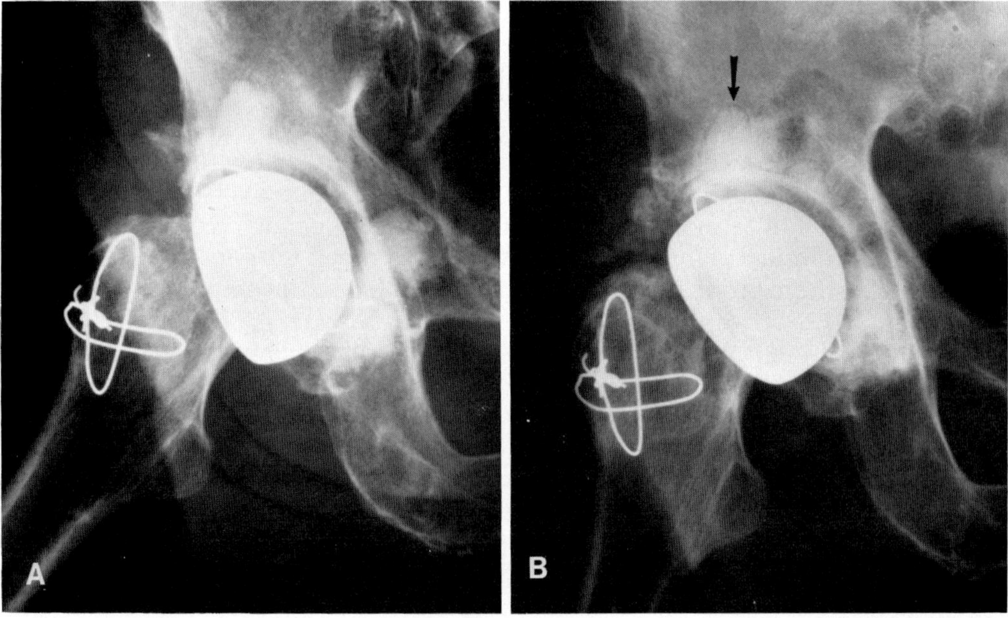

Figure 3.17. Loosening or heat of polymerization? *A,* Femoral total surface replacement shortly after surgery satisfactorily seated. *B,* Six months later a thin radiolucent zone has developed between the acrylic cement and bony acetabulum (*arrow*). This is probably due to bone necrosis from the heat of polymerization of the acrylic cement. Patient had no symptoms to suggest loosening or infection.

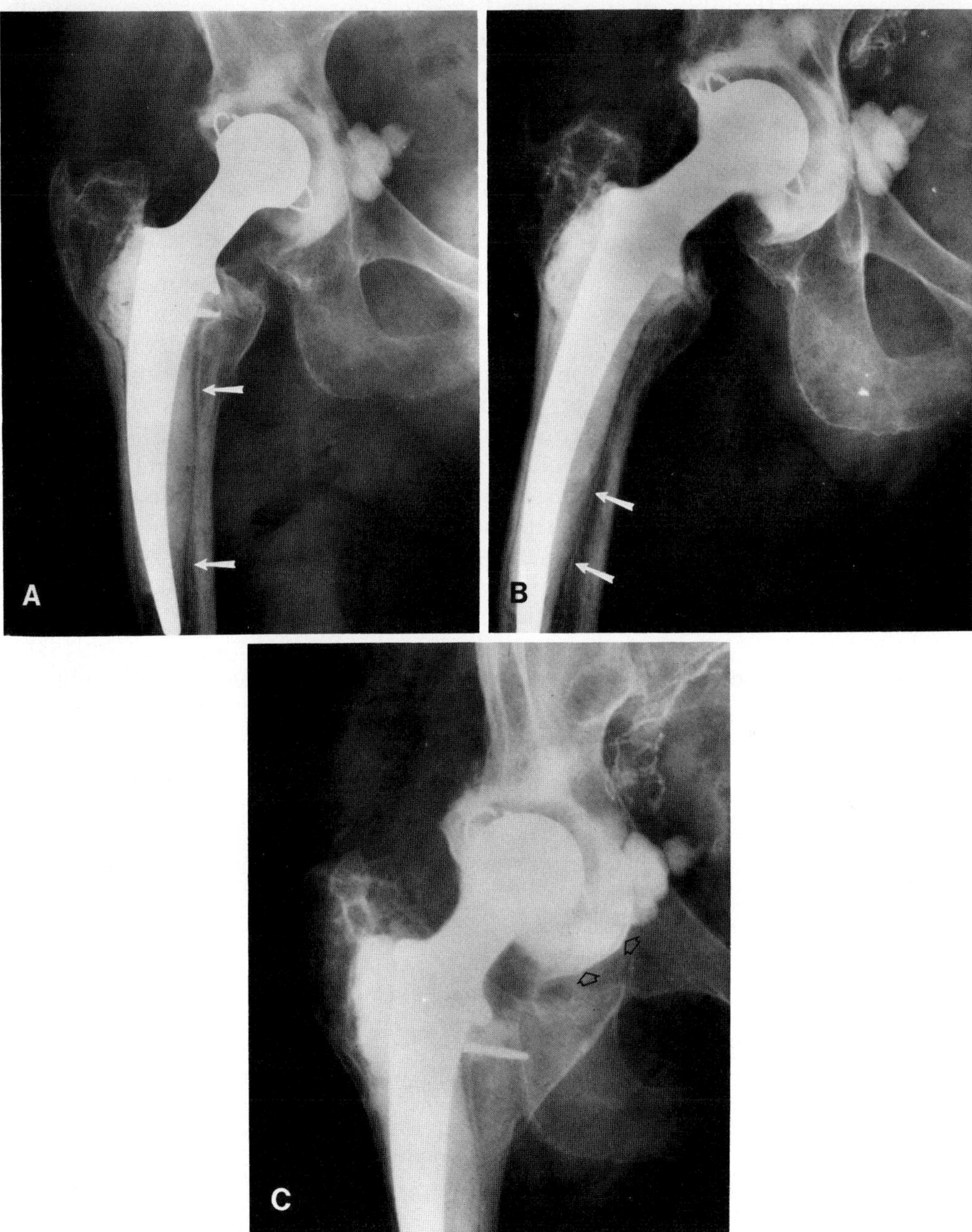

Figure 3.18. Abnormal hip arthrogram: loose total hip prosthesis. *A*, Preliminary film shows radiolucent border between acrylic cement of stem and bone (*arrows*). *B* and *C*, Arthrogram reveals interposition of iodinated contrast material between acrylic cement of stem and femur medially (*arrows*) and between cup and acetabulum (*open arrows*).

films carries more significance as an indicator of loosening or infection.

One or more fractures of the cement implies loosening, and results from the mechanical effects of prosthesis movement upon the cement. Toggling of the metallic femoral stem may cause a radiolucent zone on one side of the metal-cement interface superiorly and on the other side inferiorly. Seepage of the contrast agent between the cement and bone at arthrography is the primary radiological sign confirming the clinical impression of loosening (Fig. 3.18).

Method of Arthrography

The arthrogram on a patient with a total hip prosthesis is begun by placing a metallic marker on the skin over the medial or lateral edge of the metallic femoral neck under fluoroscopy. This is necessary because a prosthetic joint is usually further cephalad than the normal hip joint (Fig. 3.19). A 20-gauge spinal needle is advanced perpendicular to the tabletop, down toward the medial or lateral aspect of the metallic femoral neck. A metallic prosthesis interferes with fluoroscopic visualization of the needle, thus the approach to either side of the neck is easier than puncturing directly over the metallic component. Metal to metal contact between the needle tip and the prosthesis is clearly felt. The bevel of the needle is then turned toward the prosthesis and the needle tip is advanced 2 to 3 mm gliding off the side of the neck and into the residual synovial recess. Joint fluid may be aspirated at this time. If no fluid is obtained, saline or contrast agent is injected, reaspirated, and a bacterial culture obtained. Contrast is injected slowly and is first identified on the undersurface of the acetabular cup forming a collar at the base of the metallic head. Careful fluoroscopic observa-

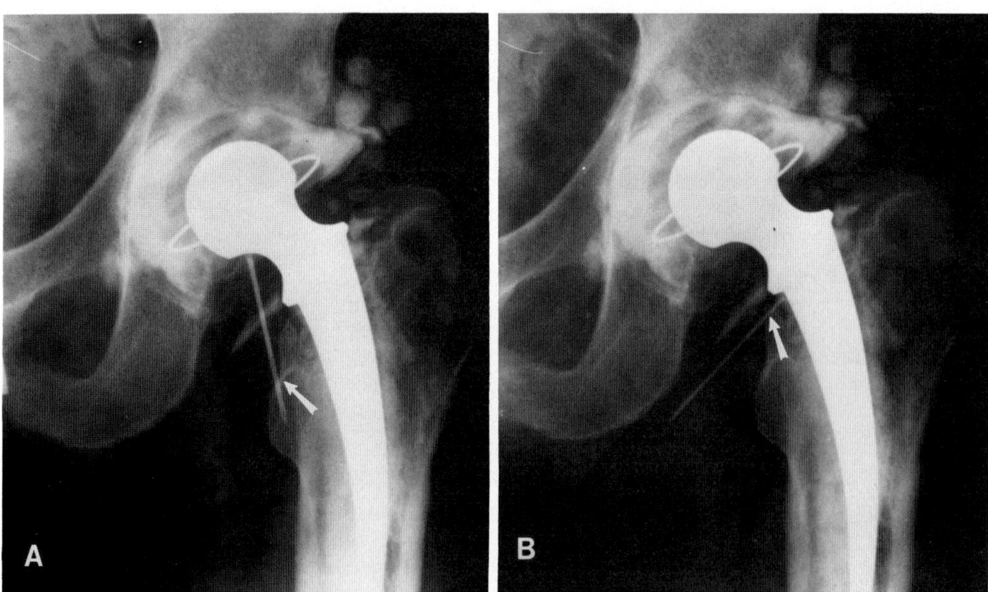

Figure 3.19. Total hip prosthesis. *A,* Needle shaft (*arrow*) denotes course of femoral artery relative to neck of prosthetic stem. *B,* Needle shaft indicates location of inguinal ligament (*arrow*). Note that neck of femoral stem, and thus site of arthrocentesis is above inguinal crease.

tion is necessary since the extreme radiodensity of metal and acrylic cement may mask the iodinated contrast medium. The capacity of the hip joint varies from 5 cc to more thn 30 cc. The patient is often unable to sense the gradual distention of the joint with contrast agent. After withdrawal of the needle and a brief interval of passive or active exercise, filming is begun. The routine projections are obtained using identical technique for pre- and postinjection films.

Arthrographic Findings

The normal joint recesses are of course absent following total hip replacement. Instead, a neocapsule forms around the rim of the acetabular cup and envelops

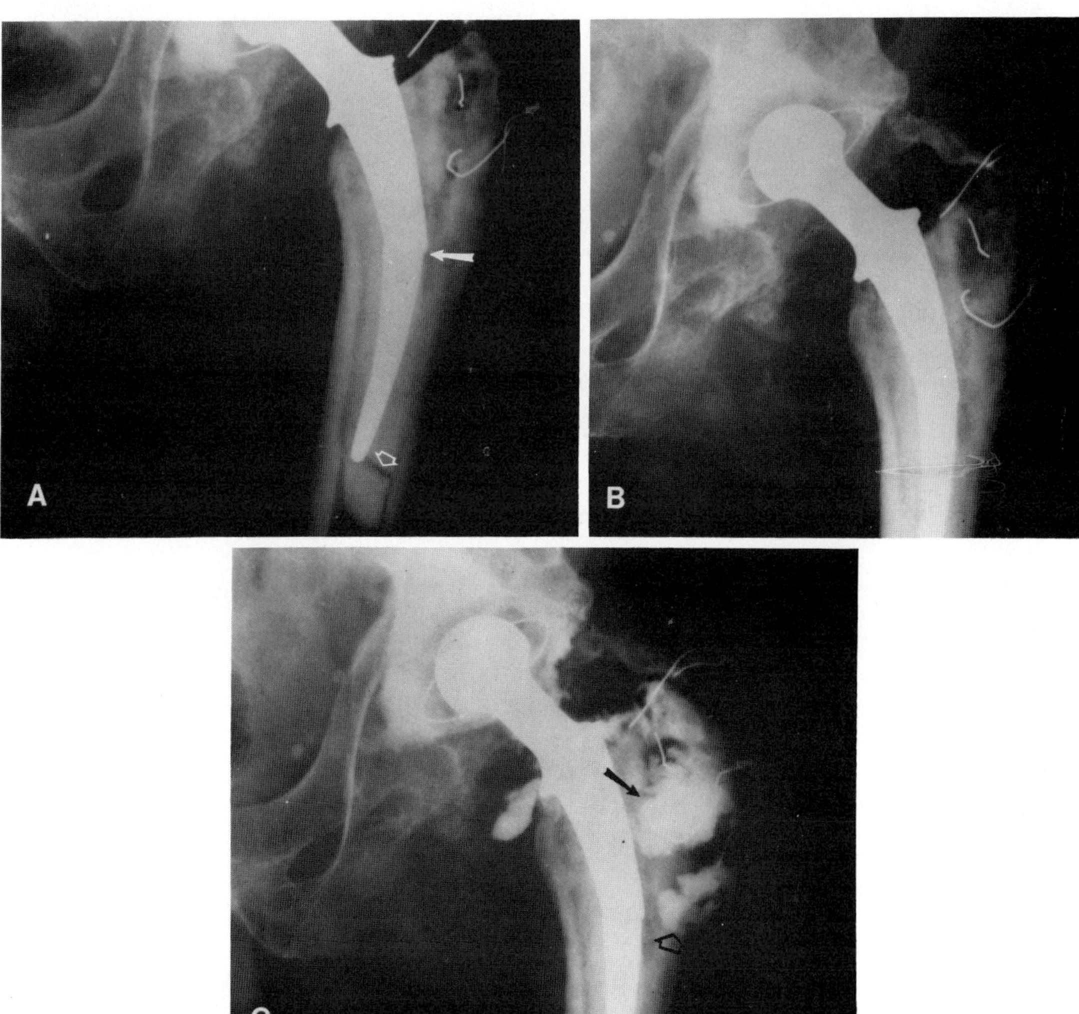

Figure 3.20. Abnormal hip arthrogram: total hip replacement loose, fractured, and infected. *A,* Note fracture through acrylic cement (*open arrow*) and metallic stem (*arrow*). *B,* Bridging heterotopic bone superolaterally restricted range of motion. *C,* Arthrogram reveals severe retraction of neocapsule, communication with trochanteric bursa (*arrow*) and dissecting synovial cyst laterally (*open arrow*).

the metallic femoral neck. This neoarticular recess does not normally communicate with surrounding tissues or bursae, except occasionally the trochanteric bursa (Fig. 3.20). The metal-cement-bone bond of the femoral and acetabular prosthetic components are open to the neoarticular space. The tight bond between bone and cement does not normally allow entry of contrast between

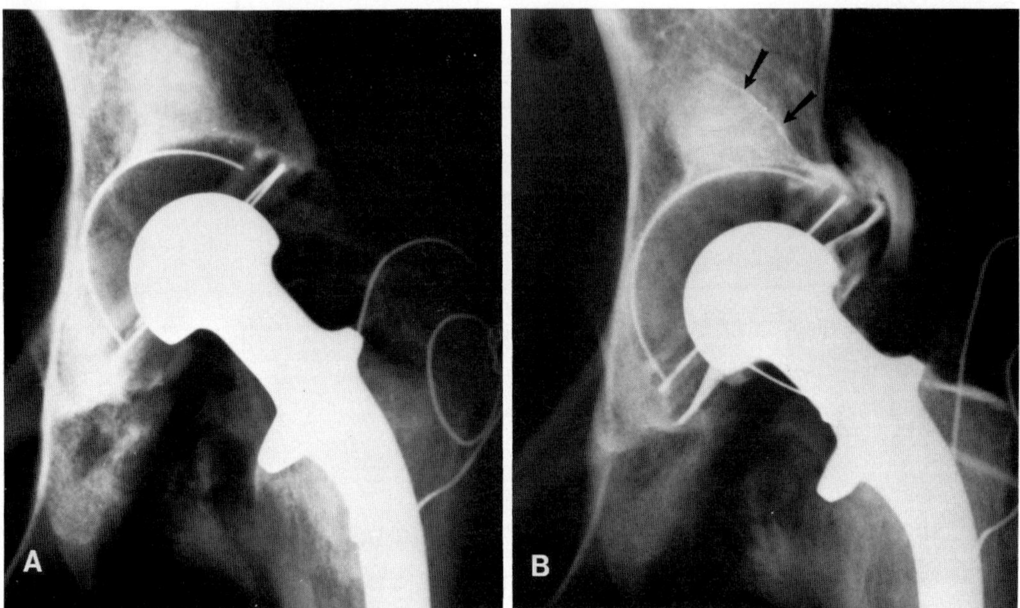

Figure 3.21. Abnormal hip arthrogram: loose total hip replacement. *A,* Preliminary film shows no abnormality. *B,* Arthrogram reveals contrast leak between cement and bone of acetabular cup indicating loosening and/or infection (*arrows*).

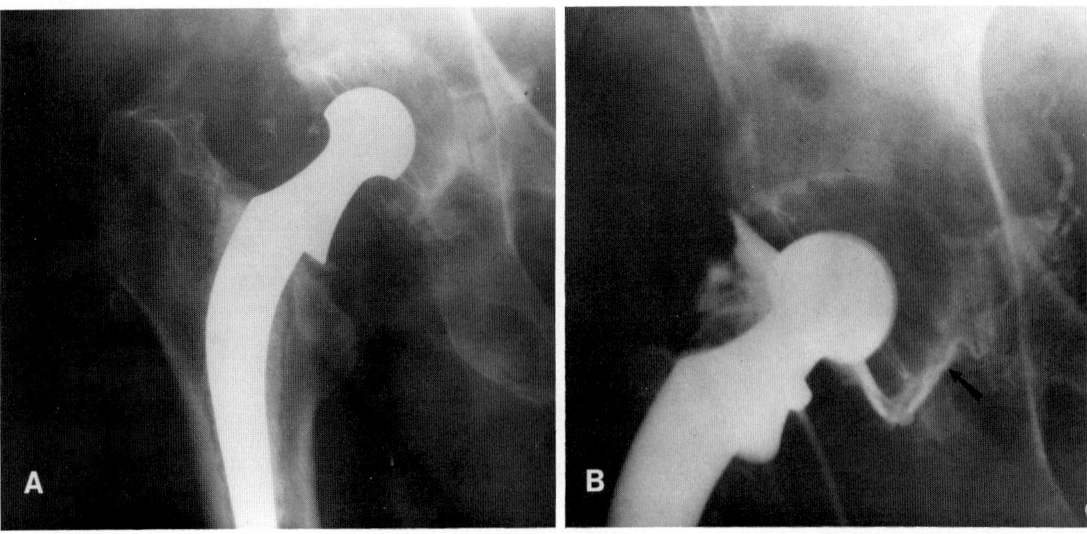

Figure 3.22. Abnormal hip arthrogram: loose total hip replacement. *A,* Preliminary film shows no evidence of loosening. *B,* Arthrogram reveals obvious interposition of contrast material between acrylic cement of cup and acetabulum (*arrow*).

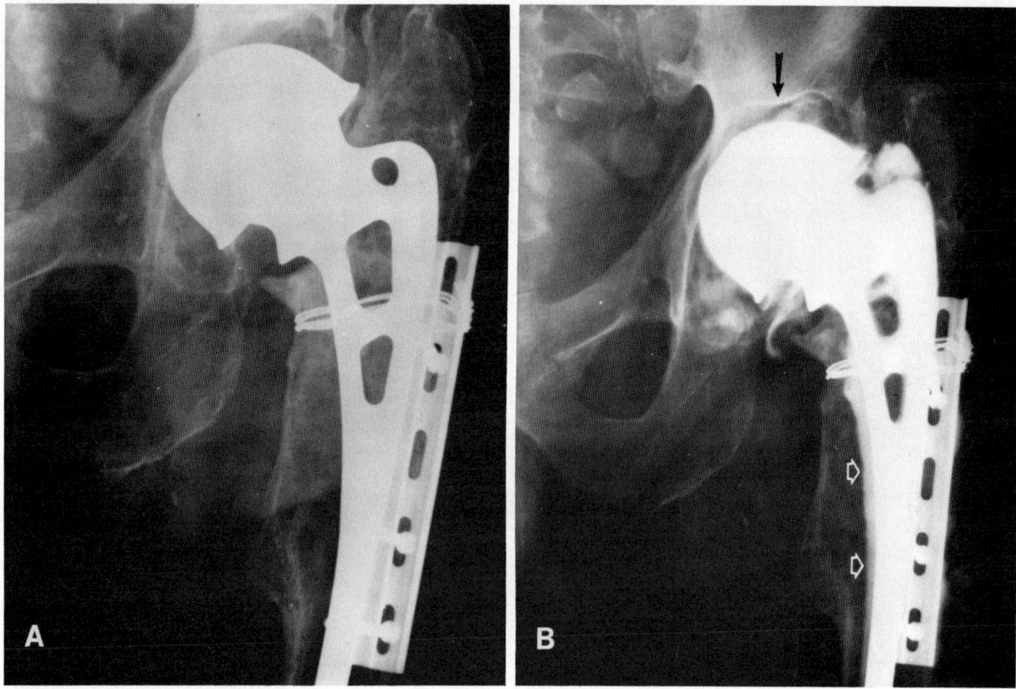

Figure 3.23. Abnormal hip arthrogram: loose total hip replacement. *A,* Preliminary film of earlier type of total hip replacement including buttressing device for stem. *B,* Arthrogram reveals contrast leak between bone and earlier nonopaque cement of acetabular cup (*arrow*) and femoral stem (*open arrows*) indicating massive loosening.

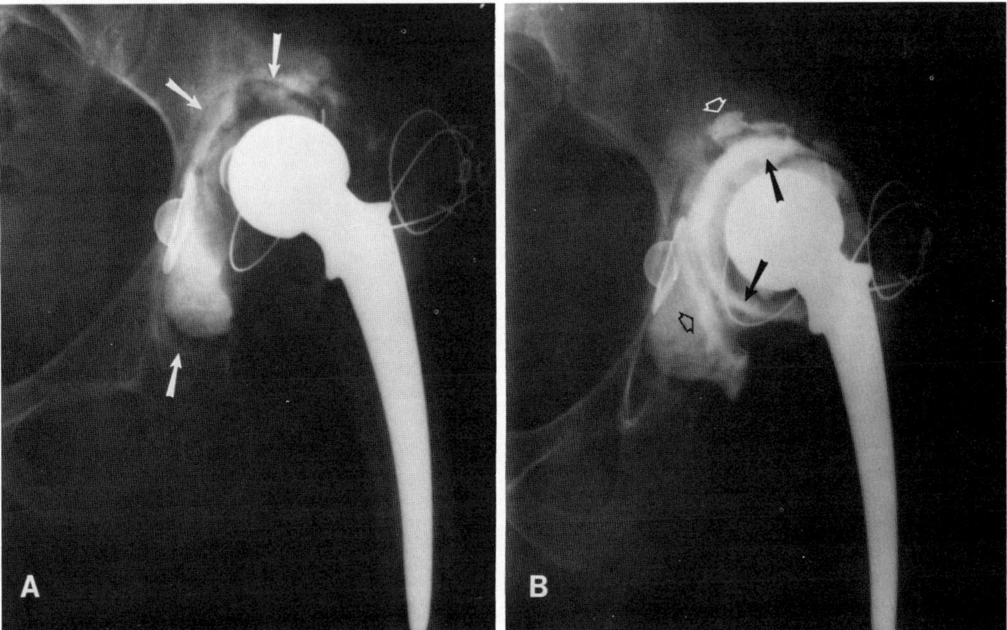

Figure 3.24. Abnormal hip arthrogram: loose total hip replacement. *A,* Preliminary film shows wide radiolucent zone between acrylic cement and acetabulum (*arrows*). *B,* Arthrogram reveals contrast leak between cup and cement (*arrows*) as well as between cement and bony acetabulum (*open arrows*) indicating compound loosening.

them. A loose bond, however, results in contrast seeping between the acrylic cement and bone and this can be demonstrated on roentgenograms. The identification of a thin line of contrast interposed between the cement-bone interface determines the diagnosis of loosening by arthrography (Figs. 3.21 to 3.23). It is

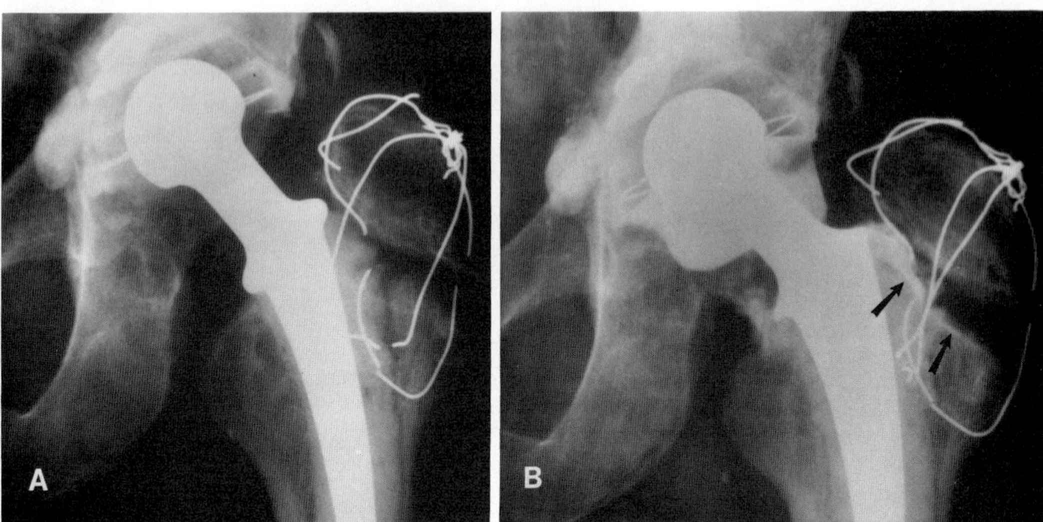

Figure 3.25. Abnormal hip arthrogram: loose total hip replacement. *A*, Preliminary film. Fractures of wires retaining greater trochanter usually do not indicate loosening since fibrous union has occurred, but in this case opposing bony margins are sclerotic. *B*, Arthrogram confirms contrast seeping over the entire femoral shaft surface (*arrows*) verifying a loose, and clinically mobile, greater trochanter.

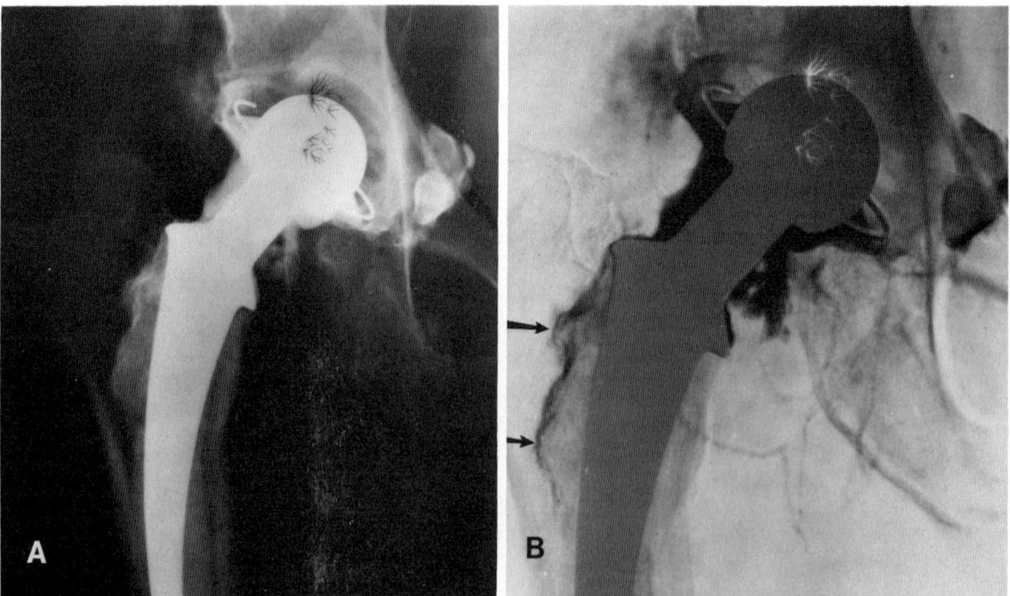

Figure 3.26. Abnormal hip arthrogram: loose total hip replacement. *A*, Contrast material dissects between acrylic cement and bone along lateral aspect of stem. *B*, Subtraction film enhances this finding (*arrows*).

exceedingly important that identical techniques and positioning are used for the pre- and postinjection films, otherwise the thin zone of interposed contrast may not be distinguishable from the edge of the radiopaque cement (Figs. 3.24 and 3.25). Films obtained during traction (push and pull) on the joint are sometimes best for demonstrating seepage of contrast material into the cement-bone interface.

Subtraction techniques may be of help in detecting bone-cement contrast seepage. Obtaining subtraction films during hip arthrography poses some dif-

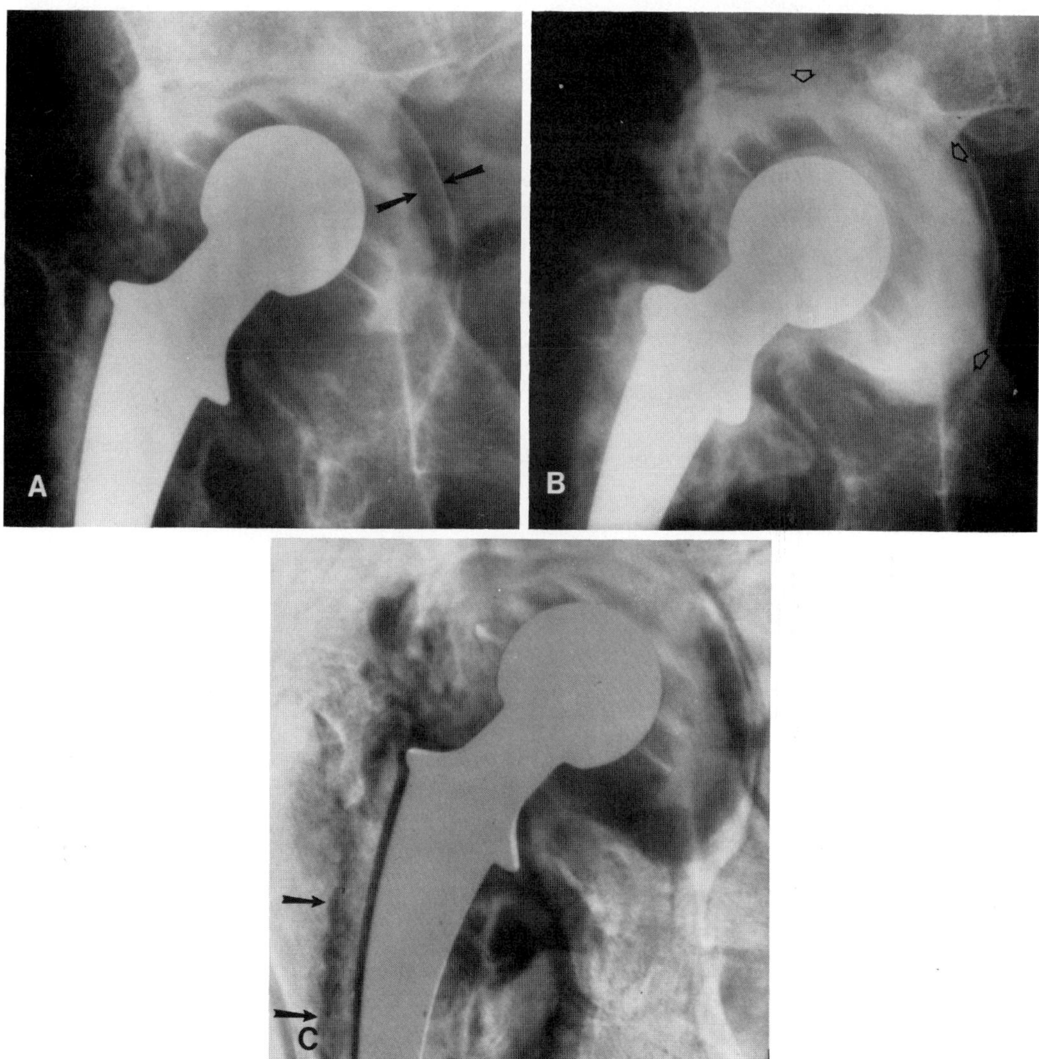

Figure 3.27. Abnormal hip arthrogram: loose total hip replacement. *A,* Preliminary film reveals wide radiolucent zone between acrylic cement and bone of acetabular cup (*arrows*). Arthrogram shows nearly all injected contrast medium seeping into this space (*open arrows*). C, Subtraction film of arthrogram confirms contrast interposed between cement and bone of acetabulum, but also between stem and femur (*arrows*). The latter was not recognized on the nonsubtracted arthrogram.

ficulty because of patient or x-ray tube movement during arthrocentesis and joint exercising prior to filming. It is helpful to place two or more centering marks on the skin with ink to allow accurate centering of the overhead tube by light collimator for the preliminary and postinjection films. When possible, a second preliminary film should be obtained with the needle tip intraarticular prior to injection of contrast agent. This yields a good subtraction mask film. Contrast is then injected and further films are obtained without moving the patient or x-ray tube. This method is easier in a remote control fluoroscopy unit. Even with careful technic, however, subtraction films in hip arthrography may turn out less than optimal, and more often than not the diagnostic information must be obtained from the original positive contrast films, demanding that they be of highest quality (Figs. 3.26 and 3.27).

As indicated earlier in this chapter, the radiologist is occasionally requested to perform a hip joint aspiration under fluoroscopic guidance for bacterial culture of the joint fluid. To guarantee the aspirate was indeed from the joint, iodinated contrast medium should be injected prior to withdrawal of the needle and a film exposed to assure the intraarticular location of the needle tip. Saline, sterile water, or contrast agent may be injected and reaspirated in the event of a "dry" joint. If the joint is distended with contrast agent, an arthrogram should be obtained.

References

Anderson, L.S., Staple, T.W., Arthrography of total hip replacement using subtraction technique. Radiology, 109:470–472, 1973.

Armbruster, T.G., Guerra, J., Resnick, D., et al., The adult hip: An anatomic study. Radiology, 128:1–10, 1978.

Bassett, L.W., Hip Arthrography, Clinical Teachings, No. 1425. Westport, Connecticut, Medical Education Programs Ltd., 1979.

Brown, C.S., Knickerbocker, W.J., Radiologic studies in the investigation of the causes of total hip replacement failures. J Can Assoc Radiol, 24:245–253, 1973.

Charnley, J., Low-friction arthroplasty of the hip joint: Symposium of joint biomechanics and joint replacement. J Bone Joint Surg, 53B:149–151, 1971.

Daffner, R.H., Carden, T.S., Gehweiler, J.A., Complications of unrecognized dislocation of the Charnley-Mueller hip prostheses. Radiology, 108:323–324, 1973.

Dolinkas, C., Campbell, R.E., Rothman, R.H., The painful Charnley total hip replacement. AJR, 121:61–68, 1974.

Gelman, M.I., Arthrography in total hip prosthesis complications. AJR, 126:743–750, 1976.

Gelman, M.I., Coleman, E.R., Stevens, P.M., et al., Radiography, radionuclide imaging, and arthrography in the evaluation of total hip and knee replacement. Radiology, 128:677–682, 1978.

Glassberg, G.B., Ozonoff, M.B., Arthrographic findings in septic arthritis of the hip in infants. Radiology, 128:151–155, 1978.

Grant, J.C.B., An Atlas of Anatomy, Ed. 5, Figs. 282–284. Williams & Wilkins, Baltimore, 1962.

Grant, J.C.B., A Method of Anatomy, Ed. 6, pp. 468–474. Williams & Wilkins, Baltimore, 1963.

Grech, P., Hip Arthrography, Ed. 1, pp. 64–98. J.B. Lippincott, Philadelphia, 1977.

Katz, J.F., Arthrography in Legg-Calve-Perthes disease. J Bone Joint Surg, 50A:467–472, 1968.

Kaye, J.J., Winchester, P.H., Freiberger, R.H., Neonatal septic "dislocation" of the hip: True dislocation or pathological epiphyseal separation? Radiology, 114:671–674, 1975.

Lachman, R.S., Rimoin, D.L., Hollister, D.W., Arthrography of the hip, a clue to the pathogenesis of epiphyseal dysplasias. Radiology, 103:317–322, 1973.

Lazansky, M.G., Complications in total hip replacement with the Charnley technique. Clin Orthop, 72:40–45, 1970.

Lewis, M.S., Norman, A., The earliest signs of postoperative hip infection. Radiology, 104:309–312, 1972.

Melson, G.L., McDaniel, R.C., Southern, P., et al., In vitro effects of iodinated arthrographic contrast media on bacterial growth. Radiology, 112:593–595, 1974.

Mitchell, G.B., Arthrography in congenital displacement of the hip. J Bone Joint Surg, 45:88–95, 1963.

Mullins, M.F., Sutton, R.N., Lodwick, G.S., Complications of total hip replacement, a roentgen evaluation. AJR, *121*:55–60, 1974.

Ogden, J.A., Jensen, P.S., Roentgenography of congenital dislocation of the hip. Radiology, *119*:189–192, 1976.

Ozonoff, M.B., Controlled arthrography of the hip: A technique of fluoroscopic monitoring and recording. Clin Orthop, *93*:260–264, 1973.

Pepper, H.W., Noonan, C.D., Radiographic evaluation of total hip arthroplasty. Radiology, *108*:23–30, 1973.

Salvati, E.A., Freiberger, R.H., Wilson, P.D., Arthrography for complications of total hip replacement. J Bone Joint Surg, *53*:701–709, 1971.

Schinz, H.R., et al., Roentgen Diagnosis, Vol. II, The Skeleton, Part 2, Edited by James T. Case, First Edit, Grune and Stratton, New York, 1952, pp. 1238–1247.

Severin, E., Arthrography in congenital dislacation of the hip, J Bone Joint Surg, *21*:304–313, 1939.

Tanaka, S., Ito, T, Yamamoto, K., Arthrography in osteoarthritis of the hip. AJR, *124*:91–95, 1975.

4

Arthrography of the Elbow

J. W. Horns, M.D.

Elbow arthrography is not commonly performed. However, it can provide valuable information in patients with various afflictions of the elbow.

Arthrography of the elbow can be performed by either a positive contrast or a double contrast technique. The arthrographer should be familiar with both methods. The choice of the technique to be used in each patient depends on the particular clinical indication for the arthrogram. The use of only the most appropriate method in each patient is preferable to the routine use of both methods in every case. However, a combination study could be conducted if a positive contrast arthrogram were followed by aspiration of contrast from the joint and injection of air for a double contrast examination.

ANATOMY

The elbow is a compound joint, consisting of the humeroulnar and the humeroradial articulations. It is also continuous with the superior radioulnar joint which is within the capsule of the elbow joint. We will consider that part of the anatomy of the elbow which is pertinent to clinical arthrography. The important structures are the articulating bones, the hyaline cartilage of the articular surfaces, the ligaments, joint capsule, and synovial membrane.

The distal articular surface of the humerus is divided into the trochlea and the capitellum which articulate, respectively, with the semilunar notch of the ulna and head of the radius. The trochlea has the shape of a pulley and is concave from side to side to accomodate the longitudinal "guiding" ridge of the semilunar notch. The capitellum is much smaller than the trochlea and is a rounded convex projection that articulates with the superior surface of the radial head. On the anterior surface of the distal humerus are the coronoid and radial fossae which are adjacent to the trochlea and capitellum and accomodate the coronoid process of the ulna and head of the radius when the elbow is flexed. When the elbow is extended the olecranon process projects into a fossa on the posterior surface of the distal humerus. The coronoid and olecranon fossae are separated by a thin plate of bone or sometimes only by fibrous tissue.

The trochlear (semilunar) notch is located on the anterior surface of the proximal ulna. The notch is divided into medial and lateral parts by its longitudinal guiding ridge. The proximal half of the notch belongs to the olecranon process which is the beak-shaped upper end of the ulna. The distal half of the trochlear notch is the proximal surface of the coronoid process. On the lateral surface of the coronoid process is a concavity, the radial notch, that receives the circumference of the radial head. The head of the radius is disc shaped with a shallow concavity of its superior articular surface.

The surfaces of the trochlea and capitellum of the humerus, trochlear notch and radial notch of the ulna, head of the radius, and interior of the annular ligament are covered with hyaline articular cartilage. The anterior, inferior, and posterior surfaces of the trochlea are covered with articular cartilage, whereas on the capitellum the cartilage is limited to its anterior and inferior surfaces. Near the center of the trochlear notch there is normally an area where the bone is not covered with cartilage.

The ligaments at the elbow are the collateral and the annular. The ulnar collateral ligament is triangular, with the upper end attached to the medial epicondyle of the humerus, and the broad lower end attached to the ulna along the medial margin of the trochlear notch (Fig. 4.1). The triangular radial collateral ligament is attached above to the lateral epicondyle and below to the annular ligament (Fig. 4.2). The annular ligament is a band which surrounds the radial head and is attached to the margins of the radial notch of the ulna (Fig. 4.3). It retains the radius against the ulna.

The anterior and posterior portions of the joint capsule are continuous on the sides of the joint with the collateral ligaments. The anterior portion of the capsule is attached above to the humerus near the proximal margin of the coronoid fossa and below to the coronoid process and the annular ligament. The posterior portion of the capsule is attached to the humerus near the posterior edge of the capitellum and around the margin of the olecranon fossa. Distally, the attachment is to the olecranon process and annular ligament.

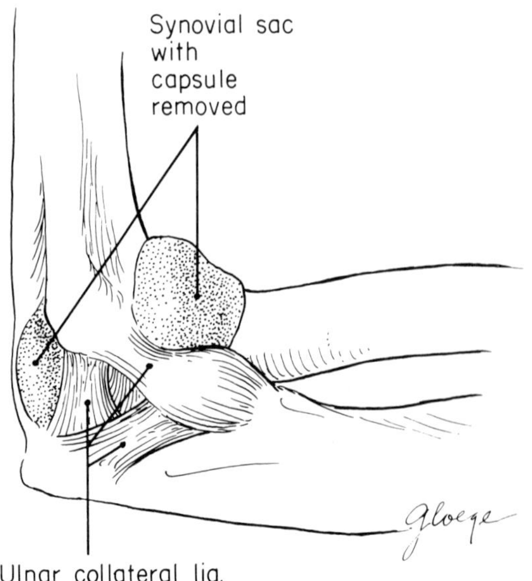

Figure 4.1. Medial side of the distended elbow joint.

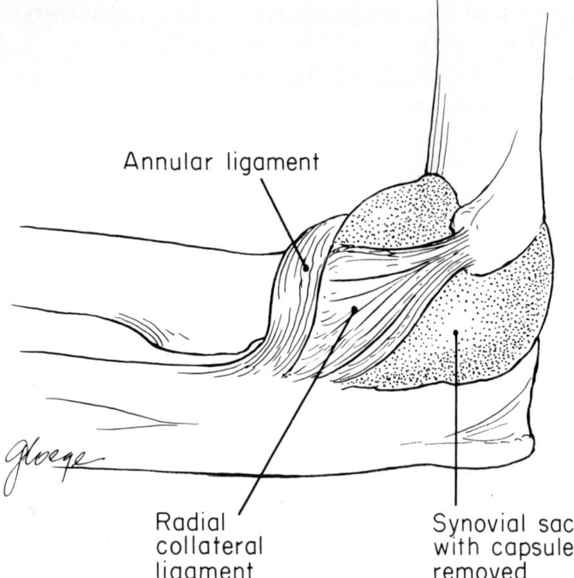

Figure 4.2. Lateral side of the distended elbow joint.

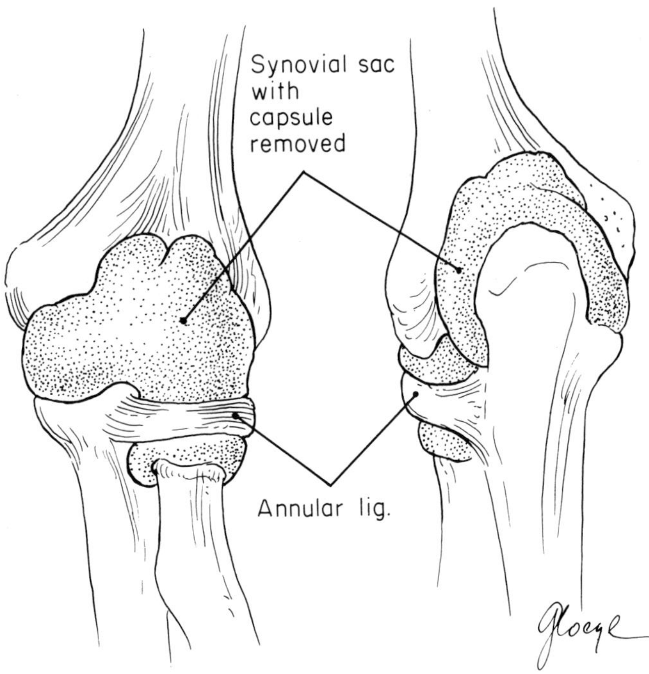

Figure 4.3. Distended elbow joint in the anterior and posterior views. Note the annular ligament surrounding the radial head and distal to this the periradial recess encircling the neck of the radius.

The synovial cavity of the elbow joint is continuous with that of the proximal radioulnar joint. The synovium lines the interior of the joint capsule and the collateral ligaments. It also covers the coronoid, radial, and olecranon fossae of the humerus and is attached to the margins of the articular cartilage of the trochlea, capitellum, trochlear notch, and annular ligament. The periradial and sacciform recesses of the joint are located distal to the annular ligament. They are lined by synovium which is attached to the cartilage of the annular ligament and to the neck of the radius. There is a fold of synovium projecting into the joint between the radius and ulna from behind. This fold contains extrasynovial fat. There are three other pads of fat between the synovium and joint capsule. They are located over the olecranon, coronoid, and radial fossae of the lower end of the humerus. These fat pads are displaced away from the humerus if the synovial sac is distended, so that elbow effusions can be diagnosed on plain radiographs.

METHOD

Prior to each arthrogram a choice is made between the positive single contrast method and the double contrast method. The selection of the technique to be used in each individual patient depends on the reason that the arthrogram is being performed. Traumatic rupture of the capsule or ligaments, stretching of the capsule from recurrent dislocation, adhesive capsulitis, synovial cyst or rupture in rheumatoid arthritis, and synovial thickening from disease are best shown by a positive single contrast arthrogram. Loose bodies within the joint space or synovial sac and abnormalities of the articular cartilage due to injury or disease are demonstrated most accurately by double contrast arthrography with tomography.

Preliminary to the arthrogram, radiographs of the elbow are exposed in the frontal, oblique and lateral projections. In many patients the plain films will display pertinent findings in the bones or soft tissues of the elbow.

Positive Contrast Arthrography

The puncture of the elbow joint and the radiographic study may be performed with the patient either seated beside the fluoroscopic table or lying prone upon the table with the arm raised above the head. The elbow is flexed about 90° and is placed on the table so that it can be punctured and fluoroscoped in the lateral position, radial side up. The skin on the lateral side of the elbow is scrubbed with antiseptic solution and the elbow is surrounded by sterile drapes. With his gloved hand, the arthrographer palpates the patients elbow and locates the depression between the radial head, olecranon, and lateral epicondyle of the humerus. The puncture site is chosen here (Fig. 4.4).

The skin is anesthetized by 1% lidocaine with a 25-gauge needle. A 22-gauge needle is usually used for the joint puncture and is connected by a plastic tube to a syringe which contains lidocaine. This needle is inserted and directed toward the interior of the joint. The needle usually enters the joint at a depth of about 1.5 cm depending on the thickness of the tissues. The passage of the needle through the capsule and into the joint can usually be felt. Any fluid existing in the joint is aspirated. If no joint fluid can be aspirated, the position of the needle is tested by the injection of about 1 ml of lidocaine. If injected lidocaine can be recovered by aspiration, the needle tip is intraarticular. If none of the injected lidocaine can be aspirated the needle tip is probably not in the joint, and the depth or direction of the needle must be changed. Once the joint is entered, diatrizoate contrast agent in 50 or 60% concentration is injected through the tubing. The filling of the joint is observed fluoroscopically; 5 or 6

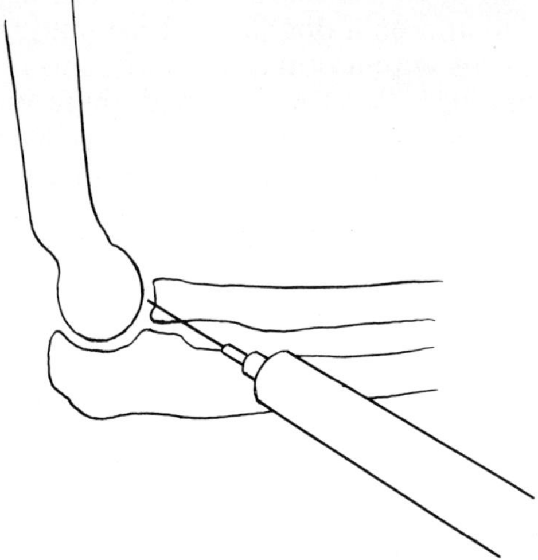

Figure 4.4. Joint puncture for elbow arthrography.

ml of contrast agent is used if the joint space is of normal size. Ten milliliters or more may be required if the capsule is stretched by effusion or recurrent dislocation, if there is a synovial cyst, or if there is rupture of the joint due to disease or trauma.

After the needle is removed the elbow is gently exercised. Radiographs are obtained in the frontal, oblique, and lateral projections with the elbow extended, plus a lateral view with 90° flexion.

The patient is advised to rest the elbow for 24 hr following the arthrogram.

Double Contrast Arthrography

The position of the patient is the same as described above for the positive contrast arthrogram. The arthrocentesis is the same, including complete removal of any effusion or blood from the joint, except that the intraarticular position of the needle is verified by the injection of 1 or 2 ml of air under fluoroscopic visualization. Diatrizoate (0.5 to 1 ml) mixed with 0.1 cc of 1:1000 epinephrine is injected. (The epinephrine delays absorption of the contrast agent while tomograms are being obtained). Filtered room air, 6 to 12 ml, is injected. The amount of air to be injected can be determined fluoroscopically. The injection is continued until there is proper distention of the recesses of the capsule.

Radiographs are obtained in the same projections as for positive contrast arthrography. The smallest focal spot available is used. Then thin section complex motion tomograms are obtained in the flexed lateral projection and in the extended frontal projection. Tomograms in an oblique view are necessary in an occasional patient.

NORMAL ELBOW ARTHROGRAM

The normal arthrogram demonstrates the boundaries of the joint cavity, namely the synovial-lined interior margins of the capsule and the surfaces of the bones covered with synovium or articular cartilage. The distended cavity will of course be filled with contrast material on a positive contrast study (Fig. 4.5) and on a double contrast study (Fig. 4.6) the distended cavity will be filled by air with a thin coating of contrast material on its synovial and cartilagenous margins. By either method, there will be only a thin layer of contrast material between the articulating surfaces where they are in contact. The articular cartilages are sharply delineated zones of decreased density located between the articular cortex of the bones and the contrast medium in the joint. The cartilage surfaces are normally smooth except for the naturally occurring defect in the cartilage near the center of the trochlear notch as previously described. Double contrast arthrography with tomography is the best technique to demonstrate the cartilages of the elbow (Figs. 4.7 and 4.8).

There are four capsular recesses of the elbow joint that are usually described. Their depth varies with the degree of filling of the joint by the injection. The largest is the anterior recess, also known as the volar or coronoid recess. It extends into the coronoid fossa. When the elbow is flexed there may normally be folds of its anterior capsular margin. The smaller posterior recess, also called the dorsal or olecranon recess, extends into the olecranon fossa. These recesses are best seen in the lateral view.

The annular recess, also called the periradial recess, extends distal to the annular ligament and surrounds the neck of the radius. The sacciform or radioulnar recess is a distal extension from the annular recess located between the ulna and radius and is seen in the frontal view. Also in the frontal view the joint space underlying the medial and lateral collateral ligaments is visible. There is normally an irregularity of the capsule beneath the medial collateral ligament.

On the lateral arthrotomograms at certain levels there may be a density within the joint space caused by a pool of contrast agent in the dependent portion of the synovial sac.

ABNORMAL DOUBLE CONTRAST ELBOW ARTHROGRAM

Osteochondritis Dissecans

The capitellum is the usual site of osteochondritis dissecans. Although the cause of the condition is controversial, it probably begins as an aseptic necrosis of the subchondral bone which later affects the overlying articular cartilage. It has been postulated that the disease is due to compressive force between the radial head and capitellum. The initial radiographic finding would be a relative lucency of the involved bone. With progression, the defect becomes better defined with sclerotic margins and there may be fracture of the overlying cartilage. The devascularized bone plug within the defect increases in density. If the plug loses all its attachments it becomes a loose osteochondral joint body, consisting of the bone fragment and attached articular cartilage. If healing occurs, the crater may be filled by fibrous tissue or fibrocartilage. Thus, a smooth articular surface may be restored.

The earliest arthrographic findings in this disease are leakage of contrast agent and air into the cartilage fracture and then around the margins of the bone plug. If the plug separates, the arthrogram will demonstrate the loose osteochondral fragment and the resultant defect in the cartilage and bone of the articular surface (Fig. 4.9).

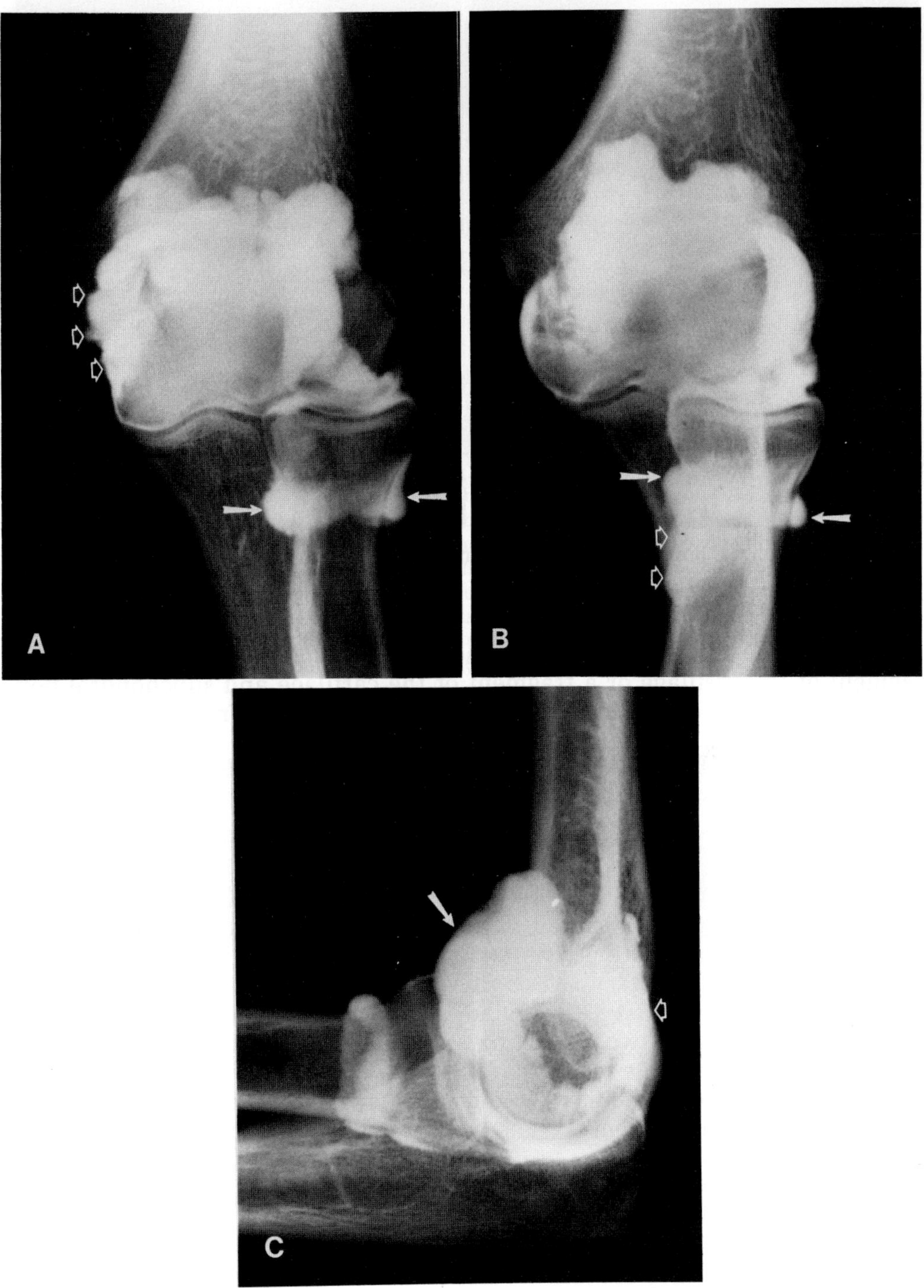

Figure 4.5. Normal positive contrast elbow arthrogram. *A*, Frontal view. Note the periradial recess (*arrows*) and the normal irregularity (*open arrows*) of the synovium beneath the ulnar collateral ligament. *B*, Oblique view. The sacciform recess (*open arrows*) is located distal to the periradial recess (*arrows*). *C*, Lateral view. The coronoid recess (*arrow*) and olecranon recess (*open arrow*) are seen separately here. They are superimposed in the frontal view.

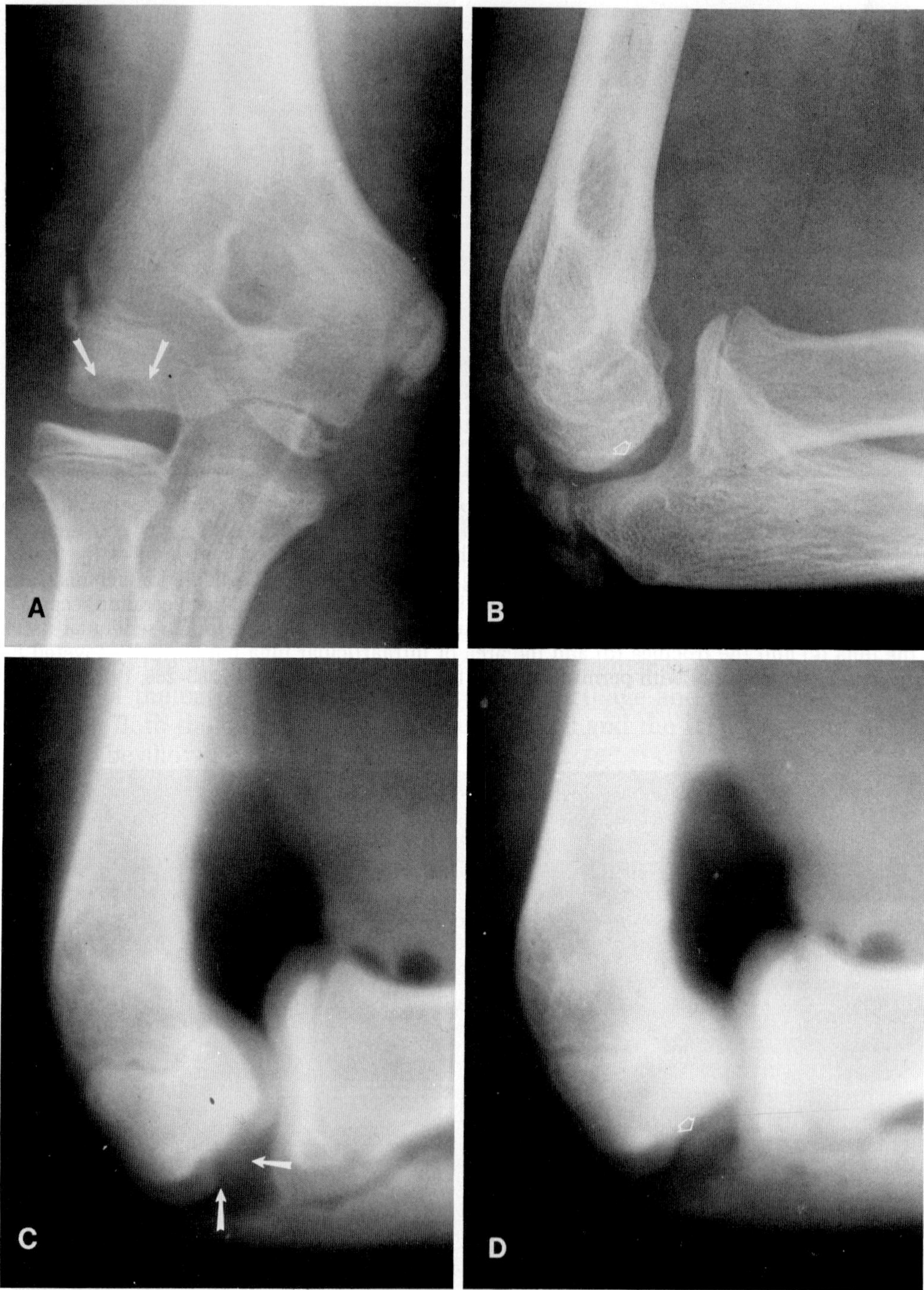

Figure 4.9. Osteochondritis of capitellum. *A* and *B*, Preliminary anteroposterior and lateral radiographs showing lytic defect (*arrows*). *C* and *D*, Same case. Lateral double contrast arthrotomograms demonstrate crater in cartilage (*arrows*) with subchondral bone defect and a loose cartilagenous fragment (*open arrow*) (Reproduced with permission from R. T. Eto: Radiology, *115*: 283–288, 1975.)

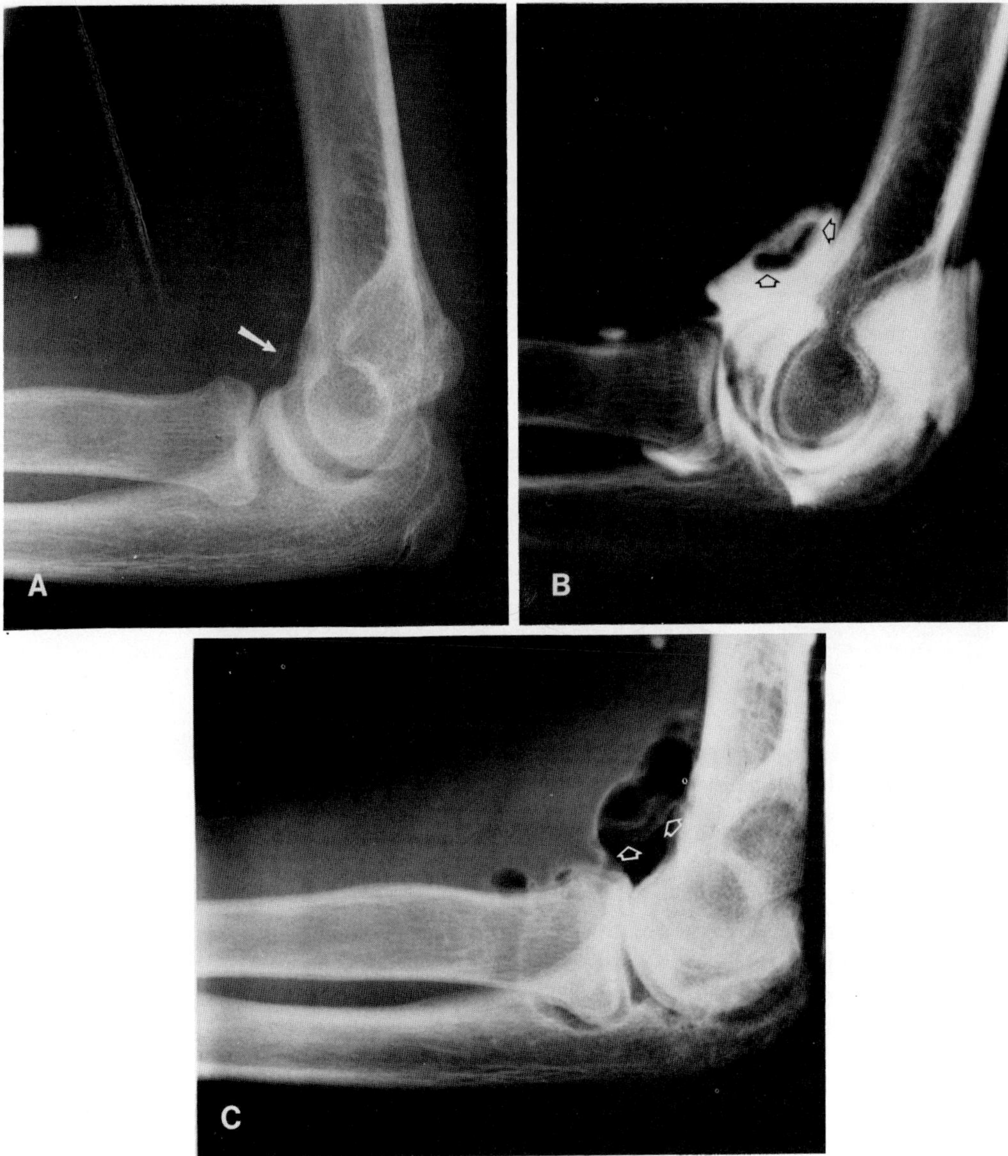

Figure 4.10. Osteochondral fracture. *A*, Preliminary film demonstrates osseous component of the loose fracture fragment (*arrow*). *B*, Osteochondral fragment in joint produces filling defect (*open arrows*) on positive contrast arthrogram. *C*, Double contrast arthrogram on same patient again demonstrates the osteochondral fragment (*open arrows*).

ABNORMAL POSITIVE CONTRAST ELBOW ARTHROGRAM

Rupture of Capsule and Ligaments

The diagnosis of traumatic ruptures of the capsule and ligaments of the elbow by arthrography can help the clinician choose the proper treatment, which might be surgical repair. These ruptures can be produced by dislocation, forced

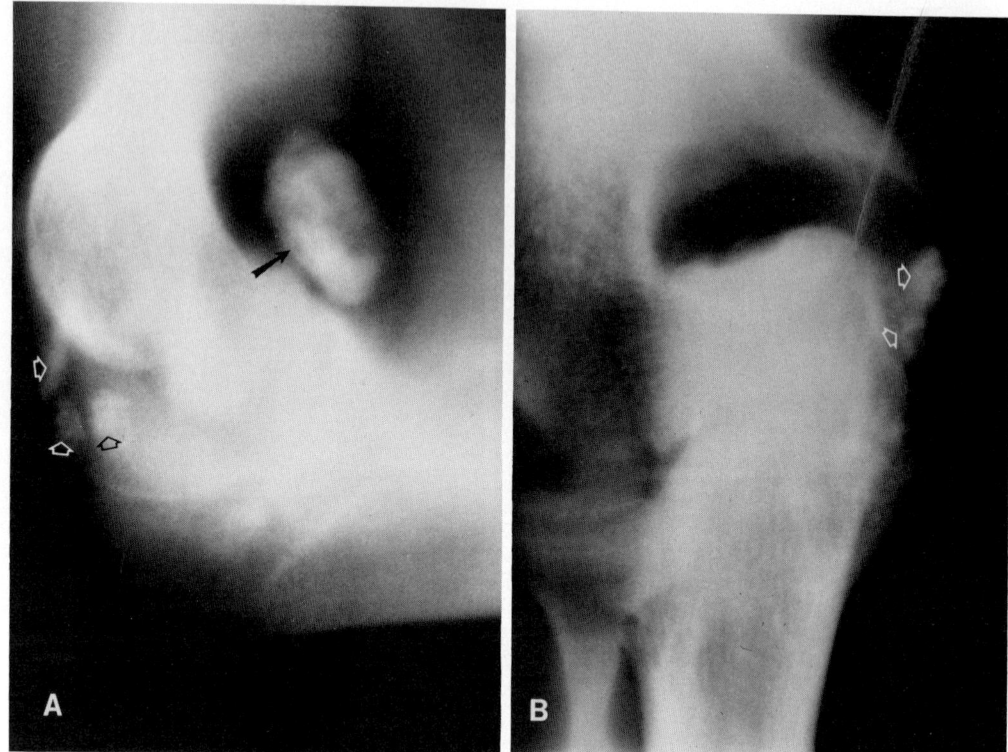

Figure 4.11. Multiple calcified joint bodies (probable osteochondromatosis). *A*, Lateral double contrast arthrotomogram demonstrates large calcific body (*arrow*) in the coronoid recess, and multiple calcifications in the olecranon recess (*open arrows*). *B*, Anteroposterior arthrotomogram of same case shows several calcified loose bodies in medial joint recess (*open arrows*). (Reproduced with permission from R. T. Eto: Radiology, *115*:283–288, 1975.)

abduction or forced adduction of the elbow, or may accompany fracture. In a comprehensive investigation of elbow injuries, which included 217 positive contrast arthrograms, Johansson found arthrography to be highly reliable in the diagnosis of collateral ligament and capsular ruptures. The ruptures are demonstrated on the arthrogram by leakage of contrast material outside the normal limits of the joint cavity. The degree of extravasation correlates with the extent of the tear (Fig. 4.13). The arthrogram should be performed soon after the injury, because there is a tendency for the ruptures to be sealed by fibrin deposits.

Rheumatoid Arthritis

Rheumatoid arthritis is primarily a disease of the synovium. The edema, inflammation, and hypertrophy cause an irregular or nodular synovial thickening that can be detected by arthrography (Figs. 4.14 and 4.15). Intrasynovial fatty masses in rheumatoid arthritis are sometimes visible on both plain film and arthrogram as reported by Weston. Chronic effusion may result in enlargement of the synovial cavity which may be shown by arthrography.

Rheumatoid arthritis may cause opacification of the lymphatics during elbow

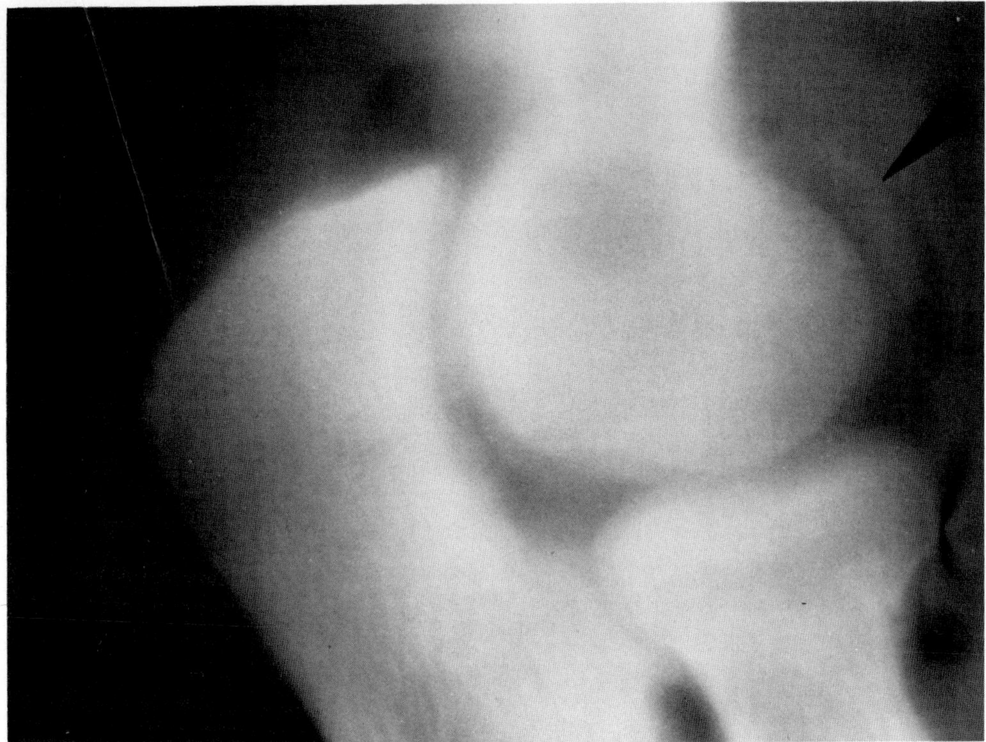

Figure 4.12. Hypertrophic synovial mass. Synovial tag over anterior surface of capitellum (*arrowhead*) causing joint locking. (Reproduced with permission from R. T. Eto: Radiology, *115:283–288*, 1975.)

arthrography (Fig. 4.14). The thinning of the articular cartilage that occurs is visible on the arthrogram (Fig. 4.16).

Synovial rupture of the elbow joint in rheumatoid arthritis was first described by Goode. The symptoms he described were pain and swelling in the forearm which sometimes spread to the hand and upper arm. Peau d'orange was sometimes seen. Arthrography reveals leakage of contrast material into the forearm from either the medial or lateral aspect of the joint (Fig. 4.17). Rheumatoid arthritis occasionally produces an expanding synovial cyst of the elbow (Fig. 4.15).

Capsular Abnormalities

Recurrent dislocation of the elbow may stretch the capsule. Arthrography will show expansion of the synovial sac (Fig. 4.18). With adhesive capsulitis the capacity of the synovial sac will be reduced as shown by arthrography with shrinkage of the recesses (Fig. 4.19).

Loose Bodies

With positive contrast arthrography loose bodies can be seen as filling defects within the opacified synovial sac (Fig. 4.10 and 4.20). However, double contrast arthrotomography is more accurate for the detection of joint bodies.

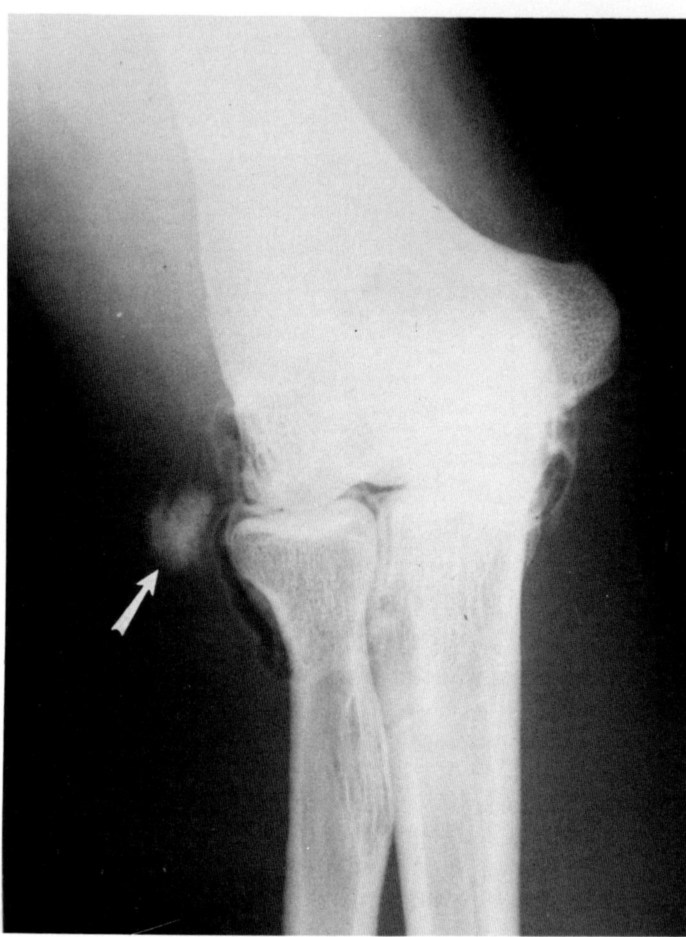

Figure 4.13. Small capsular tear with localized extravasation of contrast agent (*arrow*).

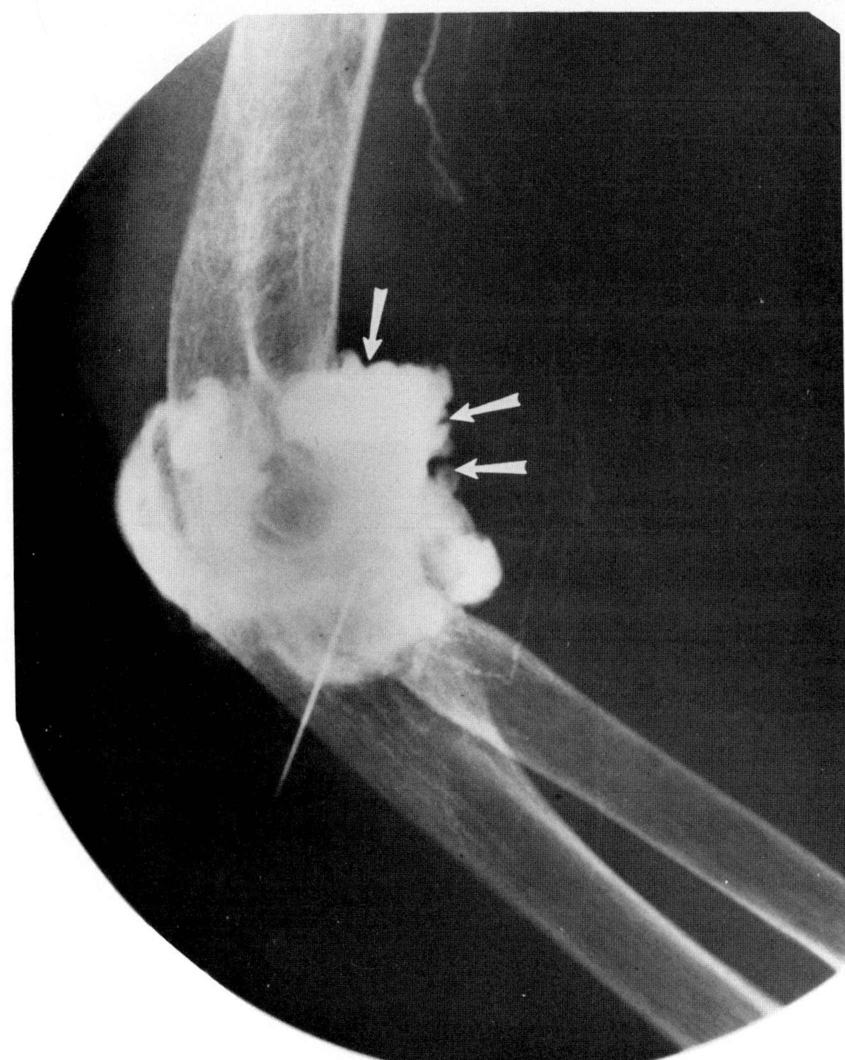

Figure 4.14. Rheumatoid arthritis. Irregular synovial thickening (*arrows*) and opacification of the lymphatics are demonstrated on positive contrast arthrogram. (Courtesy of Darwood Hance, M.D.)

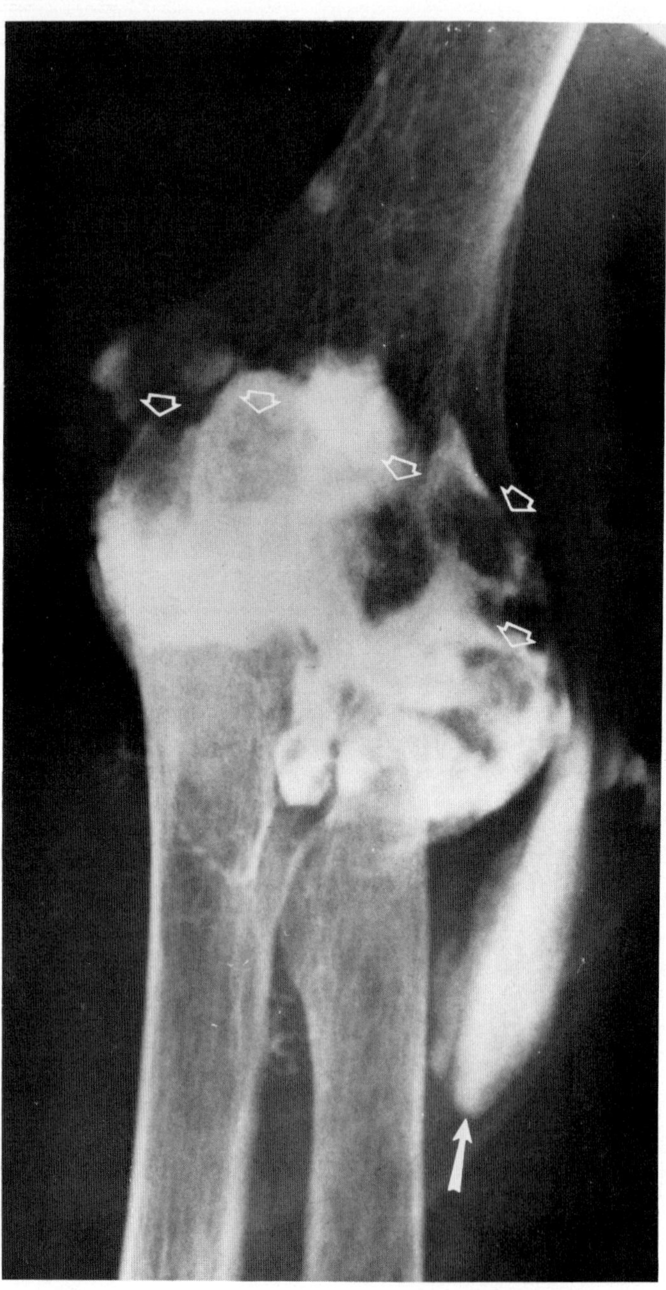

Figure 4.15. Rheumatoid arthritis. Multiple synovial nodules are demonstrated (*open arrows*). Distal to the joint there is lymphatic opacification. An antecubital cyst extends from the lateral side of the joint into the forearm (*arrow*) on the positive contrast arthrogram. (Courtesy of Darwood Hance, M.D.)

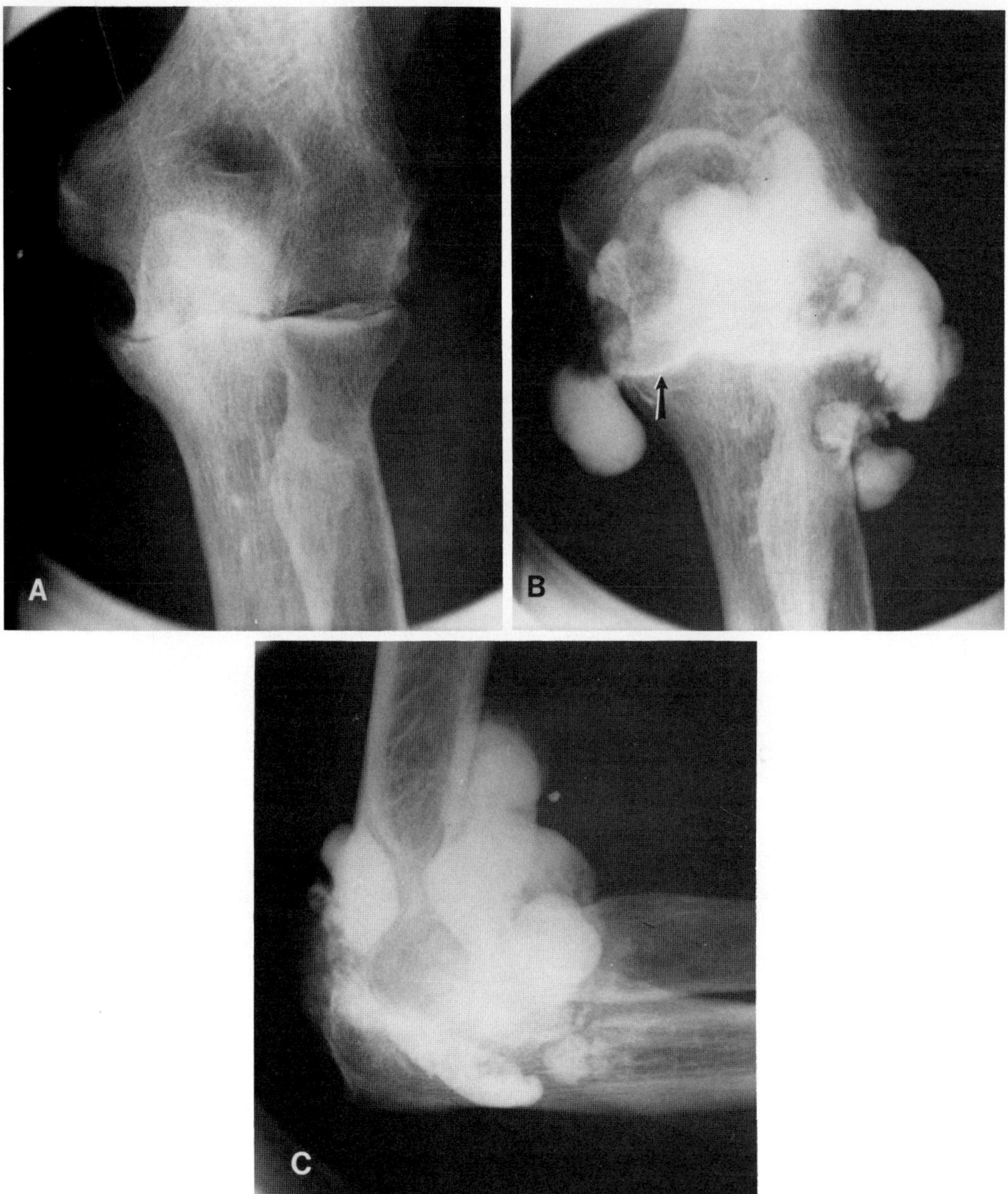

Figure 4.16. Rheumatoid arthritis. *A,* Preliminary radiograph on which marked joint space narrowing, bony sclerosis, hypertrophic change, and small erosions of the humerus are shown. *B* and *C,* Positive contrast arthrogram shows expansion of the joint recesses and multiple outpouchings. The appearance of the opacified joint space (*arrow*) indicates loss of articular cartilage.

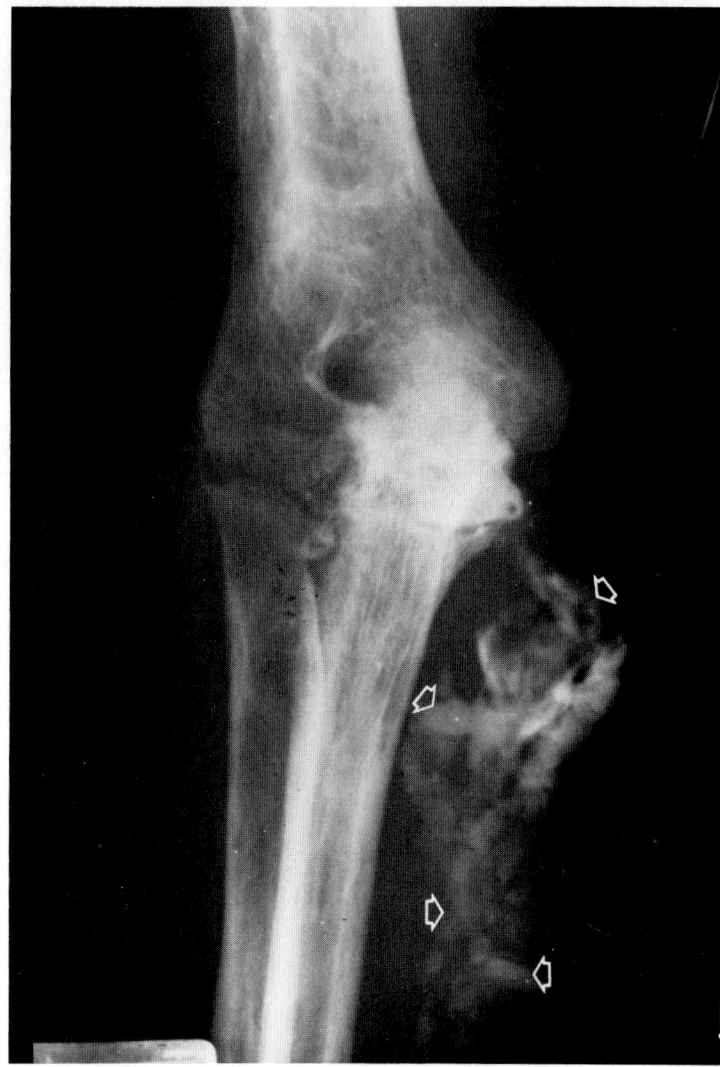

Figure 4.17. Synovial rupture in rheumatoid arthritis. Positive contrast arthrogram shows extravasation into the forearm from the medial side of the joint (*open arrows*).

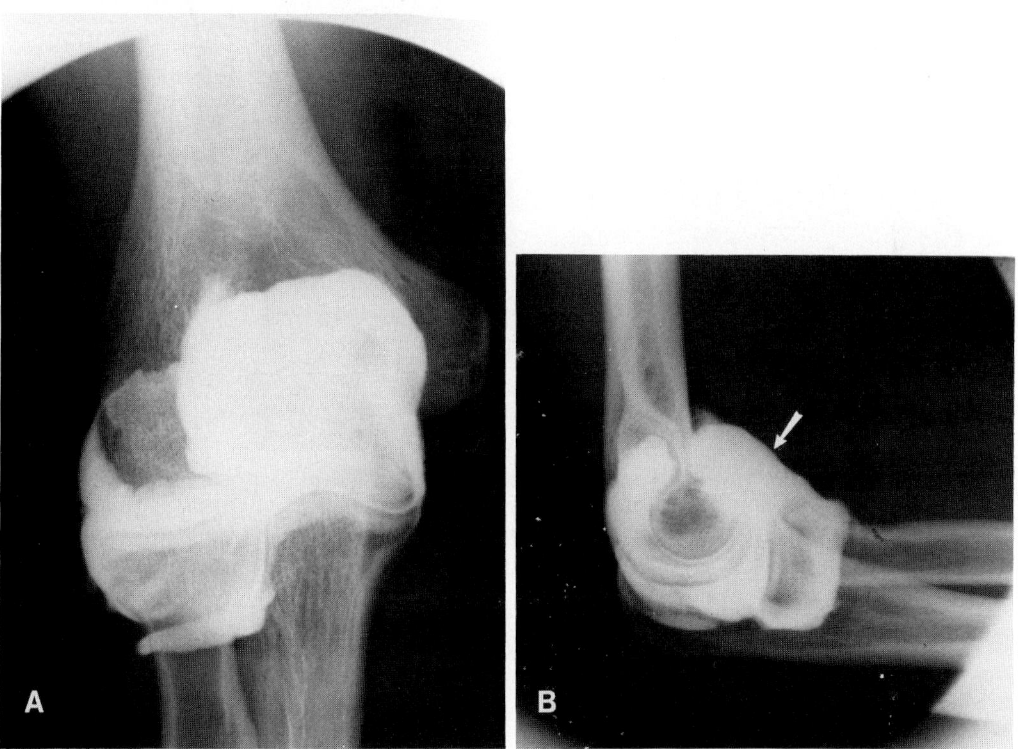

Figure 4.18. Laxity of capsule from recurrent dislocation. *A*, Frontal view. *B*, Lateral view. Note expansion of coronoid recess (*arrow*).

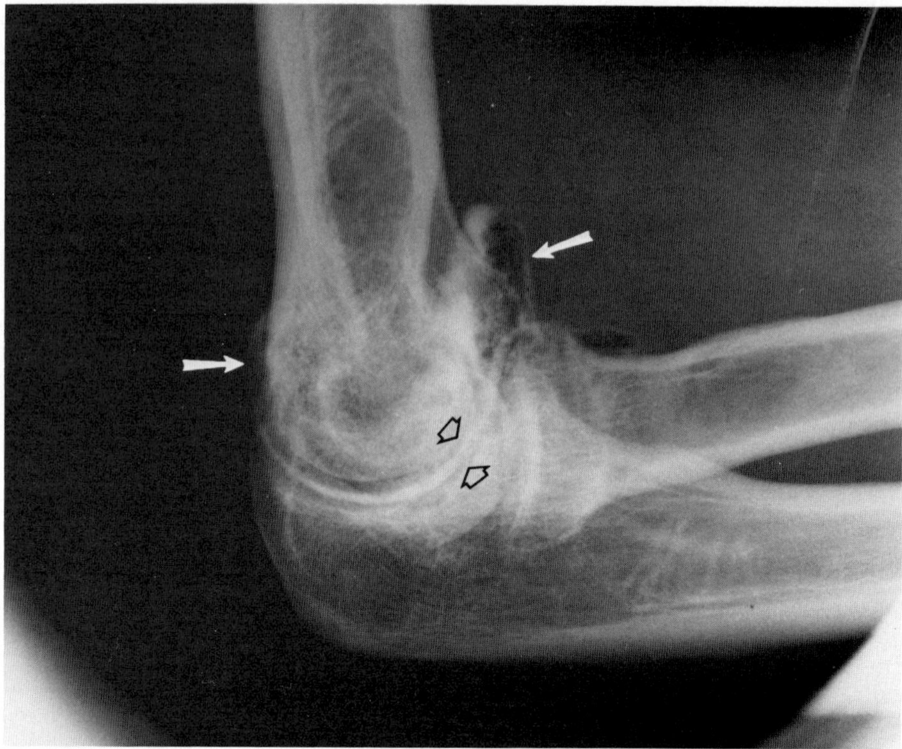

Figure 4.19. Posttraumatic arthritis with adhesive capsulitis. There is a healed fracture of the proximal ulna. The coronoid and olecranon recesses are abnormally small (*arrows*). The cartilage is thin at anterior aspect of ulnar-trochlear articulation (*open arrows*).

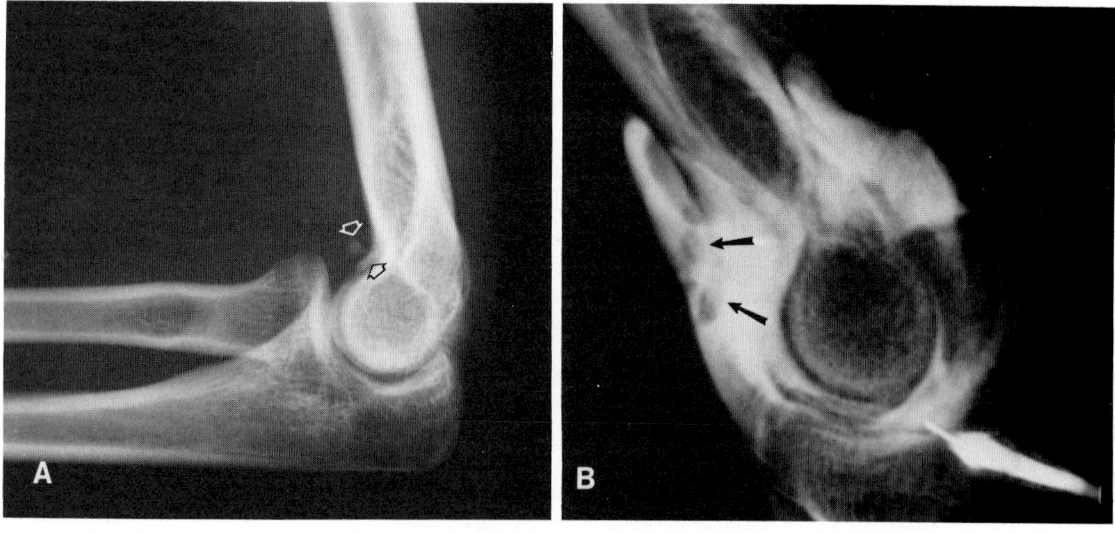

Figure 4.20. Loose joint bodies. *A*, Preliminary radiograph shows small joint calcifications (*open arrows*). *B*, Positive contrast arthrogram demonstrates filling defects caused by loose bodies in the coronoid fossa (*arrows*).

References

Bell, M.D., Loose bodies in the elbow. Br J Surg, 62:921–924, 1975.

Brown, R., Blazina, M.E., Kerlan, R.K., Carter, V.S., Jobe, F.W., Carlson, G.J., Osteochondritis of the capitellum. Am J Sports Med, 2:27–44, 1974.

Erlich, G.E., Antecubital cysts in rheumatoid arthritis—a corollary to popliteal (Baker's) cysts. J Bone Joint Surg, 54A:165–169, 1972.

Eto, R.T., Anderson, P.W., Harley, J.D., Elbow arthrography with the application of tomography. Radiology, 115:283–288, 1975.

Giustra, P.E., Furman, R.S., Roberts, L., Killoran, P.J., Synovial osteochondromatosis involving the elbow. AJR, 127:604, 1968.

Goode, J.D., Synovial rupture of the elbow joint. Ann Rheum Dis, 27:604, 1968.

Johansson, O., Capsular and ligament injuries of the elbow joint, a clinical and arthrographic study. Acta Chir Scand, [Suppl]287, 1962.

Pavlov, H., Ghelman, B., Warren, R.F., Double-contrast arthrography of the elbow. Radiology, 130:87–95, 1979.

Weston, W.J., The synovial changes at the elbow in rheumatoid arthritis. Australas Radiol, 15:170–174, 1971.

Weston, W.J., The intra synovial fatty masses in chronic rheumatoid arthritis. Br J Radiol, 46:213–216, 1972.

5

Arthrography of the Ankle

R. D. Arndt, M.D.

Arthrography of the ankle, although not as common as other joints, is becoming increasingly important as an accurate diagnostic examination of serious ankle injury with or without fractures which are clinically beyond simple sprains. Arthrography is far more reliable than stress films for determining ligamentous tears; it is safe and well tolerated by most patients.

FUNCTIONAL ANATOMY

For purposes of simplification, as suggested by Grant, supratalar joint may be used to denote the ankle joint (the articulation of the talus, tibia, and fibula), and infratalar joint to denote the combined talocalcaneal (subtalar) and talo-calcaneo-navicular joints. The supratalar joint is a hinge joint and executes the movements of plantarflexion and dorsiflexion. The movements of inversion and eversion take place at the infratalar joint. Inversion is a combination of supination and adduction; eversion combines pronation and abduction. During inversion the ankle joint is plantarflexed, whereas it is dorsiflexed during eversion. It is during forced inversion or eversion that the majority of ankle injuries occur.

The supratalar joint maintains its stability largely as a consequence of the anatomy of its "ankle mortise" whereby, in accordance with the vernacular of carpentry a press fit is achieved between the talus, representing the tenon, and the malleoli representing the inverted mortise. Further support is provided by the surrounding tendons and the joint capsule itself. The capsule is greatly strengthened by the lateral and medial collateral ligaments which are intimately associated and actually blend with the capsular membrane in most instances. The inner surface of the capsule is lined with synovium. The joint has lateral and medial pouches or recesses which extend slightly below the inferior surface of the tips of the malleoli. Slightly larger anterior and posterior pouches are present (Fig. 5.1). With injury or aging the pouches tend to enlarge and become somewhat irregular in outline. The anterior pouch flattens and diminishes in volume with the foot in plantarflexion, while dorsiflexion causes flattening of the posterior pouch. The medial and lateral pouches vary little in size or contour with movement.

141

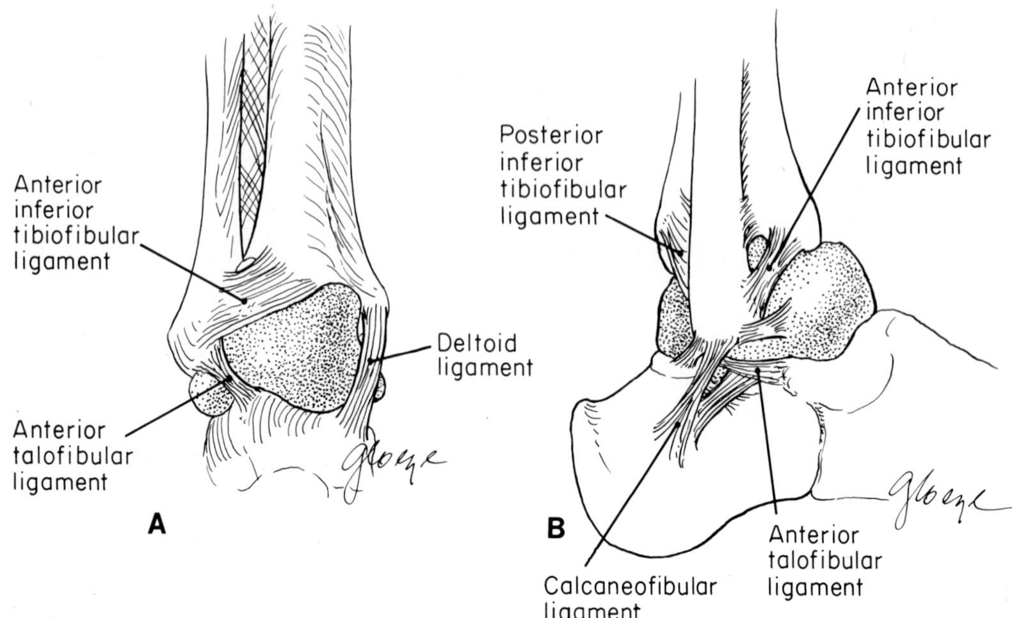

Figure 5.1. Joint capsule of the ankle. *A*, Anteroposterior. *B*, Lateral. (Modified from Grant, J.C.B., *An Atlas of Anatomy*, Ed. 5. Williams & Wilkins, Baltimore, 1962.)

During ankle arthrography the supratalar or ankle joint is opacified. The infratalar joint complex is usually not opacified. It has already been stated that the supratalar joint executes only flexion and extension, whereas inversion and eversion take place at the infratalar joints. When the latter movements are extreme as a result of trauma various ligaments may tear and the malleoli may fracture. Since most of the ligaments are intimately blended with the capsule of the supratalar joint, the capsule may be torn. Upon injection of radiopaque contrast, leakage may occur at the site of the torn ligament. Thus, arthrography of the supratalar joint allows identification of ligamentous tears, even though the free movement causing the injury, inversion, and eversion actually took place at the infratalar joint which is not directly opacified.

It is not uncommon for the supratalar joint to communicate with the synovial sheath of several of the adjacent tendons, particularly the flexor digitorum longus and flexor hallucis longus on the medial side, the tibialis posterior posteromedially, and the subtalar joint posteriorly and inferiorly. Communication with the tendon sheaths of the peroneus longus and brevis on the lateral side of the joint is not normal and most likely reflects a tear, old or new, of the calcaneofibular ligament. A minority viewpoint is that communication with these lateral muscle sheaths may be a normal variant, because at surgery it is sometimes impossible to demonstrate a tear of the calcaneofibular ligament, and moreover, some patients deny antecedent trauma. The final arthrographic interpretation of ankle joint communication with the lateral peroneus longus and brevis tendon sheaths, therefore, requires close clinical correlation. Most authorities agree, however, that communication of the supratalar joint with the sheaths of the medial tendons occurs as a normal variant in 10 to 15% of the population.

The collateral ligaments are in close association and partially fuse with the fibers of the supratalar joint capsule (Fig. 5.2). Anteriorly there is the anteroinferior tibiofibular ligament, posteriorly the posteroinferior tibiofibular ligament, laterally the anterior and posterior talofibular ligaments, and medially the deltoid ligament which is composed of multiple diverging fibers originating from the medial malleolus and extending to the calcaneous and talus. Another lateral structure, the calcaneofibular ligament is usually less intimately associated with the supratalar joint capsule but instead adheres closely to the single shared synovial sheath of the peroneus longus and brevis tendons. The intimate association of all these ligaments with the various synovial recesses allows ankle arthrography to be used in the identification of injuries.

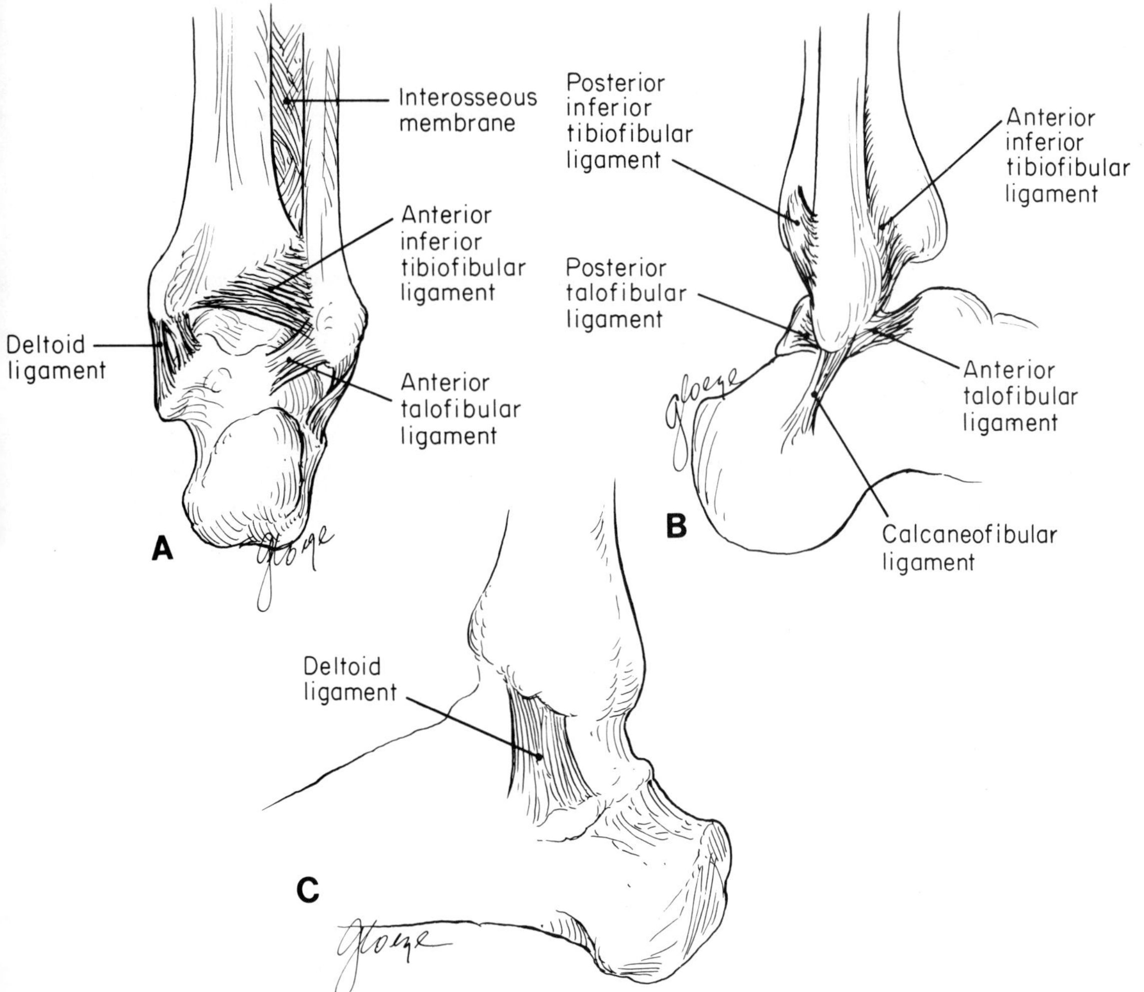

Figure 5.2. Anatomy of the ligaments of the ankle joint. *A*, Anterior. *B*, Lateral. *C*, Medial.

METHOD OF ARTHROGRAPHY

Anteroposterior and lateral preliminary films are obtained and inspected for abnormalities and especially for evidence of old or recent trauma. The patient lies supine with the supratalar joint under the fluoroscope. Although the supratalar joint can usually be palpated, it is more accurate to mark its location as viewed under fluoroscopy with a metallic object such as a needle tip. After sterile preparation and draping, the skin is anesthetized with 1% lidocaine injected through a 25-gauge needle. The site of arthrocentesis is anterior, and along the lateral or medial aspect of the joint as demarcated by the articulating surfaces of tibia and talus (Fig. 5.3). To prevent the possibility of obscuring the area in question by any leakage of contrast from the puncture site, the side opposite the painful side is punctured. Arthrocentesis is performed by penetrating the anesthetized skin with a conventional 22-gauge needle, 1.5 in in length attached to a 10-cc syringe containing 1% lidocaine or saline and then slowly progressing in depth while exerting slight pressure on the plunger. When tissue resistance to the injected fluid disappears, the needle tip may be assumed to be intraarticular. This is easily verified by turning the ankle into the lateral position at fluoroscopy. As much joint fluid as possible should be aspirated and 1 cc of lidocaine injected into the joint through the same needle. Intraarticular anesthesia may be helpful in allowing stress films or exercise of a recently injured joint. The syringe is removed from the needle, and extension tubing connected to a 10-cc syringe containing dilute diatrizoate meglumine (Renografin 60 diluted with an equal amount of saline or sterile water) is attached to the indwelling needle. Under fluoroscopy, the contrast agent is gently injected. Contrast agent that flows away from the needle tip and outlines the articular surface of the talus confirms the intraarticular placement of the needle tip. The usual capacity of the joint is 6 to 10 cc. After injection, the extension tubing is removed and any excess of contrast material is allowed to drip from the needle hub under its own hydrostatic pressure into a gauze sponge. This aids in preventing leakage from the injection site during the subsequent filming. Thereafter, the needle is withdrawn and the joint is passively or actively exercised in

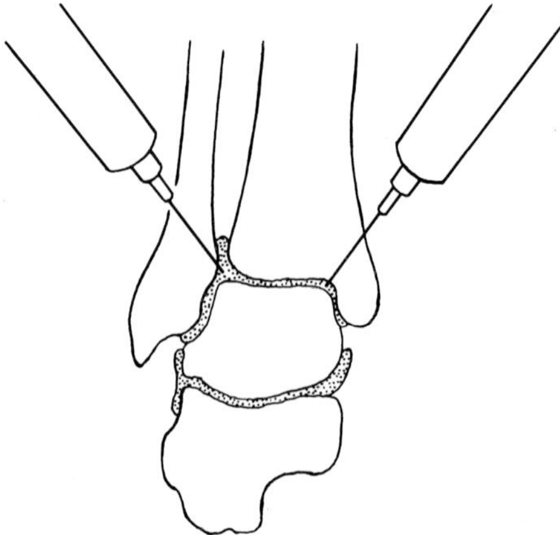

Figure 5.3. Sites of arthrocentesis, ankle joint.

all ranges of motion for 30 seconds. Anteroposterior, lateral plantarflexion, dorsiflexion, and neutral, and right and left anterior posterior oblique overhead films are exposed. In the patient with osteochondritis dissecans, immediate anteroposterior and lateral tomograms are recommended as a valuable supplement to the routine arthrogram to ensure optimal visualization of the articular cartilage over the necrotic subchondral bone fragment. Anteroposterior right and left stress films may be obtained if necessary and if they are not too painful for the patient. All films must be obtained as quickly as possible after injection before dilution and absorption of the contrast material takes place. Following the arthrogram, the patient usually experiences a sense of fullness in the joint. A mild burning sensation may be felt at the site of injury, but severe pain is rare. The patient should be advised to refrain from heavy exercise or running for 24 hours after the arthrogram, but can resume normal ambulation immediately, unless this has been restricted by the primary physician.

NORMAL ANKLE ARTHROGRAM

The lateral and medial recesses of the supratalar joint are small, smoothly marginated pouches extending to and slightly below the inferior tips of the malleoli. The anterior and posterior recesses extending from the articular space between the tibia and talus are slightly larger and somewhat sacculated, especially in older individuals and in those with joints subjected to previous acute or chronic trauma (Fig. 5.4). The anterior recess is flattened, and the posterior recess is enlarged on the lateral radiograph made in plantarflexion (Fig. 5.5). This is reversed with dorsiflexion. The capsule extends approximately 1 cm superiorly into the articulation between the tibia and fibula, and contrast should not reach beyond this level (Fig. 5.6). The joint space between the tibia, fibula,

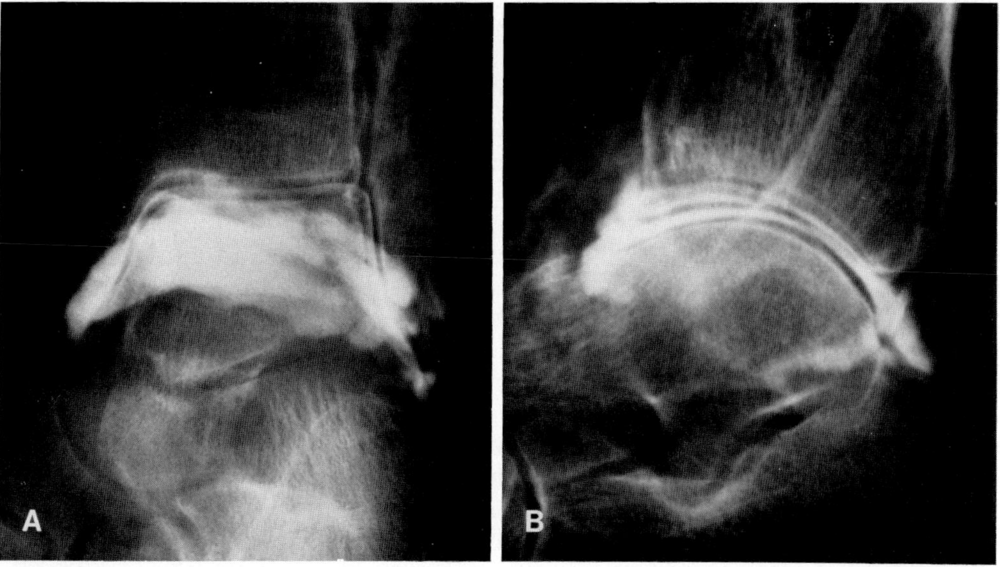

Figure 5.4. Normal ankle arthrogram. Anteroposterior (A) and lateral projections (B) show extent of joint recesses and articular cartilage.

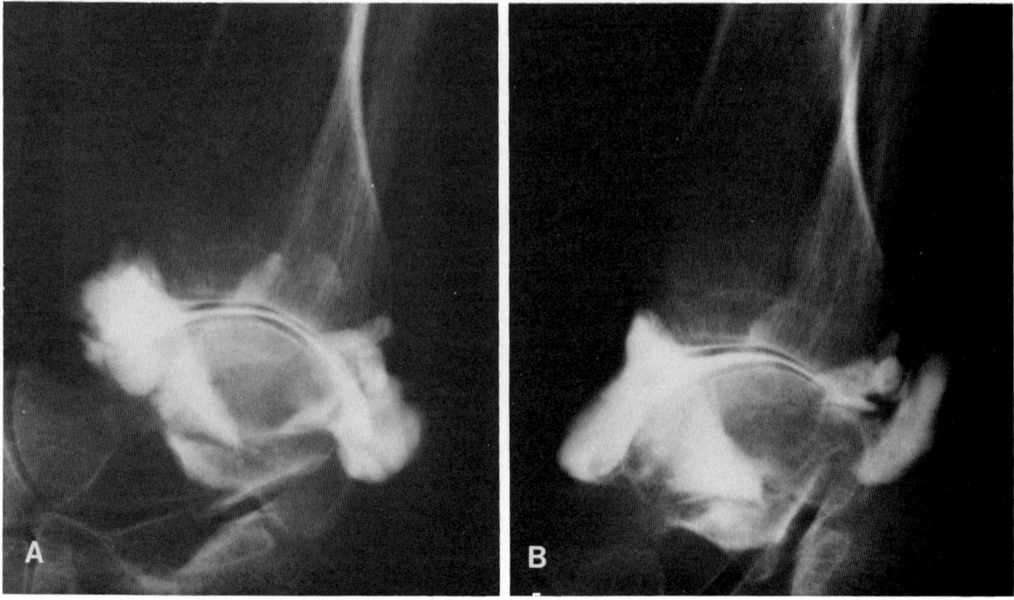

Figure 5.5. Normal ankle arthrogram. *A*, Lateral projection, dorsiflexion, anterior recess is expanded, posterior recess contracted. *B*, Plantarflexion reverses this relationship.

and talus is opacified as a thin line (Fig. 5.7). Filling of the synovium-lined tendon sheaths of the flexor digitorum longus and flexor hallucis longus along the medial surface of the supratalar and infratalar joints is seen in 10 to 15% of normal individuals (Fig. 5.8). Contrast entering the subtalar joint occurs in fewer than 10% of the population but is probably a normal variant.

ABNORMAL ANKLE ARTHROGRAM

Ligament Injuries

The usual indication for ankle arthrography is clinical suspicion of a medial or lateral collateral ligament tear especially if films exposed during stress maneuvers are equivocal or unobtainable because of extreme pain. The ankle arthrogram may also reveal a tear of the anterior inferior tibiofibular ligament, an injury usually accompanied by other ligamentous tears, or a tear of the interosseous membrane between tibia and fibula leading to tibiofibular diastasis.

Several authors have demonstrated the arthrographic findings in collateral ligament injuries. Kaye and Bohne have shown excellent correlation of arthrographic pathology with anatomical locations of the collateral ligaments in cadaver specimens. Knowledge of the origins and insertions of these ligaments leads to easier understanding of the arthrographic findings in ligamentous injury. The basis of an abnormal arthrogram in ligamentous injury is a tear in the capsule of the supratalar joint where the injured ligament fuses with or intimately adheres to the fibers of the capsule. Since these tears in most instances will undergo spontaneous although sometimes incomplete healing, it is of prime importance that arthrography be performed as soon as possible, ideally within 2 days and not later than 1 week after injury. Beyond this time,

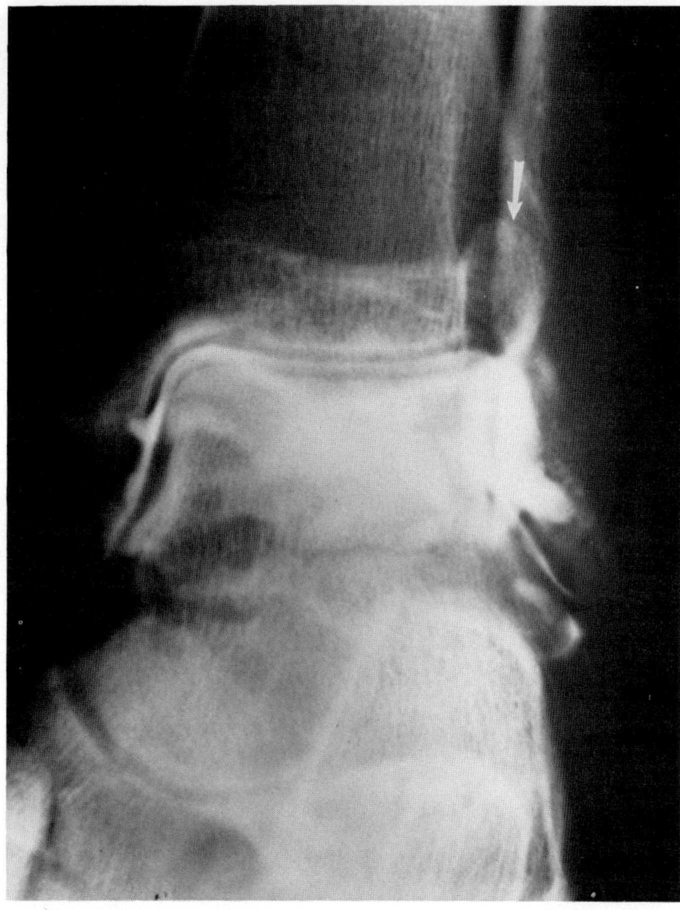

Figure 5.6. Normal ankle arthrogram.   Anteroposterior projection reveals normal limits of extension of joint recess between tibia and fibula (*arrow*).

healing may seal the leak, and arthrography may lead to a false negative diagnosis.

The lateral ligaments, specifically the anterior talofibular and the calcaneofibular ligaments, are most commonly torn. In the case of an anterior talofibular ligament tear, an anteroposterior view reveals leakage of contrast material from the supratalar joint beneath and lateral to the lateral malleolus, and extending upward to a varying extent along the lateral aspect of the fibula. On the lateral view, contrast will be seen anterior and superior to the distal head of the fibula (Fig. 5.9). A tear of the posterior talofibular ligament, although rare, reveals similar findings, except the contrast extravasation is posterior on the lateral film (Fig. 5.10). The calcaneofibular ligament, the strongest of the lateral ligaments, tears less easily. On the arthrogram a leak into the common sheath of the peroneal tendons on the lateral aspect of the joint may be identified (Fig. 5.11). The peroneous longus and brevis share a common sheath at the level of the calcaneofibular ligament, but the sheath subdivides in the tarsal area, the peroneus longus inserting on the medial cuneiform and first metatarsal, and the peroneus brevis at the base of the fifth metatarsal. This communication between the subdivided sheaths and the supratalar joint is best appreciated on the anteroposterior and lateral views (Fig. 5.12). Since the tendon sheaths and the

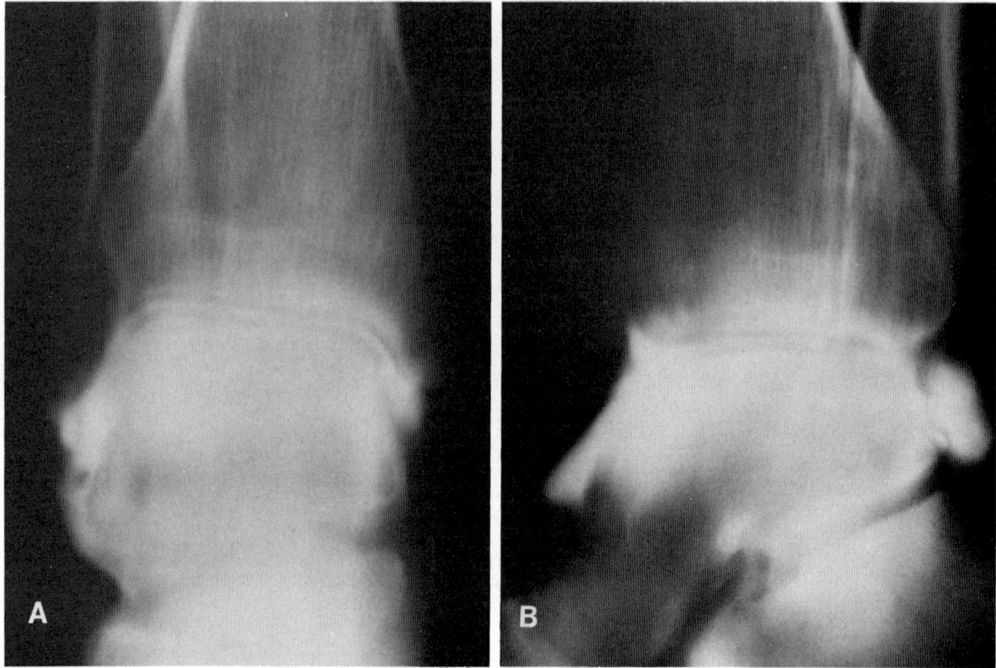

Figure 5.7. Normal ankle arthrotomogram. Anteroposterior (*A*) and lateral projections (*B*) reveal detail of articular cartilage of supratalar joint.

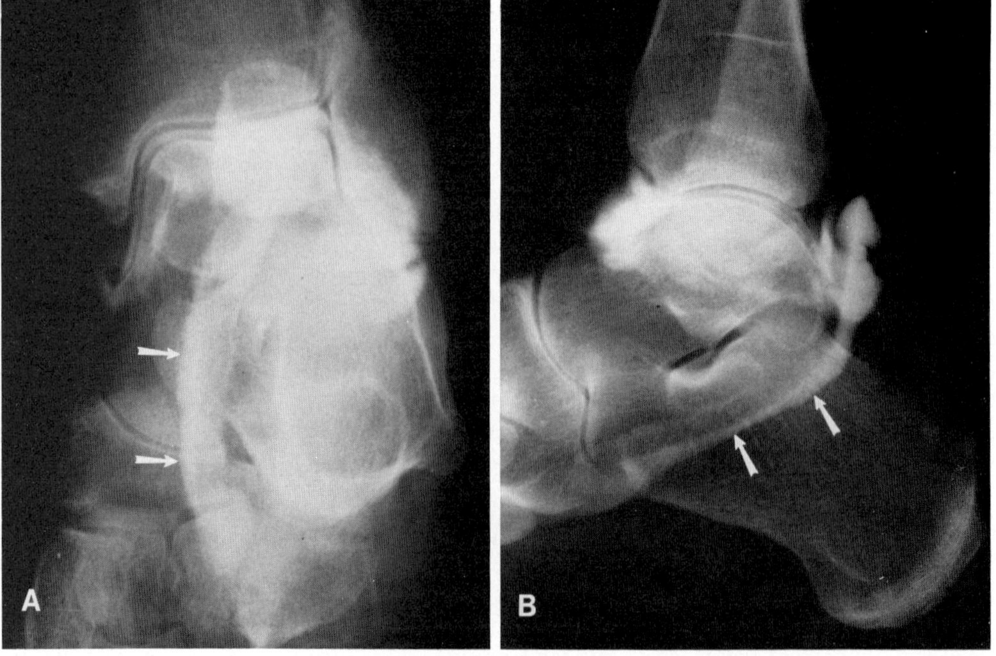

Figure 5.8. Normal ankle arthrogram. Anteroposterior (*A*) and lateral projections (*B*) reveal communication with flexor hallucis longus tendon sheath, a normal variant (*arrows*).

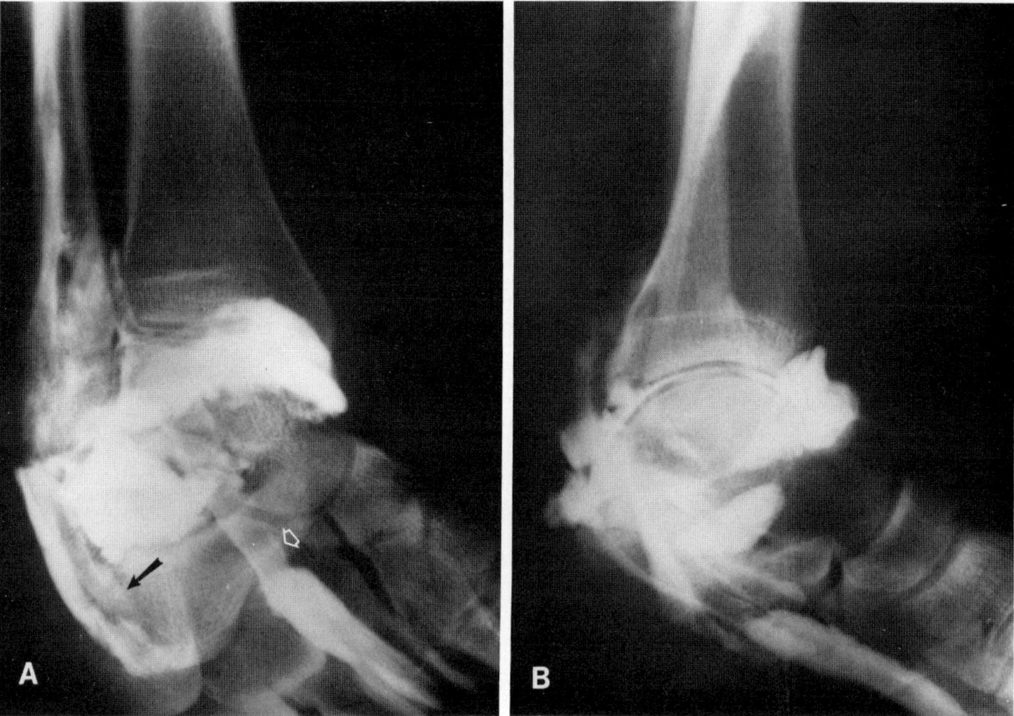

Figure 5.9. Combined anterior talofibular and calcaneofibular ligament tears. *A,* Anteroposterior, internal rotation view demonstrates contrast extravasation beneath and lateral to distal fibula (anterior talofibular ligament tear), and contrast within the peroneal tendon sheath (calcaneofibular ligament tear) (*arrow*). Contrast also fills flexor hallucis longus tendon sheath medially, a normal variant (*open arrow*). *B,* Lateral projection. Note that the medial and lateral tendon sheaths are superimposed.

supratalar joint are all lined with synovium, communication between the joint and the peroneal tendon sheath, once established, tends to persist. Unlike other ligamentous tears of the ankle, a tear of the calcaneofibular ligament may be demonstrated arthrographically long after the original injury and even after the ligament itself has healed (Fig. 5.13). Thus, identification of peroneal sheath communication at arthrography merits close clinical correlation before the final diagnosis is made. If the clinical findings do not suggest an acute tear, then the arthrographic findings should be assumed to imply an old injury.

The strongest ligament on the ankle joint medially is the deltoid ligament. This structure is rarely torn, but if so usually requires surgical repair. As revealed in an anteroposterior view, a tear of the deltoid ligament results in leakage of contrast beneath and medial to the medial malleolus, with extension upward along the medial edge of the tibia. In the lateral view the contrast agent may be seen anterior to the medial malleolus (Fig. 5.14). The diagnosis of deltoid ligament injury may be mistakenly made or masked by normal opacification of the sheaths of the flexor hallucis longus and flexor digitorum longus tendons which course beneath the medial malleolus on both the anteroposterior and lateral views. Identification of the outline of the tendon within the sheath should differentiate the normal from the pathological condition.

Tears of the anterior inferior tibiofibular ligament, which is situated on the

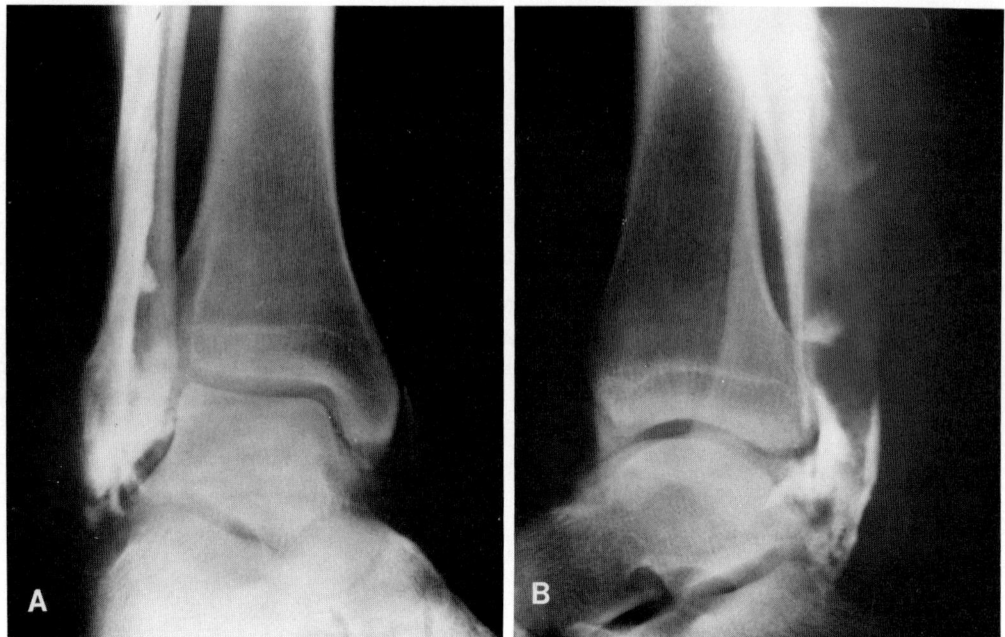

Figure 5.10. Probable posterior talofibular ligament tear. *A,* Anteroposterior projection, contrast extravasates from supratalar joint inferior and lateral to distal fibula. *B,* Lateral film shows contrast leaving joint posteriorly (not surgically proved).

upper aspect of the supratalar joint and spans the tibiofibular joint, and the interosseous membrane between the shafts of the tibia and fibula are injuries resulting in varying degrees of tibiofibular diastasis. They are often accompanied by tears of other structures, especially lateral ligaments. In the arthrogram this injury is detected in the anteroposterior view by noting contrast leaking between the tibia and fibula above the supratalar joint into and above the tibiofibular joint (Fig. 5.15). The latter joint is very small, consisting of a tiny articulating facet on the tibia and a syndesmosis between the very distal tibia and fibular shafts. The supratalar joint capsule normally extends approximately 1 cm above the level of the articulation between the tibia and fibula. The presence of contrast higher than this, above the tibiofibular joint and especially if outlining the fibers of the interosseous membrane, is consistent with a tear of the anterior inferior tibiofibular ligament (Fig. 5.16). In the lateral projection the contrast material leak is identified superior to the anterior and midportion of the supratalar joint. If the contrast agent is entirely posterior in this projection, caution is advised, because it may represent contrast in a normal communication with the flexor hallucis longus tendon, but this should be readily distinguishable on other views (Table 5.1).

Osteochondritis Dissecans

Another use of supratalar arthrography is in the evaluation of osteochondritis dissecans which occurs most commonly along the medial aspect of the subchondral bone on the superior articular surface of the talus. The determination of the integrity of the overlying cartilage is useful in planning treatment. This is easily accomplished during a single or double contrast ankle arthrogram by

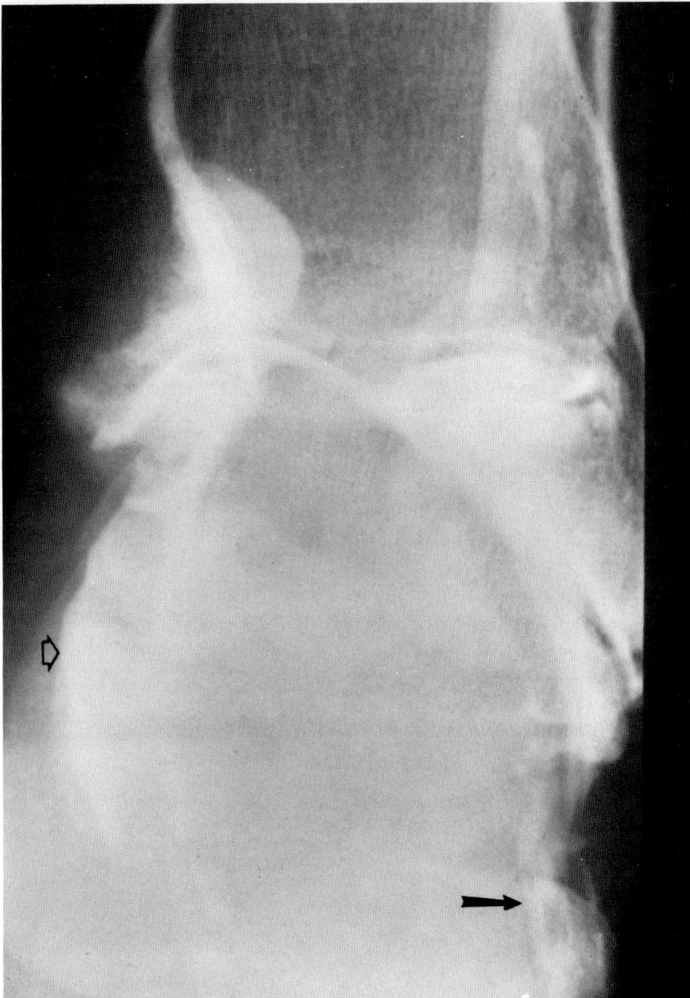

Figure 5.11. Calcaneofibular ligament tear. Anteroposterior projection reveals contrast filling the peroneal tendon sheath laterally (*arrow*) and also normal communication with flexor hallucis tendon medially (*open arrow*).

performing anteroposterior and lateral arthrotomography, which allows detailed examination of the cartilagenous surface as outlined by contrast material (Fig. 5.17). Lateral tomograms are particularly helpful if the area of osteonecrosis is on the very anterior or posterior downward curving articular surface of the talus. If the overlying cartilage is destroyed or has fractured off, a small niche of contrast material may be seen in the cavity. A smooth surface indicates intact articular cartilage. Occasionally, a loose cartilagenous or bony fragment may be detected in the opacified joint recess (Fig. 5.18). The latter makes the arthrogram useful in the evaluation of osteochondral fractures (Fig. 5.19).

Adhesive Capsulitis

Adhesive capsulitis may result from infection or trauma and is diagnosed by observing retracted, scalloped edges of the joint recesses, associated with decreased joint capacity and a higher resistance to injection of contrast media (Fig. 5.20 and 5.21). It is helpful to aspirate joint fluid, saline, or contrast and obtain appropriate bacteriological culture in such an instance.

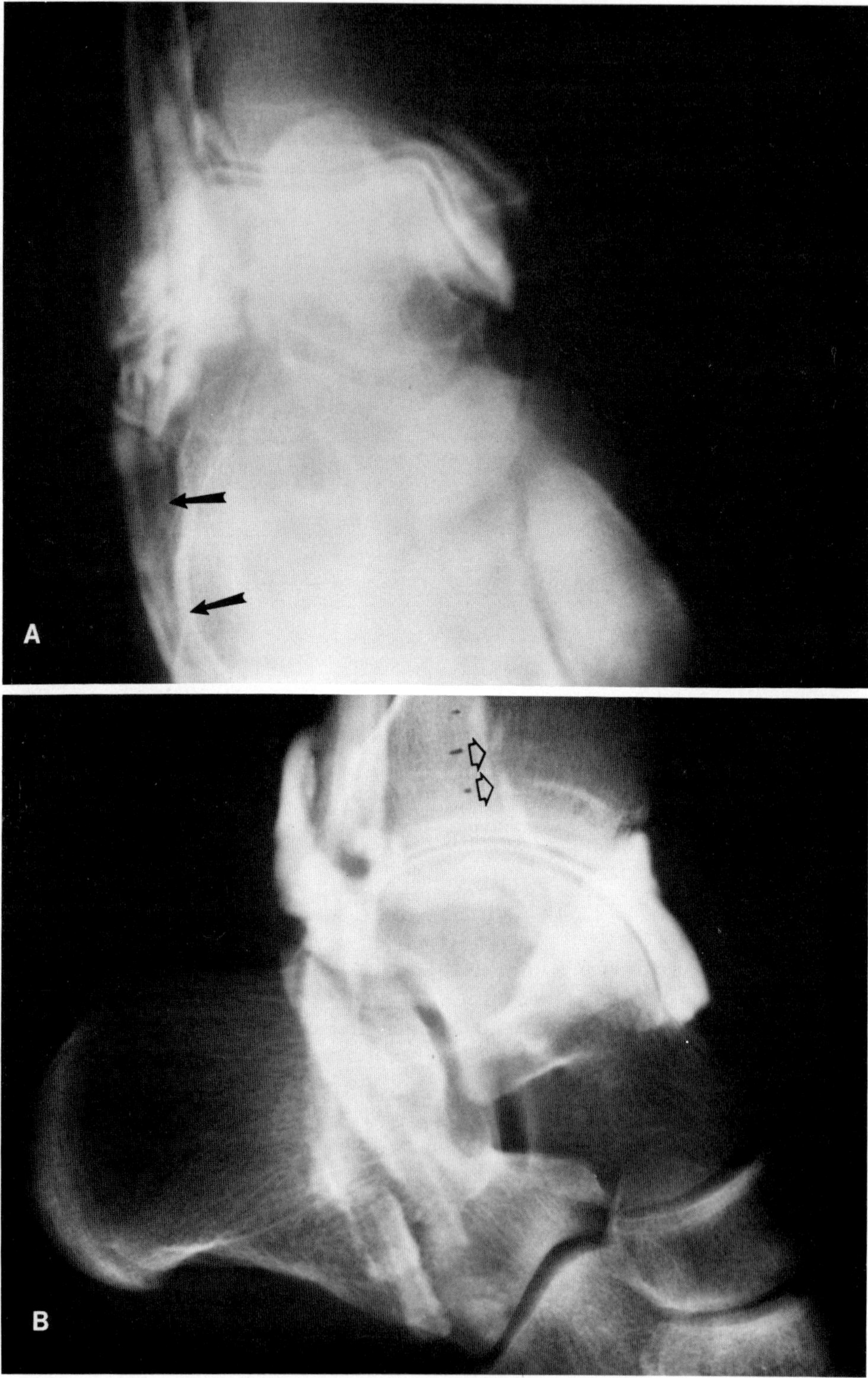

Figure 5.12. Calcaneofibular ligament tear. *A,* Anteroposterior projection shows contrast filling peroneal tendon sheaths on lateral aspect of joint (*arrows*). *B,* Lateral view confirms tendon sheath communication and also reveals small anterior inferior tibiofibular ligament tear (*open arrows*).

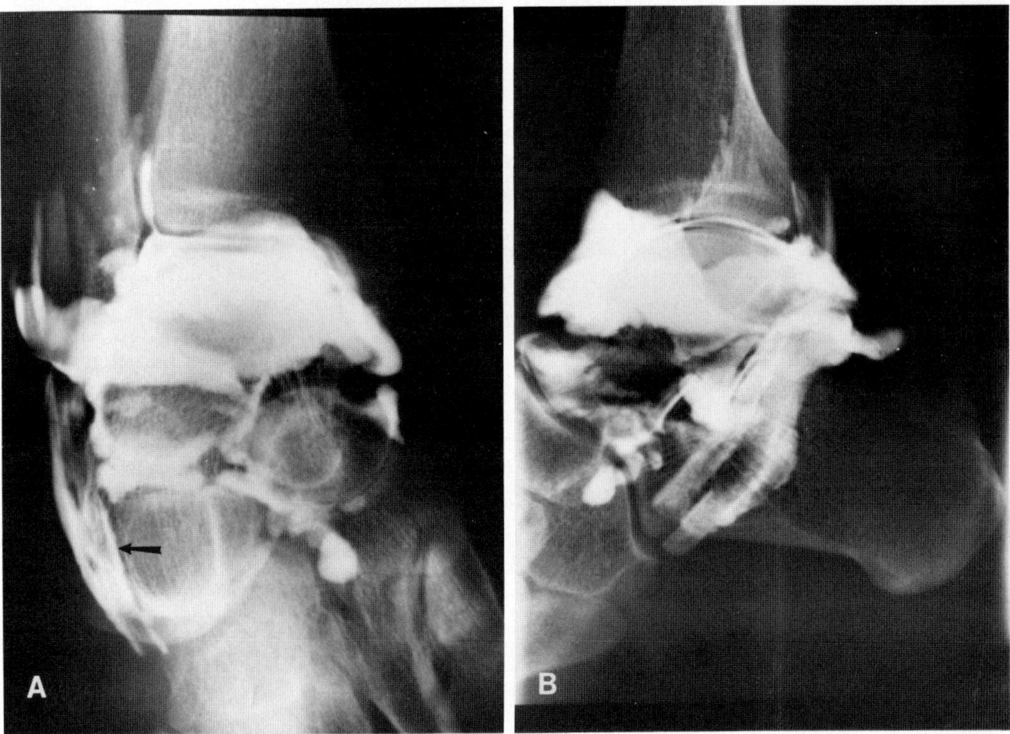

Figure 5.13. Calcaneofibular ligament tear, subacute. *A*, Anteroposterior projection. Note communication between supratalar joint and peroneal tendon sheaths laterally (*arrow*). The supratalar joint also communicates with the infratalar joint, best seen on the lateral film (*B*); this is a normal variant.

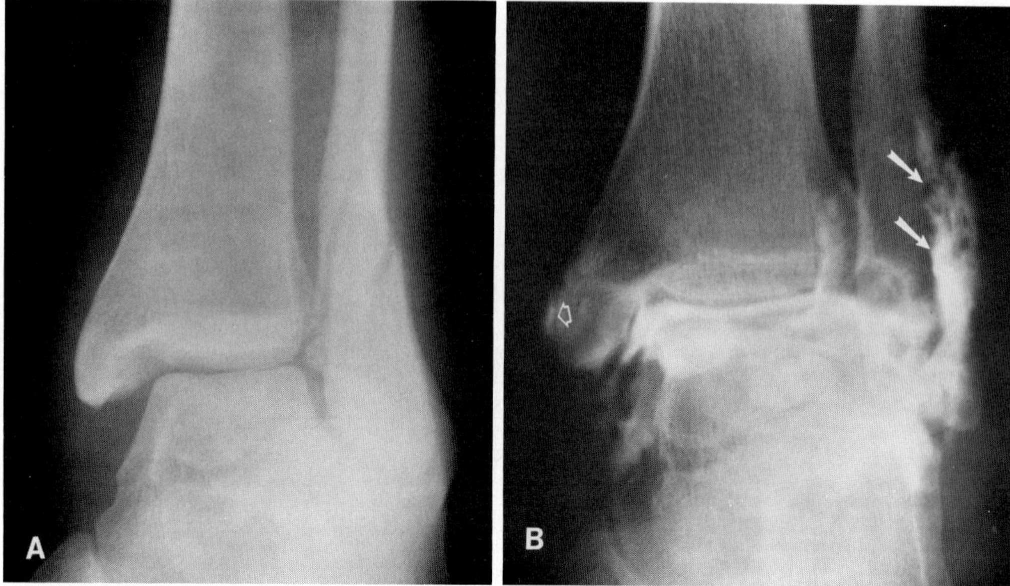

Figure 5.14. Combined anterior talofibular, anteroinferior tibiofibular, and deltoid ligament tear. *A,* Preliminary film indicates marked tibiofibular diastasis and a spiral fracture of fibula. *B,* Arthrogram reveals contrast leak inferiorly and superiorly along lateral aspect of lateral malleolus (*arrows*) (anterior talofibular ligament tear), above distal tibiofibular syndesmosis (tibiofibular ligament tear), inferiorly and superiorly along medial aspect of medial malleolus (*open arrow*) (deltoid ligament tear).

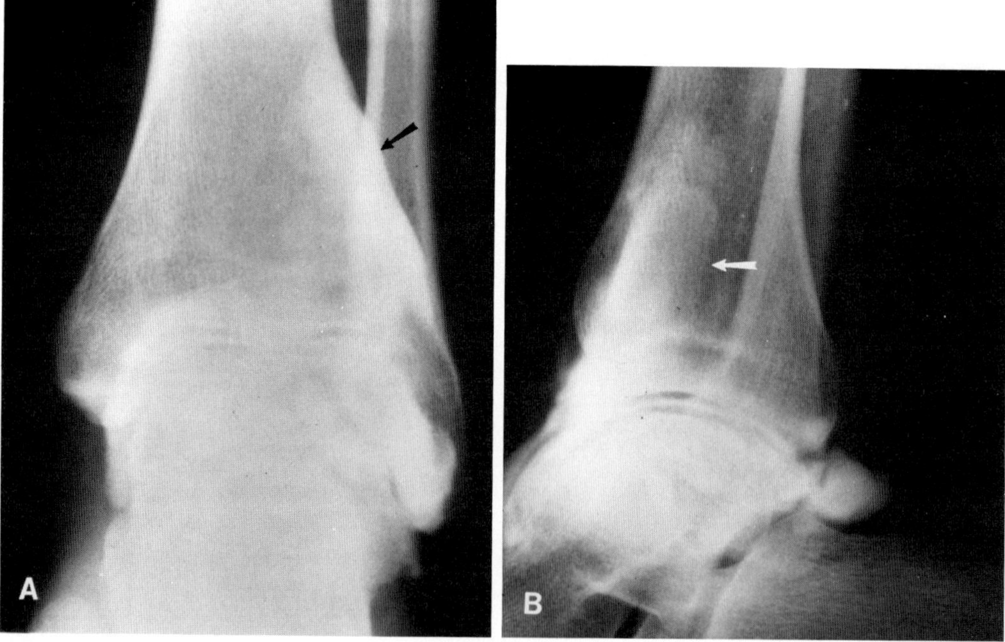

Figure 5.15. Anterior inferior tibiofibular ligament and interosseous ligament tear. *A,* Anteroposterior film reveals contrast extravasation high above tibiofibular syndesmosis into interosseous membrane (*arrow*). *B,* Lateral film verifies that contrast is between tibia and fibula (*arrow*), not within tendon sheaths.

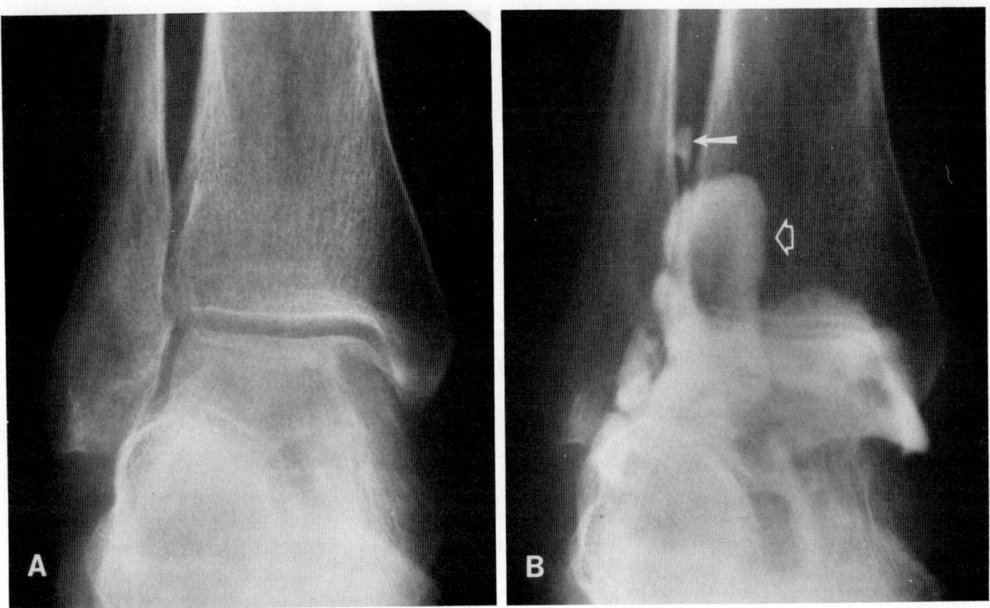

Figure 5.16. Anterior inferior tibiofibular ligament tear. *A*, Preliminary film shows moderate tibiofibular diastasis. *B*, Arthrogram confirms contrast high above tibiofibular syndesmosis (*arrow*). Contrast-filled sheath of flexor hallucis tendon overlaps posteriorly (*open arrow*).

Table 5.1
Summary of Important Ankle Collateral Ligament Tears

Injury	Contrast Leak	Comment
Calcaneofibular ligament	Into peroneal tendon sheaths along lateral aspect of ankle	Largest of lateral ligaments; commonly torn; joint-sheath communication tends to persist after tear has healed
Anterior talofibular ligament	Laterally, anteriorly, and upward around lateral malleolus	Most common lateral collateral ligament tear
Anterior-inferior tibiofibular ligament	Upward between distal tibia and fibula	Usually accompanied by tears of other ligaments
Deltoid ligament	Beneath, medially, and upward around medial malleolus	Strongest medial ligament; rarely torn, but if so requires surgical repair; normal filling of medial flexor tendon sheaths can cause erroneous diagnosis

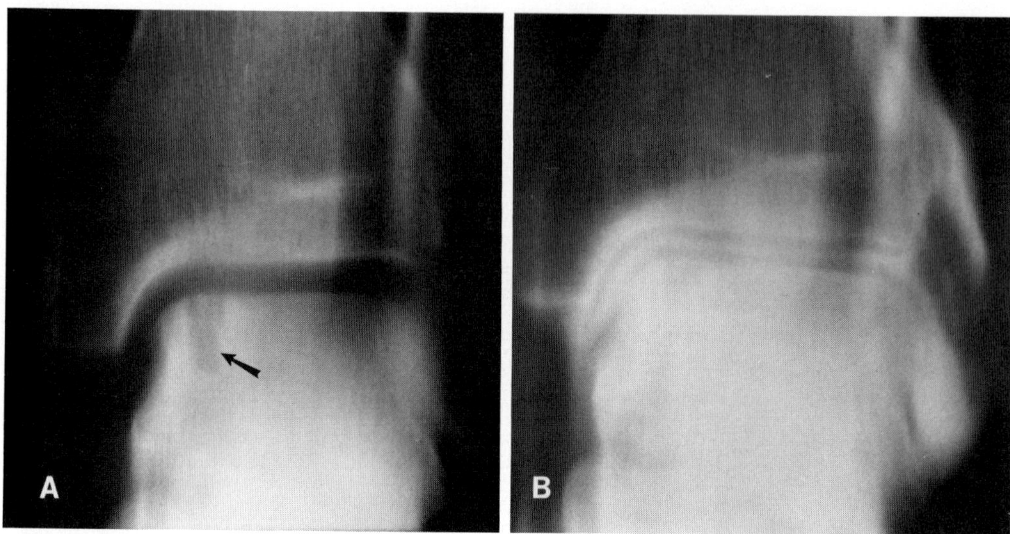

Figure 5.17. Osteochondritis dissecans, medial aspect of talus. *A*, Noncontrast tomogram delineates the subcortical rarefaction (*arrow*). *B*, Contrast anteroposterior arthrotomogram indicates the overlying articular cartilage to be intact.

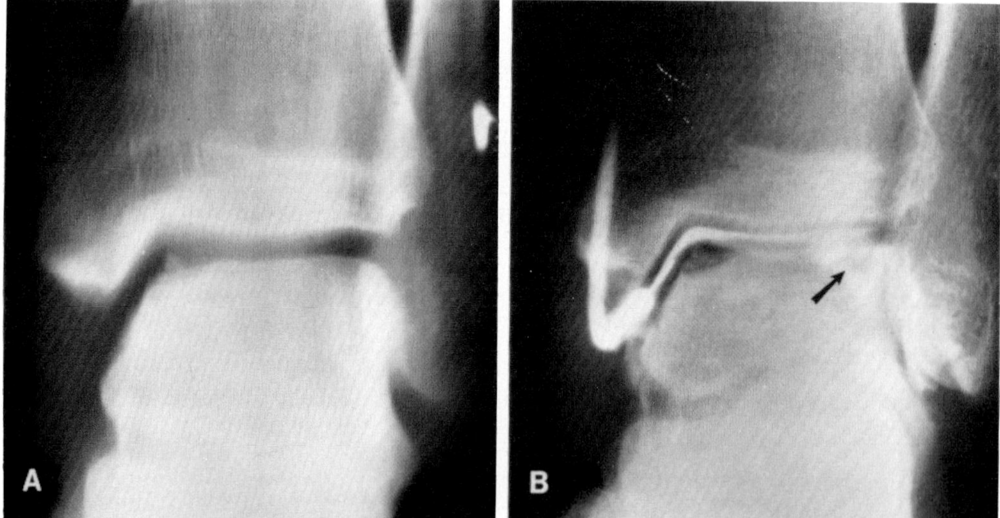

Figure 5.18. Osteochondritis dissecans with loose cartilaginous fragment. *A*, Noncontrast anteroposterior tomogram reveals irregular and fragmented medial cortical surface of talus. *B*, Arthrogram shows a cartilaginous fragment free within lateral aspect of supratalar joint (*arrow*).

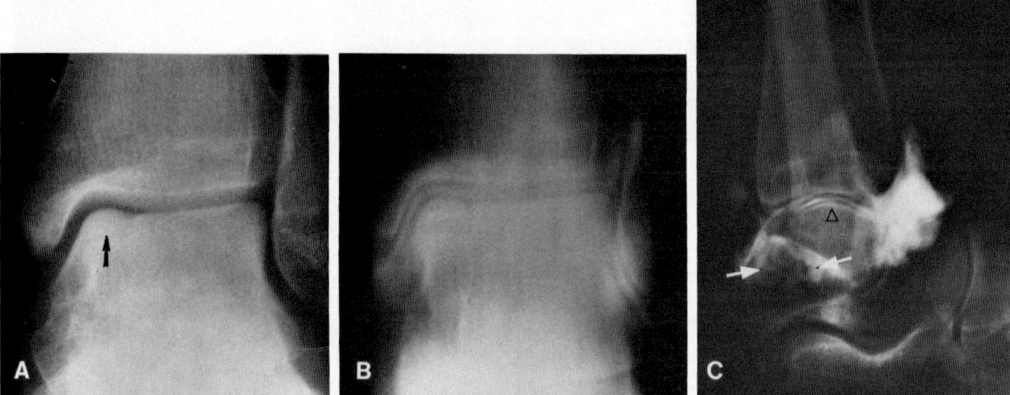

Figure 5.19. Osteochondral fracture. *A*, Preliminary anteroposterior film reveals a fissure in the cortex of the medial articulating surface of the talus (*arrow*). *B*, Contrast arthrotomogram clearly shows the undisplaced osteochondral fragment with healed, intact cartilage. *C*, Another patient with an osteochondral injury. Lateral arthrogram reveals filling defects of multiple loose bodies in posterior recess (*arrows*) and thinning of articular cartilage over talar dome (*open arrow*).

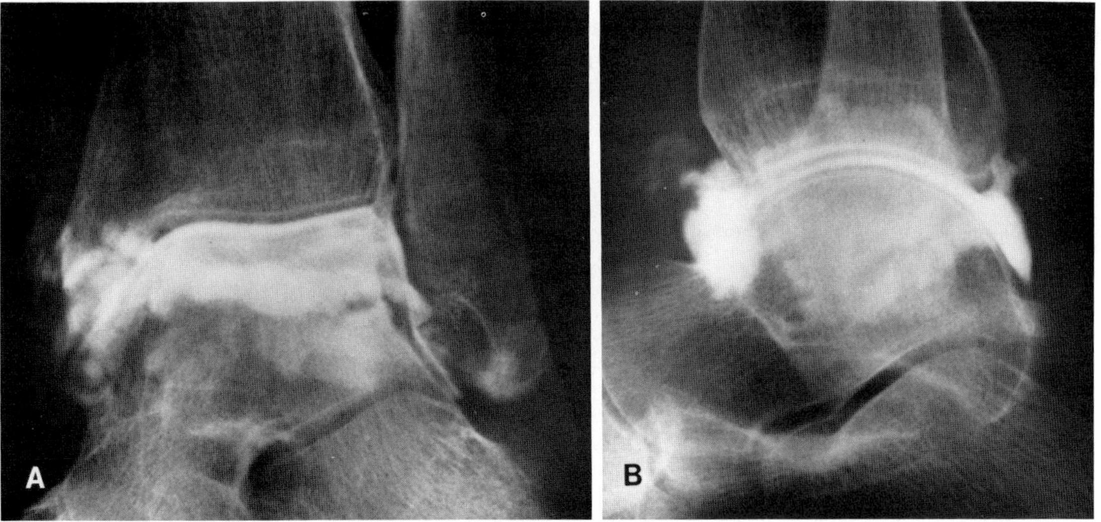

Figure 5.20. Adhesive capsulitis. *A*, Note retracted margins and diminished volume of synovial recesses. Contrast peripheral to medial malleolus is leak from anterior puncture site, *not* a deltoid ligament tear, verified by lateral film (*B*).

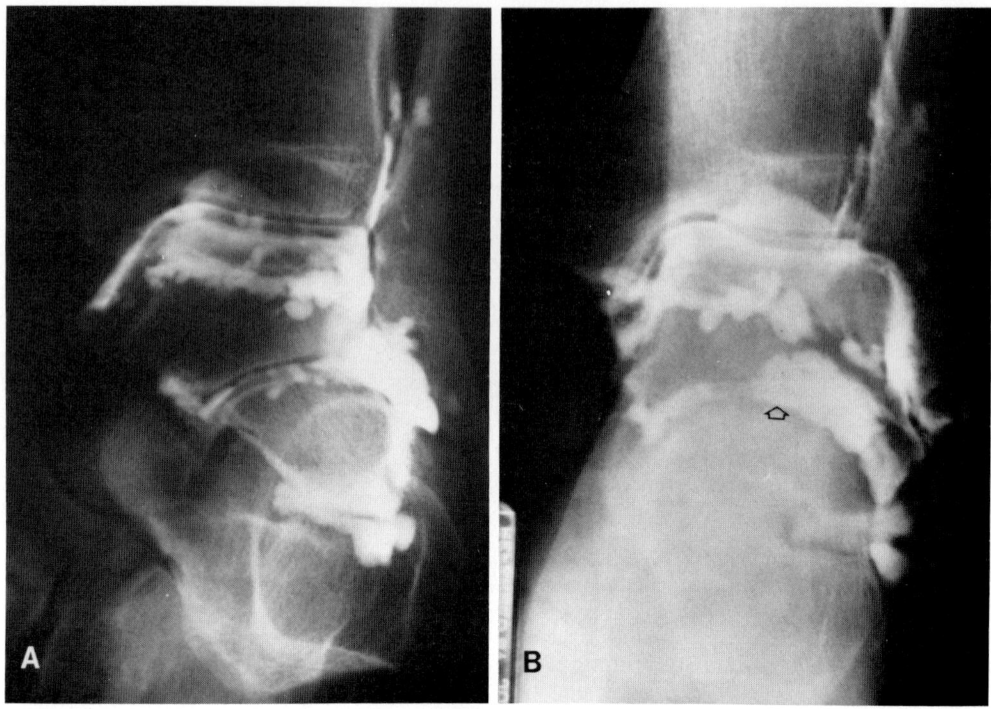

Figure 5.21. Adhesive capsulitis. *A*, Anteroposterior projection internal rotation. *B*, Anteroposterior projection, neutral. Note markedly retracted synovial recesses and decreased volume of supratalar joint. Communication with the infratalar joint, a normal finding in 10% of the population (*open arrow*).

References

Ala-Ketola, L., Puranen, J., Koivisto, E., Puuperae, M., Arthrography in the diagnosis of ligament injuries and classification of ankle injuries. Radiology, *125:* 63–68, 1977.

Brostroem, L., Liljedahl, S., Lindvall, U.N., Sprained ankles. II. Arthrographic diagnosis of recent ligament ruptures. Acta Chir Scand, *129:*485–499, 1965.

Edeiken, J., Cotler, J.M., Ankle injury, the need for stress films. JAMA, *240:*1182–1184, 1978.

Fordyce, A.J., Horn, C.V., Arthrography in recent injuries of the ligaments of the ankle. J Bone Joint Surg, *54B:*116–122, 1972.

Fussel, E.M., Godley, D.R., Ankle arthrography in acute sprains. Clin Orthop, *93:*278–290, 1973.

Goldman, A.B., Katz, M.C., Freiberger, R.H., Posttraumatic adhesive capsulitis of the ankle: Arthrographic diagnosis. AJR, *127:*585–588, 1976.

Gordon, R.B., Arthrography of the ankle joint. J Bone Joint Surg, *52A:*1623–1631, 1970.

Grant, J.C.B., *A Method of Anatomy*, Ed. 6, pp. 487–498. Williams & Wilkins, Baltimore, 1958.

Grant, J.C.B., *An Atlas of Anatomy*, Ed. 5, Figs. 332–340. Williams & Wilkins, Baltimore, 1962.

Harris, E.J., Galinski, A.W., The evaluation of ankle pathology with arthrography. J Am Podiatry Assoc, 64:202–215, 1974.

Kaye, J.J., Bohne, W.H.O., A radiographic study of the ligamentous anatomy of the ankle. Radiology, *125:*659–667, 1977.

Mehrez, M., El Geneidy, S., Arthrography of the ankle. J Bone Joint Surg, *52B:*308–315, 1970.

Olson, R.W., Arthrography of the ankle: Its use in evaluation of ankle sprains. Radiology, *92:*1439–1446, 1969.

Resnick, D., Radiology of the talocalcaneal articulations: Anatomic considerations and arthrography. Radiology, *111:*581–586, 1974.

Smith, G.R., Winquist, R.A., Allan, T., Noel, K., et al., Subtle transchondral fractures of the talar dome: A radiological perspective. Radiology, *124:*667–673, 1977.

Spiegel, P.K., Staples, S.H., Arthrography of the ankle joint: Problems in diagnosis of acute lateral ligament injuries. Radiology, *114:*587–590, 1975.

6

Arthrography of the Wrist

R. H. Gold, M.D.

Arthrography of the wrist joint is useful (1) in the persistently painful or dysfunctional wrist, especially following trauma, with or without plain radiographic abnormality, to detect tears or degeneration of the triangular fibrocartilage and ligaments and to localize osseous and cartilaginous fragments resulting from fractures or avascular necrosis; (2) to reveal the extent of synovial and articular cartilage involvement by rheumatoid arthritis when therapeutic synovectomy is being considered; (3) to localize communications between recurrent ganglia and the wrist joint, so that the communicating channels can be completely excised along with the ganglia, thus preventing further recurrence.

FUNCTIONAL ANATOMY

Traditional anatomical descriptions refer to the wrist joint as merely the articulation between the radius and the proximal row of carpal bones. For a better understanding of the functional and pathological abnormalities that take place in the region of the wrist, it is convenient to expand this definition to include the nearby radioulnar, intercarpal, carpometacarpal, and intermetacarpal articulations or compartments (Fig. 6.1). Thus, the wrist may be subdivided into nine compartments—three major compartments and six minor ones.

Compartments of the Wrist

Major compartments
    A. Radiocarpal compartment
    B. Inferior radioulnar compartment
    C. Midcarpal compartment
Minor compartments
    D. Pisiform-triquetral compartment
    E. Two carpometacarpal compartments
    F. Three intermetacarpal compartments

Radiocarpal Compartment

The proximal border of the radiocarpal compartment is formed by the distal surface of the radius and the triangular fibrocartilage. The latter, also called the

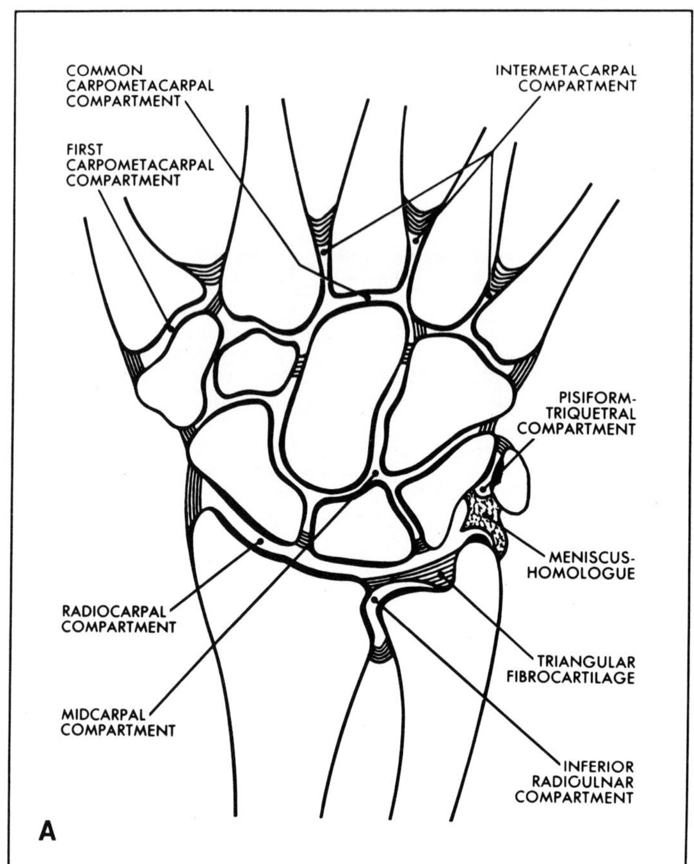
COMMON
CARPOMETACARPAL
COMPARTMENT
INTERMETACARPAL
COMPARTMENT
FIRST
CARPOMETACARPAL
COMPARTMENT
PISIFORM-
TRIQUETRAL
COMPARTMENT
MENISCUS-
HOMOLOGUE
RADIOCARPAL
COMPARTMENT
TRIANGULAR
FIBROCARTILAGE
MIDCARPAL
COMPARTMENT
INFERIOR
RADIOULNAR
COMPARTMENT
A

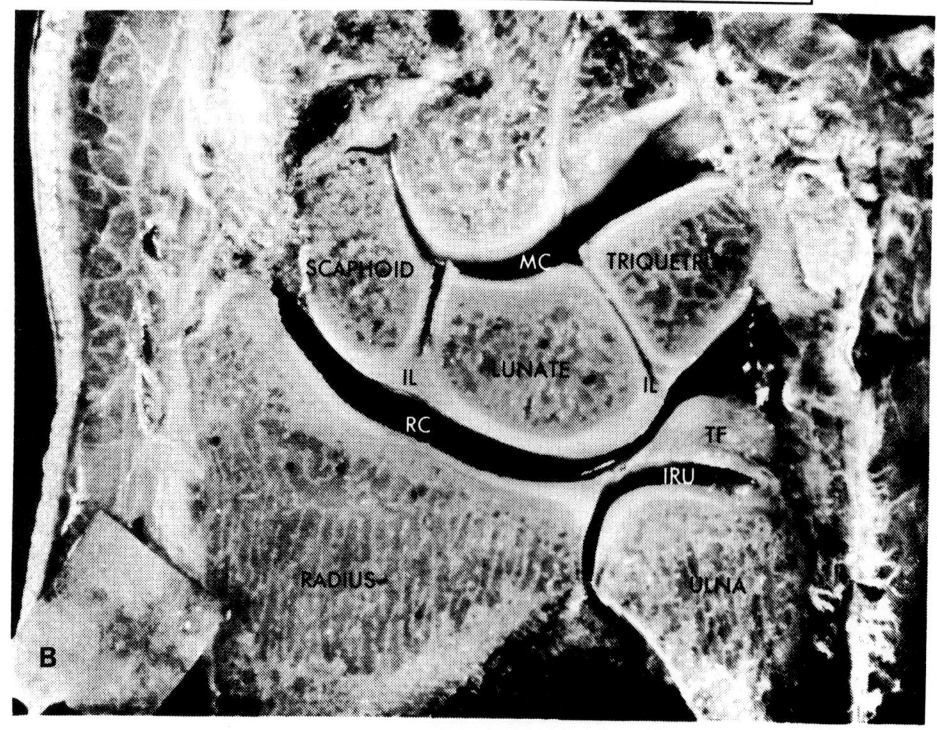
SCAPHOID
MC
TRIQUETRUM
IL
LUNATE
IL
RC
TF
IRU
RADIUS
ULNA
B

articular disk, extends laterally from the base of the styloid process of the ulna to the adjacent ulnar notch of the radius and separates the radiocarpal compartment from the inferior radioulnar compartment. The distal border of the radiocarpal compartment is formed by the proximal row of carpal bones (exclusive of the pisiform) and the interosseous ligaments that extend between them. The ligaments prevent communication between the radiocarpal and midcarpal compartments.

The ulnar or medial border of the radiocarpal compartment is formed by the meniscus-homologue which attaches proximally to the styloid process of the ulna and distally to the triquetrum. The resultant Y-shaped medial extent of the compartment consists of a proximal pouch called the prestyloid recess and a distal pouch which is bordered in part by the proximal surface of the triquetrum.

The radial or lateral border of the radiocarpal compartment is formed by the radial collateral ligament. Palmar radial recesses which vary in number and in size extend proximally from the radiocarpal compartment.

The radiocarpal joint contains certain "bare areas" of bone, so called because they lack protective articular cartilage and are instead coated with synovium, thus making them highly susceptible to early erosions by the inflammatory arthropathies. These bare areas extend over much of the proximal aspect of the triquetrum, the midportion of the scaphoid bone, and the styloid process of the radius.

Inferior Radioulnar Compartment

The proximal borders of this compartment (Fig. 6.2) are formed by the radial (or lateral) aspect of the distal end of the ulna and the ulnar notch of the radius. The distal border is formed by the triangular fibrocartilage.

Midcarpal Compartment

This compartment lies between the proximal and distal rows of carpal bones. The radial side of the compartment is known as the trapezioscaphoid articulation. A bare area on the medial portion of the distal surface of the triquetrum is covered with synovium and may be an early site of inflammatory erosion.

Figure 6.1. Compartments of the wrist. *A,* Compartmental anatomy. The radiocarpal compartment is separated from the inferior radioulnar compartment by the triangular fibrocartilage and from the pisiform-triquetral compartment by the meniscus-homologue. Between the proximal and distal rows of carpal bones lies the midcarpal compartment. The common carpometacarpal compartment is formed by the bases of the second through fifth metacarpals and the distal row of carpals, and extends distally between the metacarpals to form three small intermetacarpal compartments. The carpometacarpal compartment of the thumb or first carpometacarpal compartment lies between the trapezium and the base of the first metacarpal. (Reproduced with permission from D. Resnick: Med Radiogr Photogr Vol. 52, No. 3, 1976.) *B,* Coronal section through the wrist showing radiocarpal (*RC*), inferior radioulnar (*IRU*), and midcarpal (*MC*) compartments. The triangular fibrocartilage (*TF*) separates the radiocarpal from the inferior radioulnar compartment. The interosseous ligaments (*IL*) between the carpals in the proximal row separate the radiocarpal compartment from the midcarpal compartment. D. Resnick: Med Radiogr Photogr, Vol. 52, No. 3, 1976.)

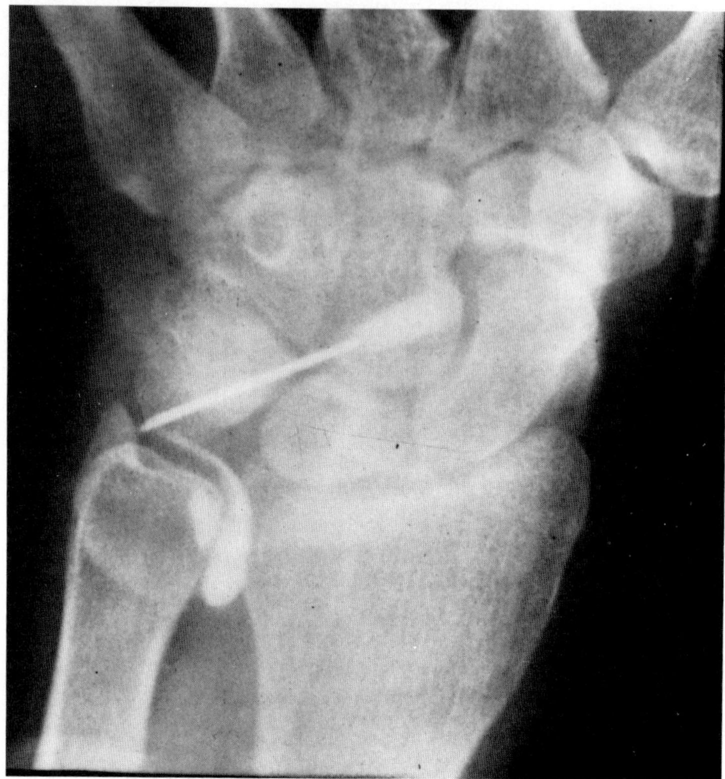

Figure 6.2. Inferior radioulnar compartment. Direct injection of contrast medium into the compartment has been performed to show its full extent. The distal border of the compartment is formed by the triangular fibrocartilage, while the proximal borders are formed by the radial (lateral) aspect of the distal end of the ulna and the ulnar notch of the radius. When injection is made into the radiocarpal joint, the inferior radioulnar compartment does not fill unless the triangular fibrocartilage has been torn or has degenerated. (Courtesy of Jerrold Mink, M.D.)

Pisiform-Triquetral Compartment

This distensible synovial-lined cavity lies between the palmar surface of the triquetrum and the dorsal surface of the pisiform and features small proximal and distal recesses. It is usually incompletely separated from the radiocarpal compartment by the attachment of the meniscus-homologue to the triquetrum.

Carpometacarpal and Intermetacarpal Compartments

The carpometacarpal compartments are two in number: the carpometacarpal compartment of the thumb—a separate cavity between the trapezium and the base of the first metacarpal, and the common carpometacarpal compartment—located between the bases of the second through fifth metacarpals and the distal row of carpals. The synovial cavity of the common carpometacarpal compartment extends proximally between the carpals of the distal row for variable distances and distally between the bases of the metacarpals to form three small intermetacarpal compartments.

Normal Intercompartmental Communication

The only compartment normally communicating with the radiocarpal compartment is the pisiform-triquetral compartment. Pathological communication with the midcarpal compartment is frequently accompanied by communication between the midcarpal and common carpometacarpal compartment. Such communication may occur by way of a normal opening between the trapezium and trapezoid. The subject of intercompartmental communications will be subsequently discussed in the section, "The Abnormal Arthrogram."

METHOD OF ARTHROGRAPHY

With the patient seated in a chair, the hand, wrist, and forearm are placed on the fluoroscopy table. A triangular radiolucent sponge-rubber support beneath the wrist is used to produce slight flexion. Following disinfection of the skin of the dorsum of the wrist and sterile preparation and draping, local anesthesia is accomplished through a 25-gauge needle at the site of arthrographic injection. This site is the dorsal aspect of the wrist at the point where the radius, scaphoid, and lunate articulate with each other (Fig. 6.3). Although it is easiest to localize

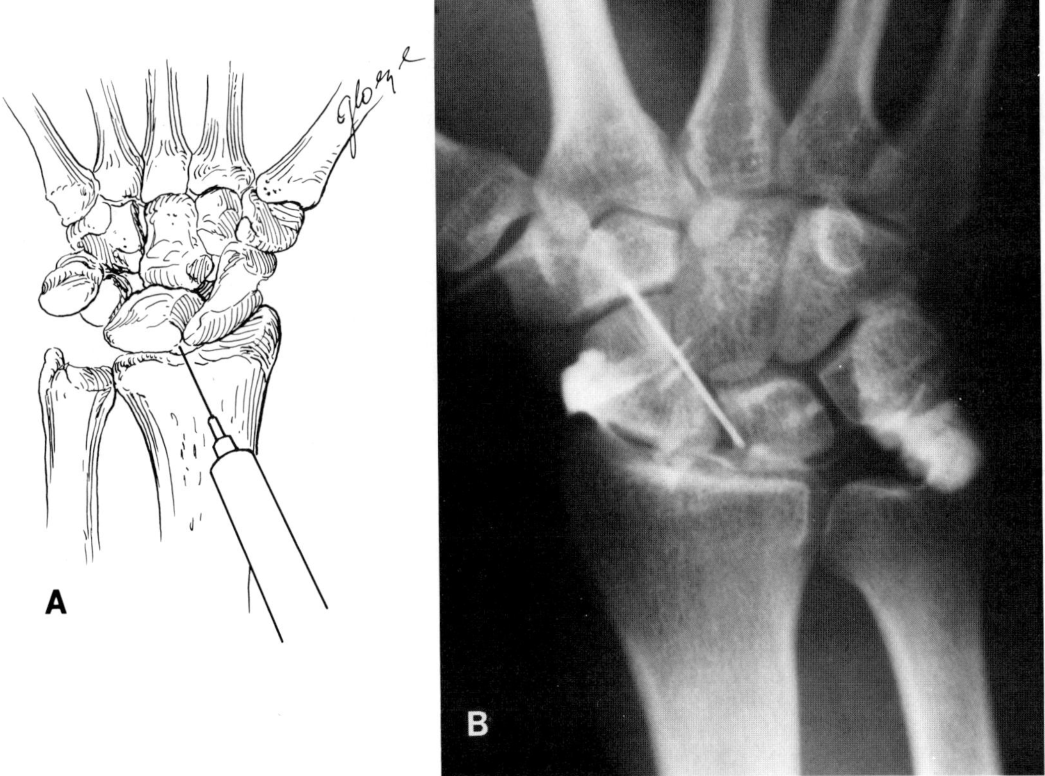

Figure 6.3. Dorsal approach for arthrography. *A*, The site of injection of the contrast medium is that point where the radius, scaphoid, and lunate articulate with each other. The wrist should be in slight flexion during introduction of the needle. *B*, Posteroanterior radiograph showing placement of needle tip. Injection of the contrast medium is incomplete.

the site of injection with fluoroscopy, localization may alternatively be achieved by using the radial aspect of the extensor indicis proprius tendon as a palpable guide; the tendon becomes prominent when the index finger is hyperextended.

A 22-gauge, 1½-in needle is introduced dorsally, angled under the radial lip and advanced along the volarly tilted radial articular surface, and 1 ml of the anesthetic is injected. Intraarticular injection is confirmed if the flow through the needle meets with no resistance or if the injected fluid can be aspirated. Thereupon, as much anesthetic and synovial fluid should be aspirated as possible. Without withdrawing the needle, the syringe of anesthetic is exchanged for one containing water-soluble iodinated contrast medium. Between 1.5 and 2.5 ml of the contrast medium are injected, ideally under fluoroscopic control. During injection the patient experiences a sensation of local pressure, but no pain.

The needle is removed and, after a minute of passive exercise of the wrist, roentgenograms are obtained in anteroposterior, lateral, and both oblique projections. Aspiration of the contrast medium is unnecessary following the examination.

NORMAL ARTHROGRAM

For an understanding of the normal arthrogram, the previous description of functional anatomy should be reviewed. Upon injection of the contrast medium into the radiocarpal compartment, the contrast, as previously mentioned, usually fills the pisiform-triquetral compartment (Fig. 6.5). Indeed, communication between the two compartments is considered to be a normal variant. However, communication between the radiocarpal and compartments other than the pisiform-triquetral is abnormal and will be considered subsequently.

The triangular fibrocartilage, which separates the radiocarpal from the inferior radioulnar compartment, forms a gentle, curvilinear filling defect at the distal end of the ulna (Figs. 6.4 and 6.5).

Numerous recesses varying in number, size, and shape may complicate the interpretation of the arthrogram. An extension of the meniscus-homologue creates a filling defect in the ulnar (or medial) border of the radiocarpal compartment, dividing it into a proximal pouch called the prestyloid recess (Figs. 6.4 and 6.5), and a distal pouch at the volar aspect of the triquetrum (Fig. 6.4). One or more palmar radial recesses may extend from the volar aspect of the radiocarpal compartment (Figs. 6.4 and 6.5), and dorsal radial recesses may extend from the dorsal aspect of the compartment.

ABNORMAL ARTHROGRAM

Intercompartmental Communications

With the exceptions of the communicating radiocarpal and pisiform-triquetral compartments and the communicating midcarpal and common carpometacarpal compartments, the compartments of the wrist are normally separated from each other. Pathological communications in patients with unexplained wrist pain

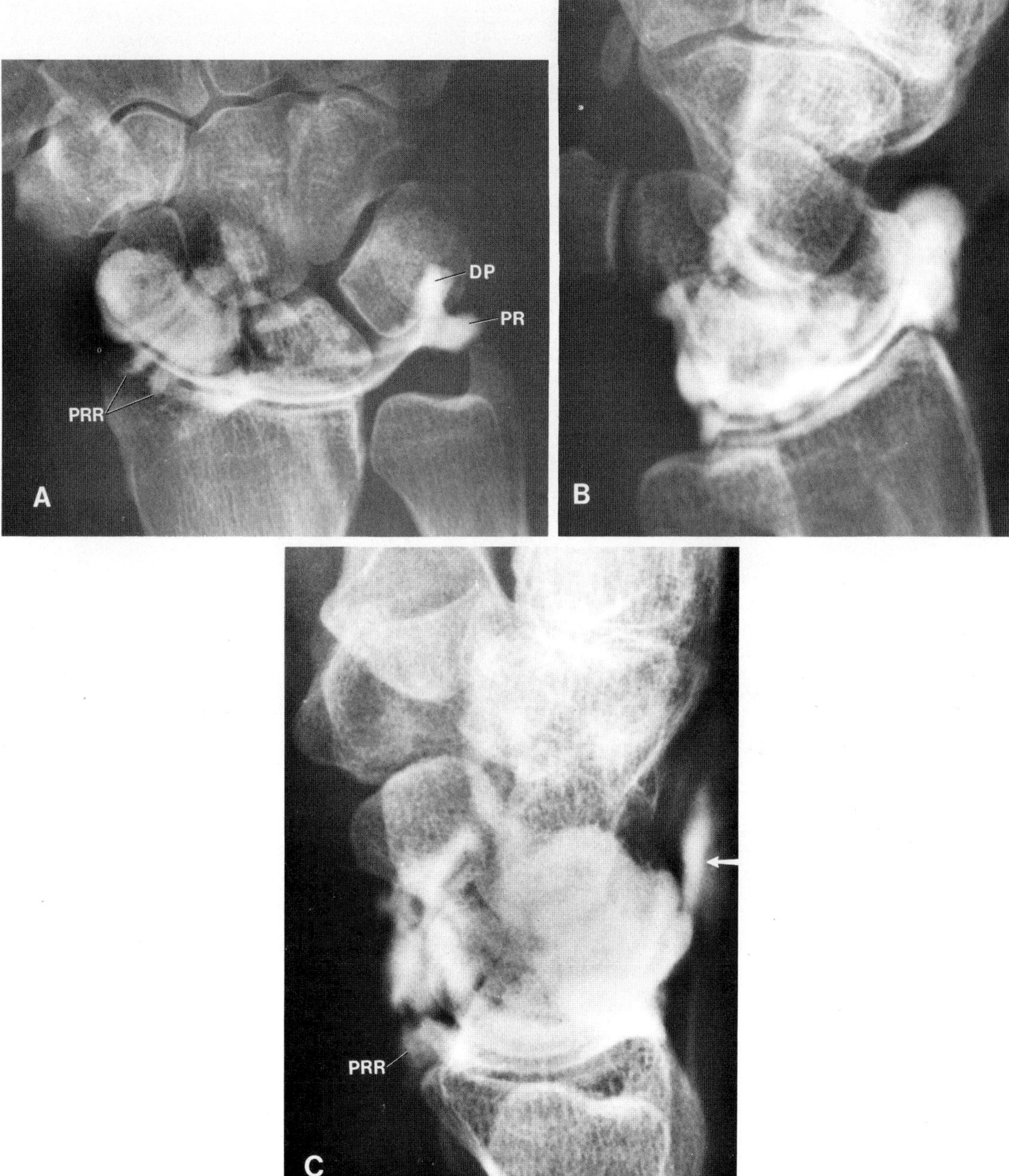

Figure 6.4. Normal wrist (radiocarpal) arthrogram. *A*, Posteroanterior projection. *B*, Oblique projection. *C*, Lateral projection. The pisiform-triquetral compartment remains unopacified, signifying absence of communication with the radiocarpal compartment. The Y-shaped radial extent of the radiocarpal compartment consists of a proximal pouch—the prestyloid recess (*PR*)—and a distal pouch (*DP*) bordered in part by the triquetrum. The palmar radial recesses (*PRR*) are not prominent. Some of the contrast medium has extravasated dorsally at the site of injection (*arrow*) in *C*.

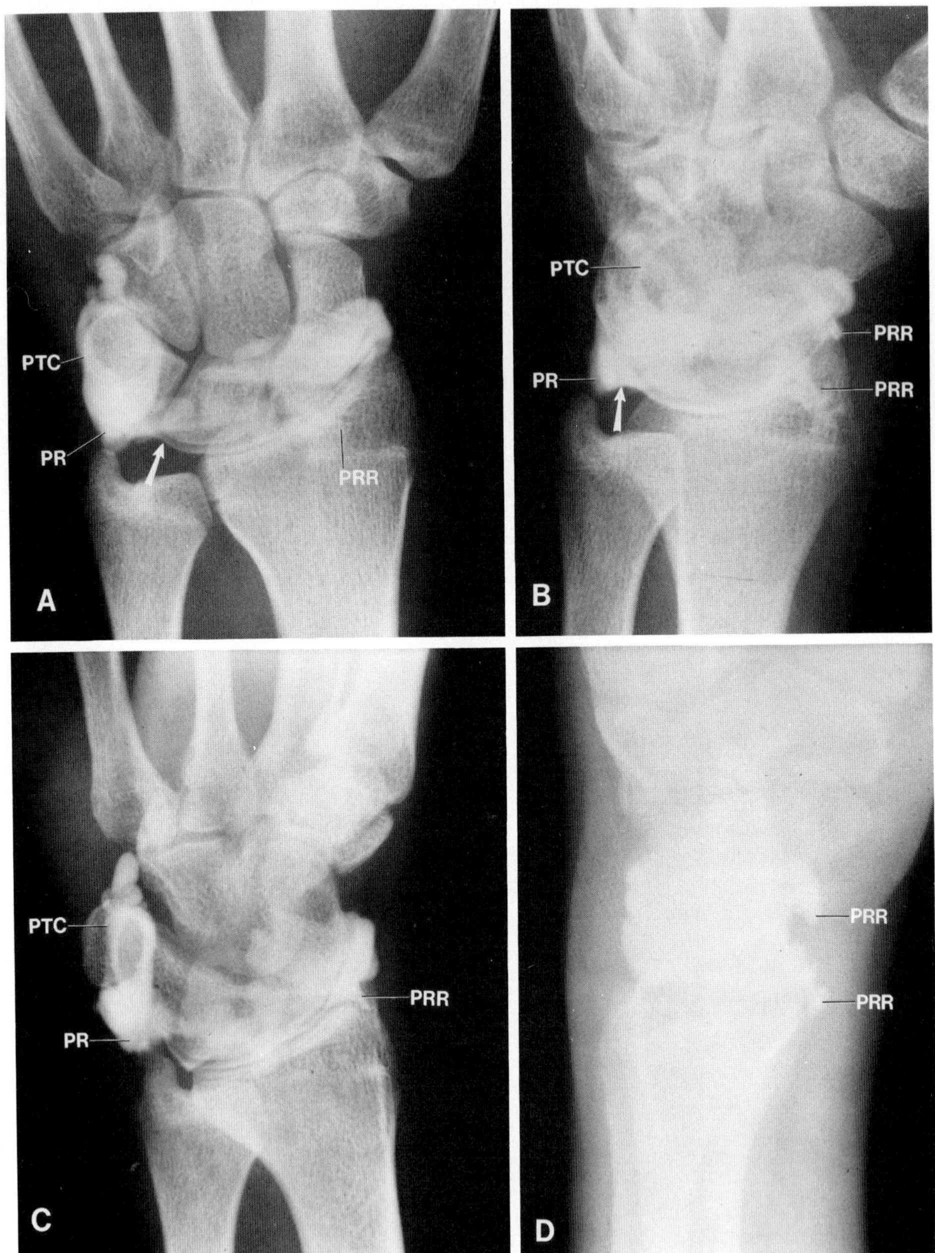

Figure 6.5. Normal wrist arthrogram with incidental opacification of pisiform-triquetral compartment. *A*, Posteroanterior projection. *B*, Posteroanterior oblique projection. *C*, Anteroposterior oblique projection. *D*, Lateral projection. The pisiform-triquetral compartment (*PTC*) has filled by way of communication from the radiocarpal compartment, a normal variation. The prestyloid recess (*PR*) and palmar radial recesses (*PRR*) are filled with contrast medium. The gentle, curvilinear filling defect in the contrast medium distal to the distal end of the ulna (*arrow*) is formed by the distal margin of the triangular fibrocartilage. (Courtesy Jerrold Mink, M.D.)

may at times be demonstrable by arthrography, although not nearly so frequently as by anatomical dissection of ostensibly normal cadavers. Equally important is the inability of arthrography to demonstrate all such communications, especially some small rents in the triangular fibrocartilage. Since the incidence of these communications increases with advancing age, it is reasonable to suppose that they are degenerative or traumatic in origin.

Communication between the radiocarpal and inferior radioulnar compartments results from a defect in the triangular fibrocartilage. The triangular fibrocartilage separating these two compartments undergoes gradually progressive degeneration and episodes of trauma, accounting for the increasing incidence of communications with advancing age. Lewis et al. found an incidence of communication as high as 60% in elderly cadavers, as determined by anatomical dissection. The existence of congenital fenestration of the triangular fibrocartilage in the absence of degeneration has been proposed, but is not generally accepted.

Communication between the radiocarpal and midcarpal compartments may result from degeneration or trauma of the interosseous ligaments between the bases of the carpals comprising the proximal row. In anatomical dissections of elderly cadavers, Lewis et al. found a defective lunate-scaphoid ligament in 40% and a defective lunate-triquetral ligament in 36%.

Communication between the radiocarpal and pisiform-triquetral compartments is a feature in arthrograms of most normal subjects and probably represents a normal variant rather than a degenerative change. The reasons for this opinion regarding the origin of this communication are 3-fold: a similar communication exists in primates other than man, the communication in man is generally broad in caliber, and the communication is present more often than not in arthrograms at all ages.

Communication between the midcarpal, common carpometacarpal, and intermetacarpal compartments is frequently demonstrable by midcarpal arthrography. The usual site of communication is a normal aperture between the trapezium and trapezoid. However, communication between the midcarpal and carpometacarpal compartment of the thumb is unusual because of the tough fibrous capsule that envelops the latter.

Posttraumatic and Degenerative Arthropathies

The persistently painful or dysfunctional wrist with or without plain radiographic abnormality, especially following trauma, is a key indication for radiocarpal arthrography. The most commonly observed abnormality in the arthrogram is a tear of the triangular fibrocartilage with resultant opacification of the inferior radioulnar compartment (Figs. 6.6 and 6.7). Rotary instability of the scaphoid results from a tear in the ligament between the scaphoid and lunate and is reflected arthrographically in opacification of the midcarpal compartment. A tear of the lunate-triquetral ligament may also result in opacification of the midcarpal compartment (Fig. 6.8) and, with or without associated injury to other intercarpal ligaments, may lead to opacification of the common carpometacarpal and intermetacarpal compartments as well (Fig. 6.9). As previously

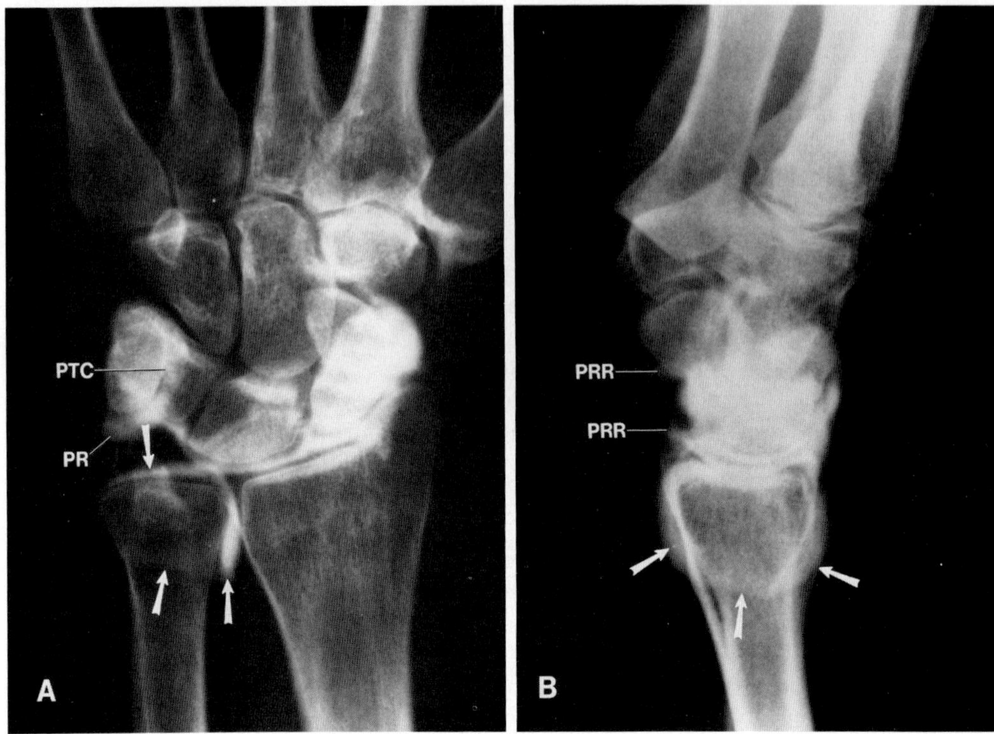

Figure 6.6. Posttraumatic arthropathy in a woman, age 26, who suffered Colle's fractures of the radius and ulnar styloid 7 months ago. *A,* Posteroanterior projection. A tear of the triangular fibrocartilage has led to abnormal opacification of the inferior radioulnar compartment (*arrows*). The prestyloid recess (*PR*) is attenuated. The pisiform-triquetral compartment (*PTC*) has filled with contrast medium, a normal variant. *B,* Lateral projection. The small palmar radial recesses (*PRR*) are normal. The inferior radioulnar joint is abnormally opacified (*arrows*). The distal articular surface of the radius has lost its normal volar slant as a result of dorsal impaction at the fracture site.

mentioned, the carpometacarpal compartment of the thumb is enveloped by a strong fibrous capsule and is thus highly resistant to communication with the midcarpal compartment, seldom opacifying even in the presence of extensive tears or degeneration of adjacent ligaments.

Posttraumatic and degenerative arthropathies, in addition to causing abnormal intercompartmental communication, may also be reflected in synovial irregularity localized to the area of trauma and resulting from synovial hypertrophy and scarring (Figs. 6.10 and 6.11). The irregularity in outline of the synovium is usually relatively mild and less striking than the corrugated pattern characteristic of rheumatoid arthritis. The abnormalities are usually localized to areas in which the synovial membrane is reflected over abnormal bone or in which osteocartilaginous fragments have become embedded in the synovium leading to secondary inflammation. Fracture and fragmentation of the scaphoid is often accompanied by radiocarpal-midcarpal communication (Fig. 6.11). Fracture of the ulnar styloid may result in communication with the inferior radioulnar compartment and/or obliteration or attenuation of the prestyloid recess

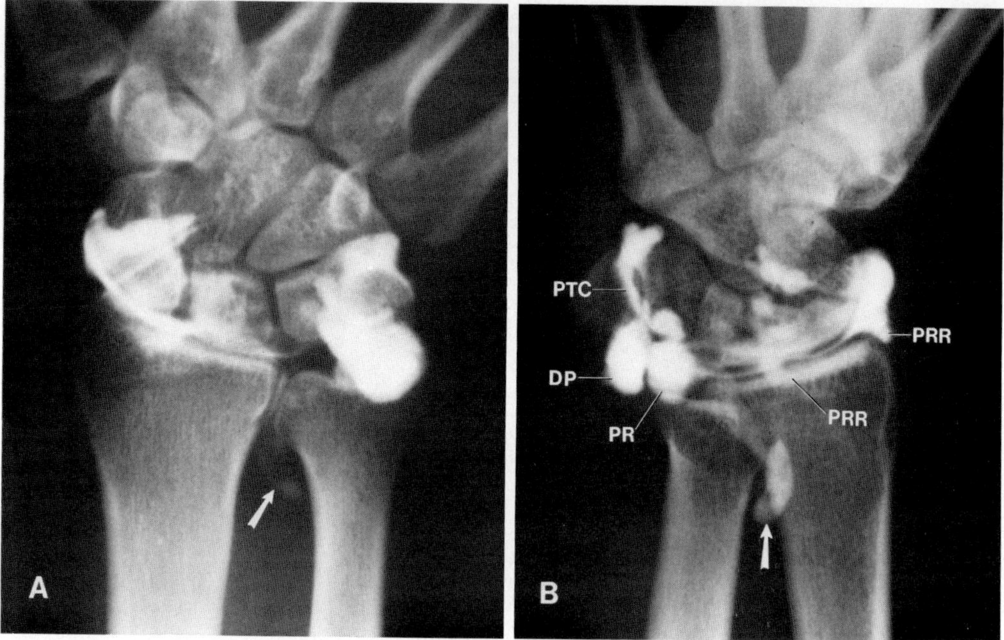

Figure 6.7. Extensive traumatic tear of the triangular fibrocartilage in a male, age 19, resulting in opacification of the inferior radioulnar compartment. *A,* Posteroanterior projection. Some air has been inadvertently injected with the positive contrast medium, accounting for the double contrast outline of the inferior radioulnar compartment (*arrow*). *B,* Oblique projection. The inferior radioulnar compartment has now filled with additional positive contrast medium (*arrow*). Palmar radial recesses (*PRR*), the prestyloid recess (*PR*), the distal pouch (*DP*) of the ulnar margin of the radiocarpal compartment, and the pisiform-triquetral compartment (*PTC*) are structures that normally opacify.

leading to its failure to opacify (Figs. 6.6 and 6.12). Communication with the extensor tendon sheaths may occur subsequent to trauma (Figs. 6.12 and 6.13), but traumatic communication with the flexor tendon sheaths is most unusual.

Pneumatic Driller's Disease

This disorder, an unusually severe degenerative arthropathy, has been described in individuals with longstanding, intense occupational trauma to the wrists. Raynaud's phenomenon may accompany bilateral arthritic changes in the wrists, elbows, or shoulders. Carpal cysts are characteristic and probably result from traumatic fissuring of articular cartilage and passage of synovial fluid, under the high hydrostatic pressure that occurs during drilling, through the fissures and into the subchondral bone, which gradually wears away. The arthrographic features (Fig. 6.14) include synovial irregularity, intercompartmental communication, and lymphatic filling simulating rheumatoid arthritis.

Filling of the volar lymphatic channels, a frequently occurring feature of rheumatoid and other chronic inflammatory arthritides and occasionally seen following trauma or in severe degenerative arthropathies such as pneumatic driller's disease and calcium pyrophosphate dihydrate deposition disease (pseu-

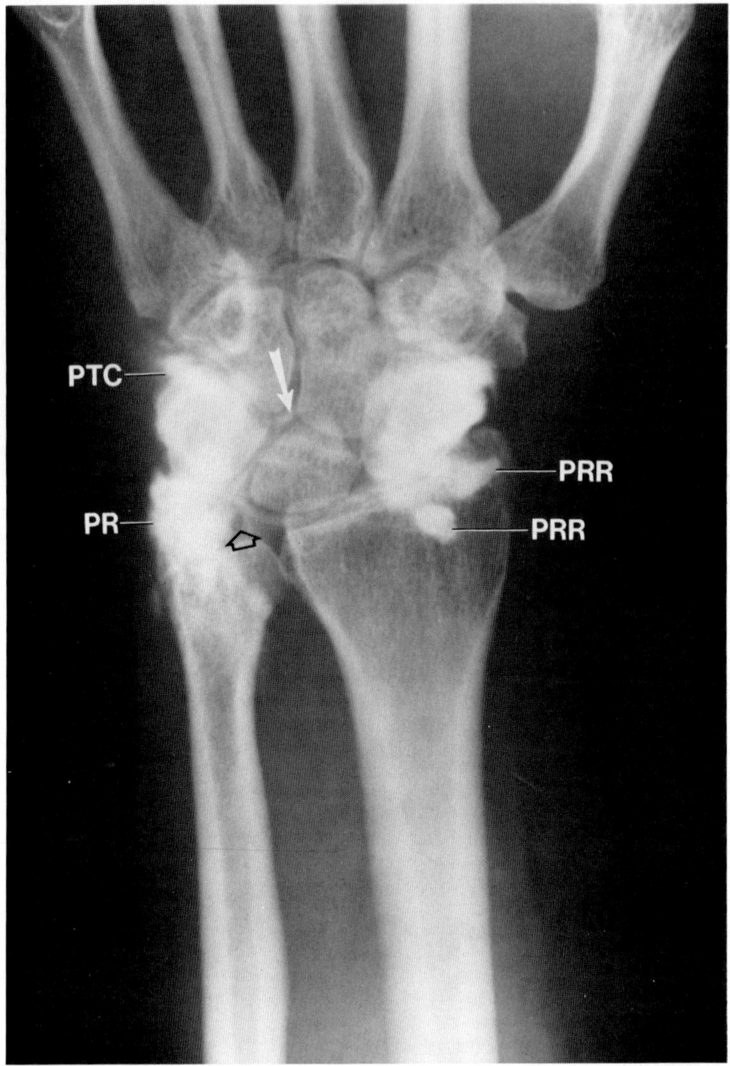

Figure 6.8. Traumatic tear of the lunate-triquetral ligament in a man, age 48, with resultant opacification of the midcarpal compartment (*arrow*). Disruption of the ulnar collateral ligament is signified by the irregular margin of the contrast medium in the regions of the pisiform-triquetral compartment (*PTC*) and the prestyloid recess (*PR*). A small filling defect (*open arrow*) represents a loose fragment of articular cartilage in the prestyloid recess. The palmar radial recesses (*PRR*) are normal.

dogout), has not yet been reported in normal subjects. Interestingly, we have seen one instance of lymphatic filling without other accompanying plain radiographic or arthrographic abnormalities in a 52-year-old man with unexplained pain in the left wrist, 6 weeks following hyperextension injury and no other joint symptoms (Fig. 6.15).

Neuropathic Joint Disease

This disorder (Fig. 6.16) leads to fragmentation of cartilage and bone, with the fragments becoming embedded within the synovium and producing secondary

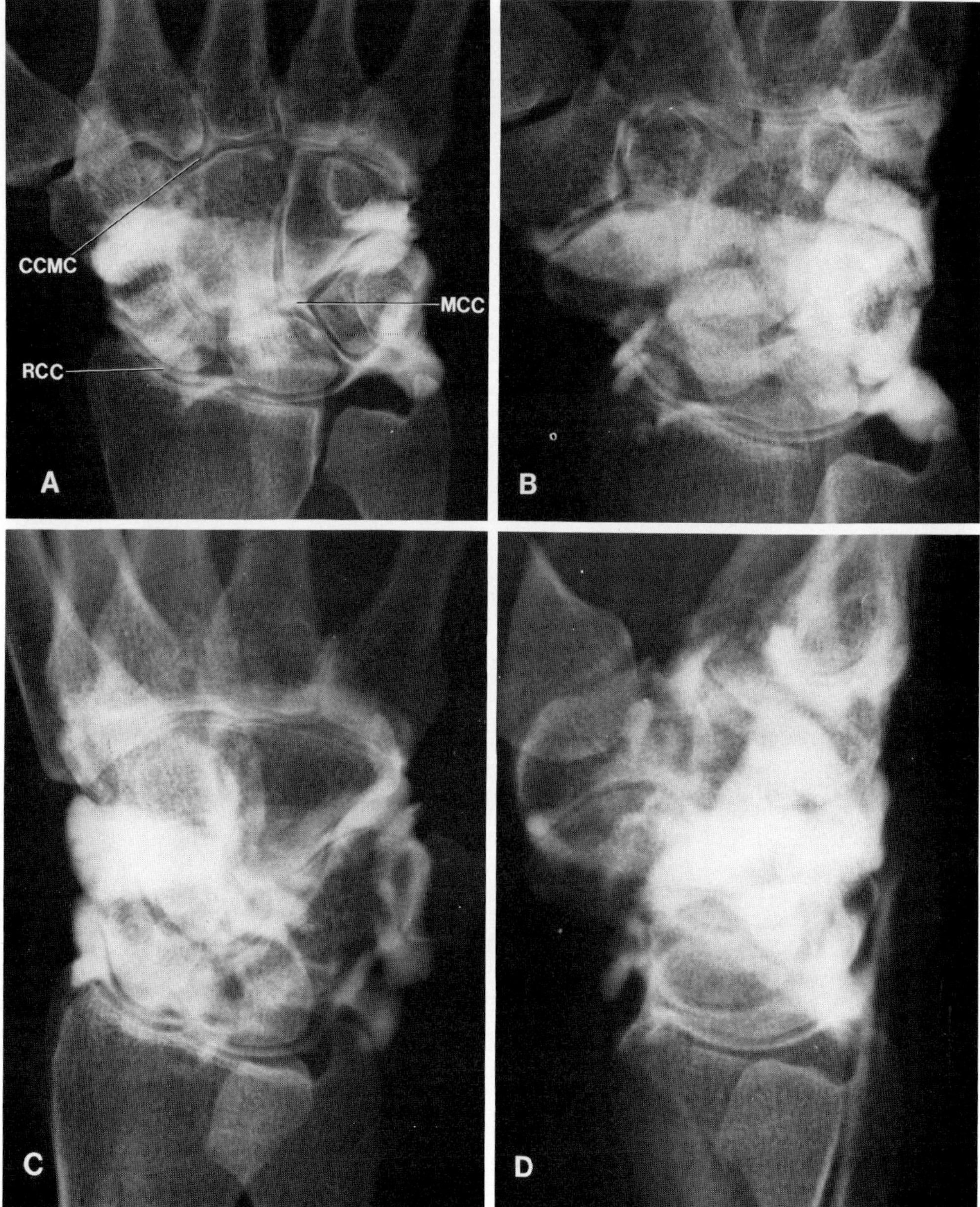

Figure 6.9. Communication between the radiocarpal compartment (*RCC*) and the midcarpal compartment (*MCC*) and common carpometacarpal (*CCMC*) has resulted from ligamentous degeneration in a 53-year-old woman with no history of trauma. *A*, Posteroanterior projection. *B* and *C*, Oblique projections. *D*, Lateral projection. Opacification of the midcarpal compartment has occurred by way of a disrupted lunate-triquetral ligament. Similarly, although communication between the midcarpal and common carpometacarpal compartments may normally occur through an opening between the trapezium and trapezoid, opacification of the common carpometacarpal compartment (*CCMC*) in this case has resulted from communications with the midcarpal compartment by way of disrupted ligaments between the trapezoid and capitate and between the capitate and hamate bones. The inferior radioulnar and first carpometacarpal compartments remain unopacified. Communication between the midcarpal and the first carpometacarpal compartment is unusual even in the presence of severe traumatic or degenerative change in the adjacent ligaments, because the first carpometacarpal compartment is enveloped by an impervious thick connective tissue capsule.

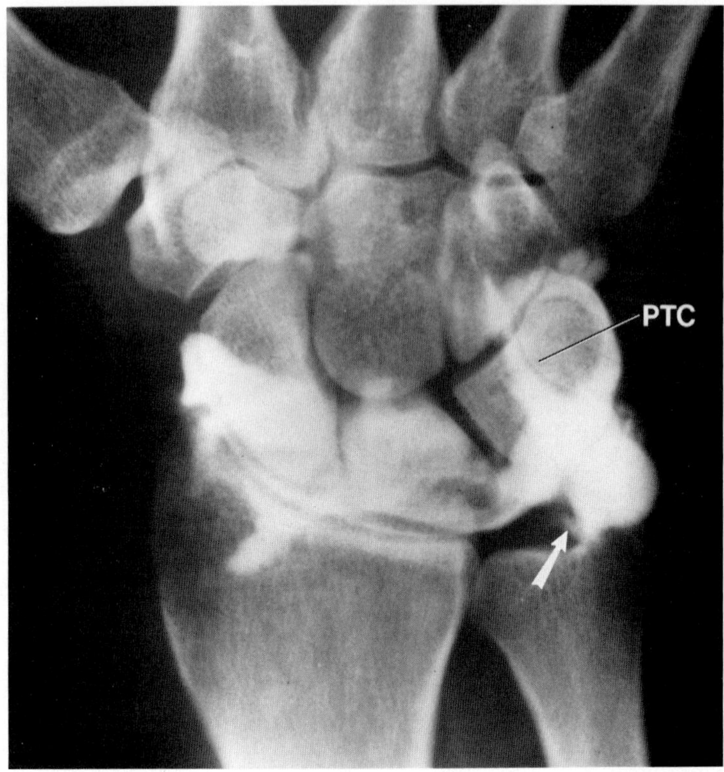

Figure 6.10. Opacification of a small traumatic tear (*arrow*) of the prestyloid recess in a man age 43. Filling of the pisiform-triquetral compartment (*PTC*) is a normal variation, but the striking irregularity of its radial border implies synovial hypertrophy and scarring resulting from previous trauma.

irritation. The resultant synovial hypertrophy is reflected in irregularity of the synovial margins. Osteochondral fragments are depicted arthrographically by filling defects in the contrast medium. Since extensive disruption of joint capsules is a key manifestation of neuropathic joint disease, intercompartmental communication and tendon sheath opacification may be extensive.

Rheumatoid Arthritis

Synovectomy is a controversial therapeutic procedure for rheumatoid arthritis. Its proponents claim that synovectomy of the wrist has a protective effect, diminishing later joint destruction and reducing the chance of rupture of the extensor tendons. But in order for it to be effective, synovectomy must be performed when destruction of articular cartilage is still minimal. The arthrogram is able to depict early abnormalities of the synovium and articular cartilage before osseous erosions are visible in plain radiographs.

The most specific arthrographic abnormalities in patients with rheumatoid arthritis are, according to Resnick (1974), in order of decreasing frequency, synovial irregularity (92%), prestyloid recess irregularity (75%), and lymphatic

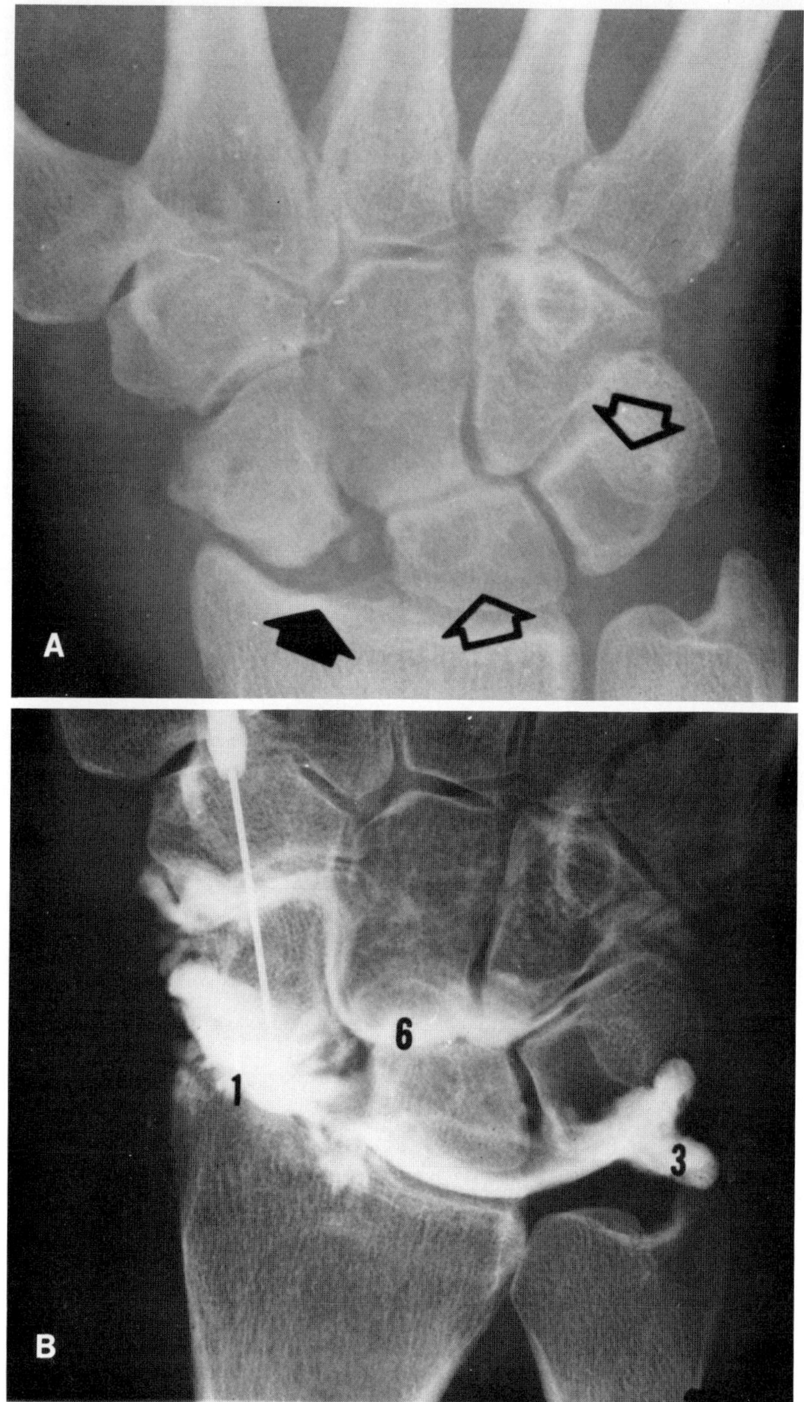

Figure 6.11. Posttraumatic arthropathy. *A,* Sclerosis and fragmentation of the scaphoid (*closed arrow*) are seen, along with partial resorption and cystic changes of multiple carpal bones (*open arrows*). *B,* Arthrography reveals synovial irregularity along the radial aspect of the wrist (*1*), a prominent, minimally irregular prestyloid recess (*3*), and a communication with the midcarpal compartment (*6*). (Reproduced with permission from D. Resnick: Radiology, *113:*331–340, 1974.)

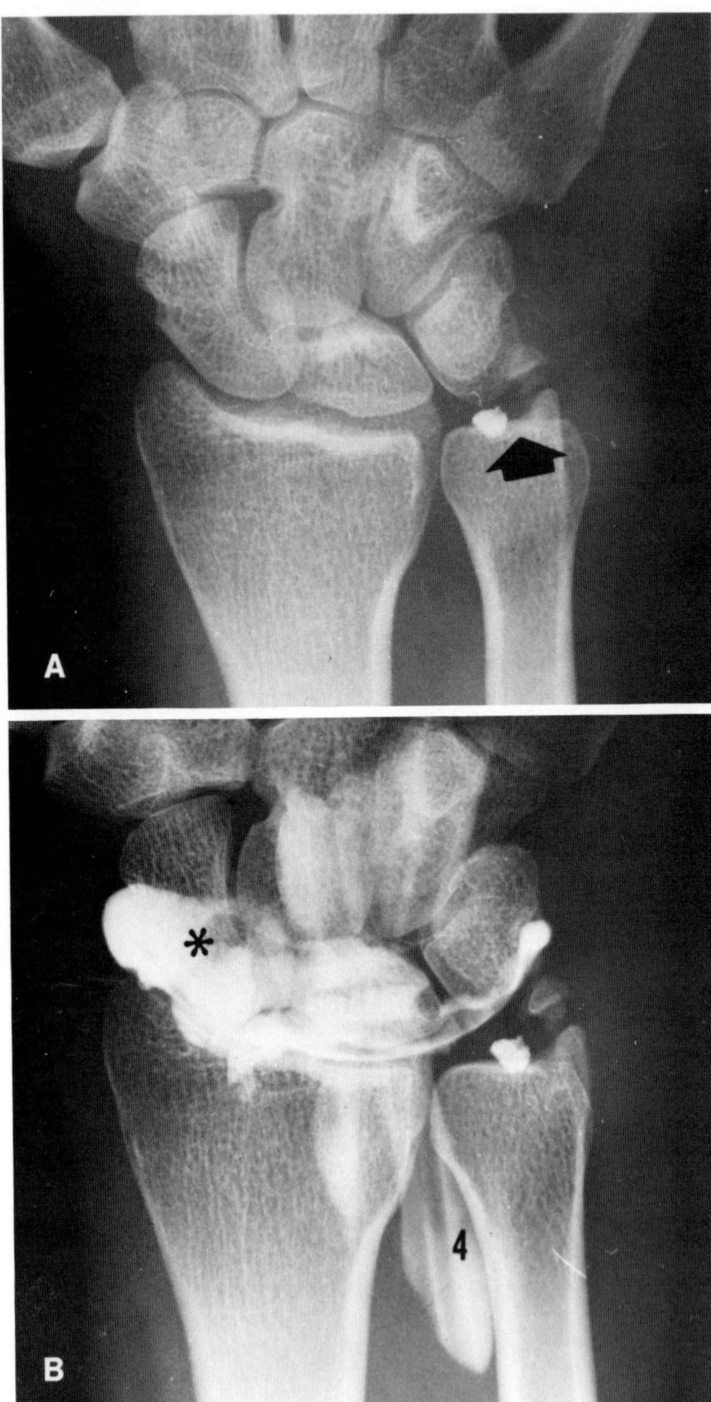

Figure 6.12. Posttraumatic arthropathy. *A,* An old fracture of the ulnar styloid and a metallic fragment are visible (*arrow*). *B,* Arthrography reveals smooth synovium within the confines of the radiocarpal compartment. The prestyloid recess is not filled, but opacification of extensor tendon sheaths is disclosed (*4*). A persistent filling defect (*asterisk*) represents an intraarticular fragment of articular cartilage. (Reproduced with permission from D. Resnick: Radiology, *113:* 331–340, 1974.)

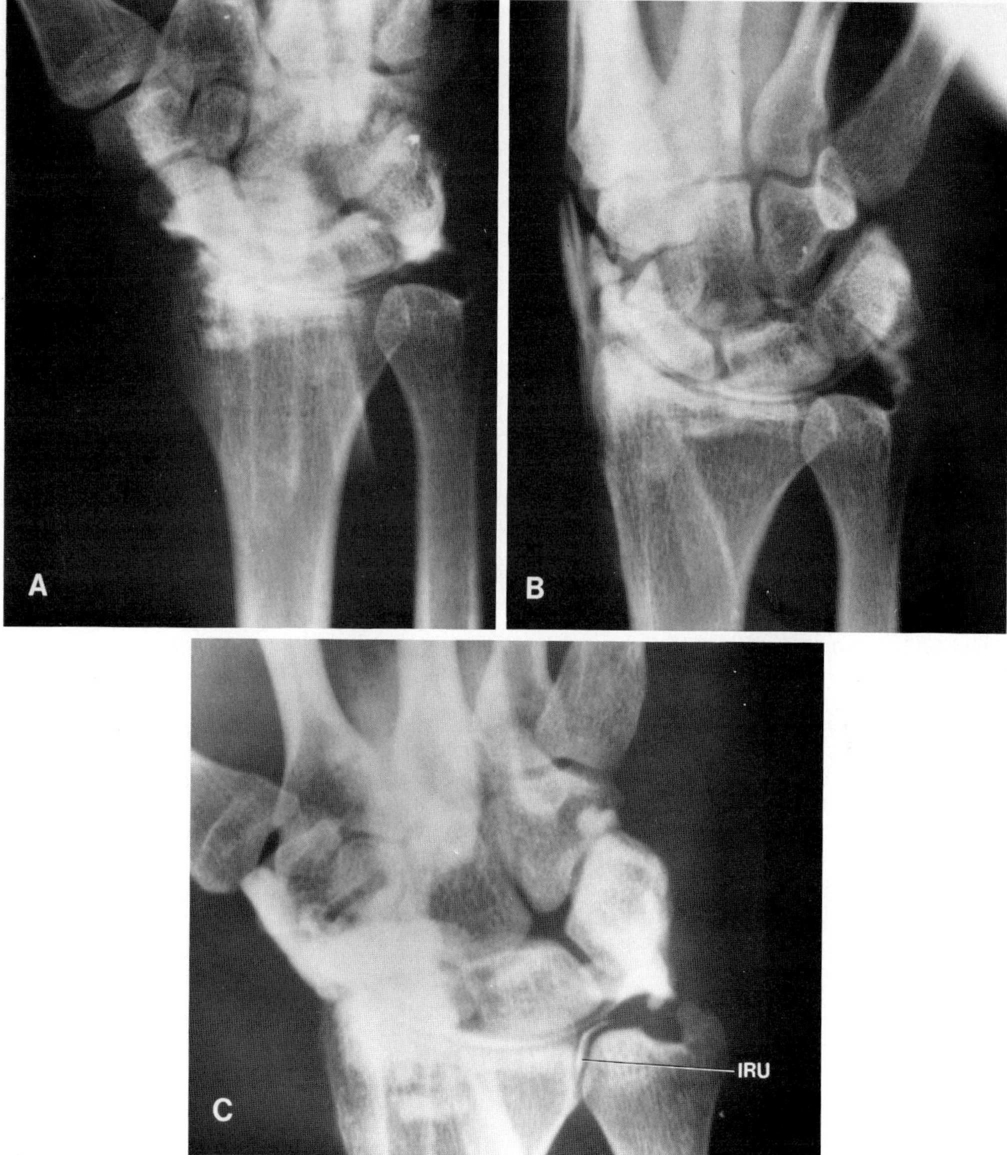

Figure 6.13. Communication between the radiocarpal compartment and the extensor tendon sheaths resulting from severe injury to the dorsal ligaments. *A* and *B*, Oblique projections. *C*, Posteroanterior projection after brief passive exercise. The inferior radioulnar compartment (*IRU*) contains contrast medium, implying a tear of the triangular fibrocartilage.

filling (42%) (Figs. 6.17 and 6.18). A nonspecific but commonly occurring feature is intercompartmental communication (92%), which is often almost total in its extent. Communication with the dorsal extensor tendon sheaths occurs in 25% of cases, but communication with the volar flexor tendon sheaths is exceedingly rare.

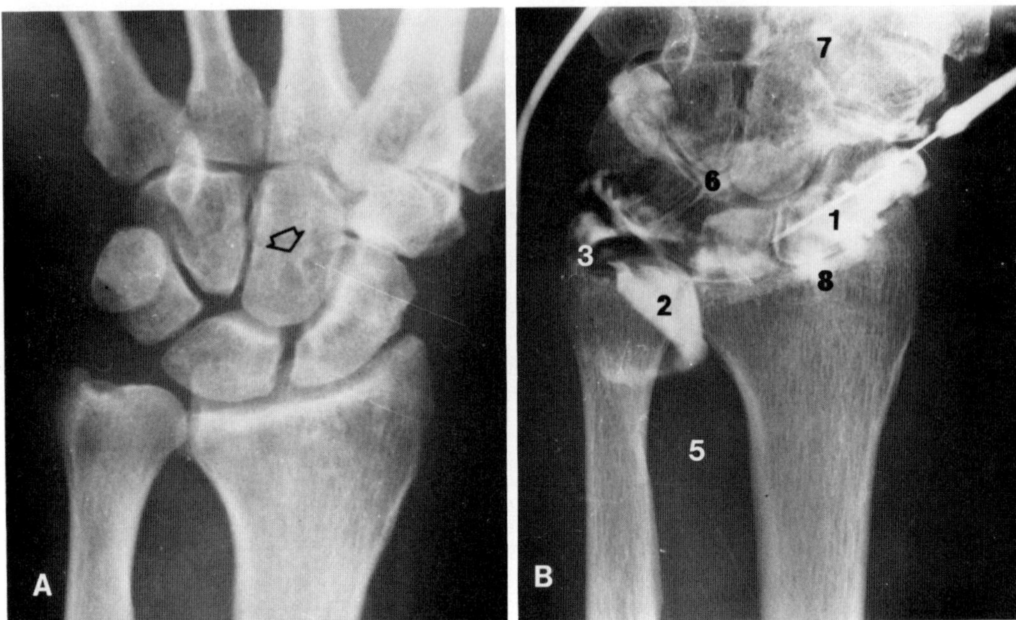

Figure 6.14. Pneumatic driller's disease. *A*, Characteristic cyst formation in the carpal bones (*open arrow*) probably results from passage of synovial fluid through minute fissures in the articular cartilage and into subchondral bone. Continued occupational trauma accompanied by increased intraarticular hydrostatic pressure during work leads to progressively severe cystic change. *B*, The synovium is irregular (1). There has been opacification in the inferior radioulnar compartment (2). Filling of the midcarpal (6) and carpometacarpal compartments (7) has also occurred. The prestyloid recess (3) is irregular. The volar recesses (8) are normal. Faint opacification of delicate, beaded lymphatic channels (5) has heretofore been reported only in pathological disorders, usually inflammatory arthropathies such as rheumatoid arthritis, but not in the normal wrist. (Reproduced with permission from D. Resnick: Radiology, *113*:331–340, 1974.)

The corrugated outline of the synovium, most prominent along the volar and dorsal surfaces and along the prestyloid recess, is caused by nodules of pannus in combination with villous hypertrophy of the inflamed synovium.

The cause of the lymphatic filling which accompanies synovial inflammation, particularly in rheumatoid arthritis, is not entirely understood. The synovial membrane contains lymphatic channels, particularly along the volar aspect of the wrist. Presumably, synovial inflammation and hypertrophy increases the permeability of the membrane, allowing greater and more rapid absorption of contrast medium by vascular and lymphatic channels.

Calcium Pyrophosphate Dihydrate Deposition Disease (Pseudogout)

According to Resnick et al., who performed radiocarpal arthrograms on nine wrists in six individuals with this disorder, the arthrographic features consist of mild to moderate synovial corrugation and communication with inferior radioul-

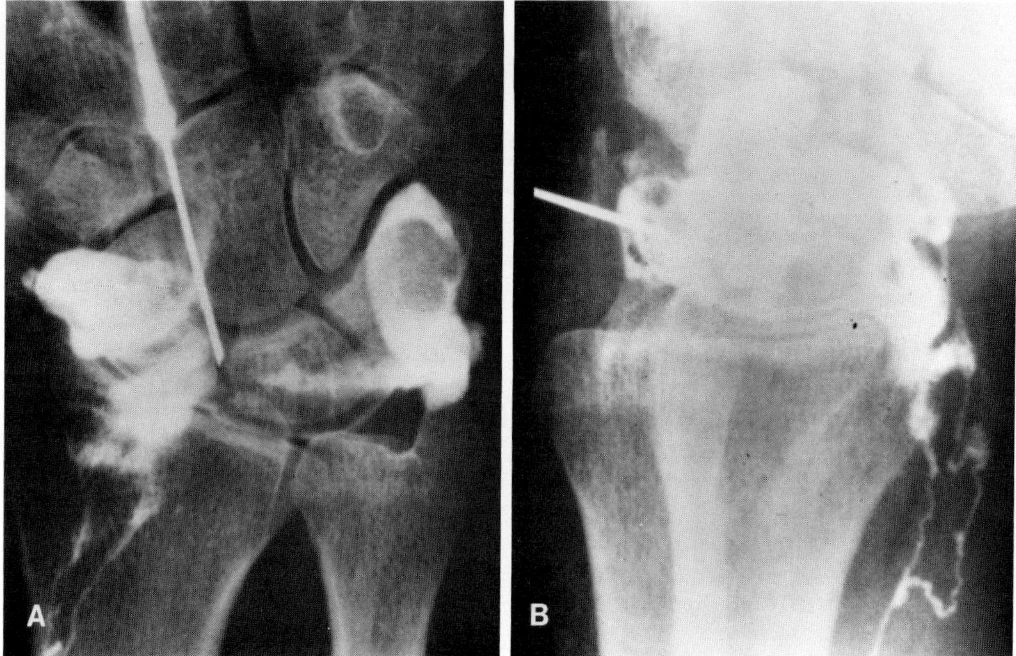

Figure 6.15. Unexplained filling of volar lymphatic channels in a man, age 52, with pain in the left wrist 6 weeks following hyperextension injury and no other joint symptoms. Posteroanterior (*A*) and lateral projections (*B*). The arthrogram and plain radiographs were otherwise normal. (Courtesy of Darwood B. Hance, M.D.)

nar, midcarpal, and common carpometacarpal compartments. Lymphatic filling was noted in two patients, and tendon sheath communication in one. Although the pattern was similar to that in rheumatoid arthritis, irregularity of the margin of contrast medium was less severe.

Recurrent Ganglion

The genesis of wrist ganglia is obscure. The most persuasive theory of origin borne out by arthrographic investigation is that ganglia represent synovial herniations from the compartments of the wrist. Nevertheless, opacification of a ganglion by injecting it directly with contrast medium usually fails to demonstrate a communication with the wrist joint because of a valve-like mechanism which prevents the contrast medium from returning to the joint. This mechanism results from the configuration of the communicating stalk, which is usually narrow and tortuous. Recurrence of a ganglion that has presumably been excised may result from any one of three factors: (1) failure to excise the lesion originally, (2) failure to excise the communicating stalk that extends between the ganglion and the wrist joint, or (3) failure to recognize and excise satellite ganglia.

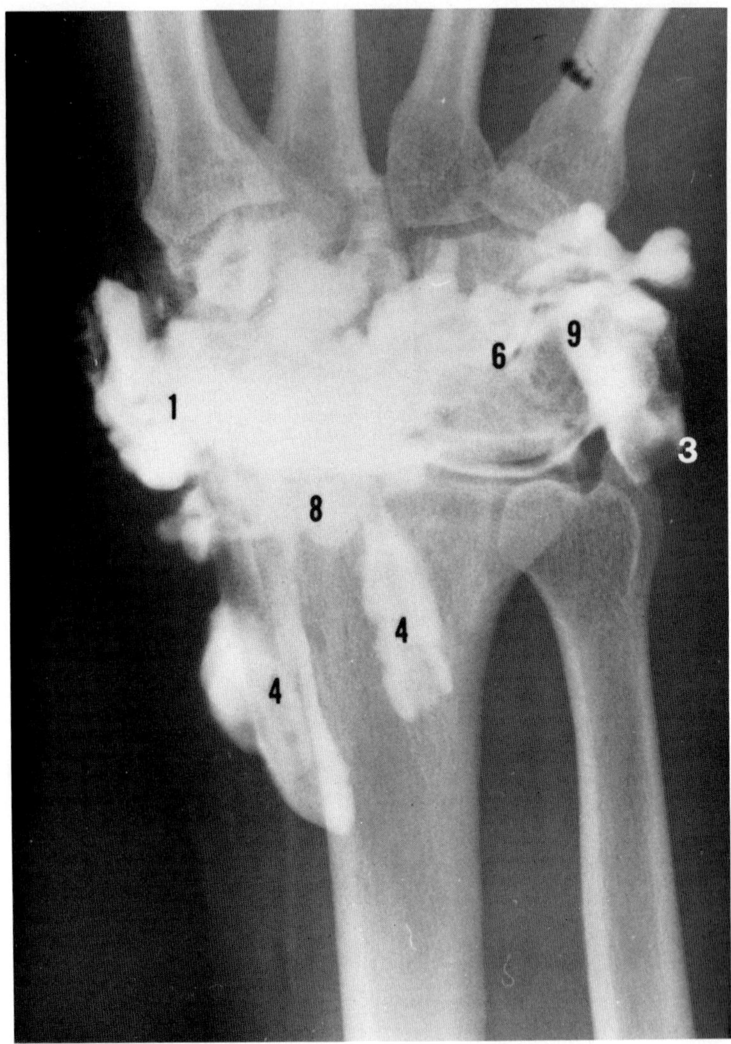

Figure 6.16. Neuropathic joint disease. Localized synovial irregularity and capsular distension (*1*) are present along with opacification of extensor tendon sheaths (*4*), communication with the midcarpal (*6*) and pisiform-triquetral compartments (*9*), and a prominent palmar radial recess (*8*). The prestyloid recess (*3*) contains a filling defect representing a loose fragment of articular cartilage. (Reproduced with permission from D. Resnick: Radiology, *113*:331–340, 1974.)

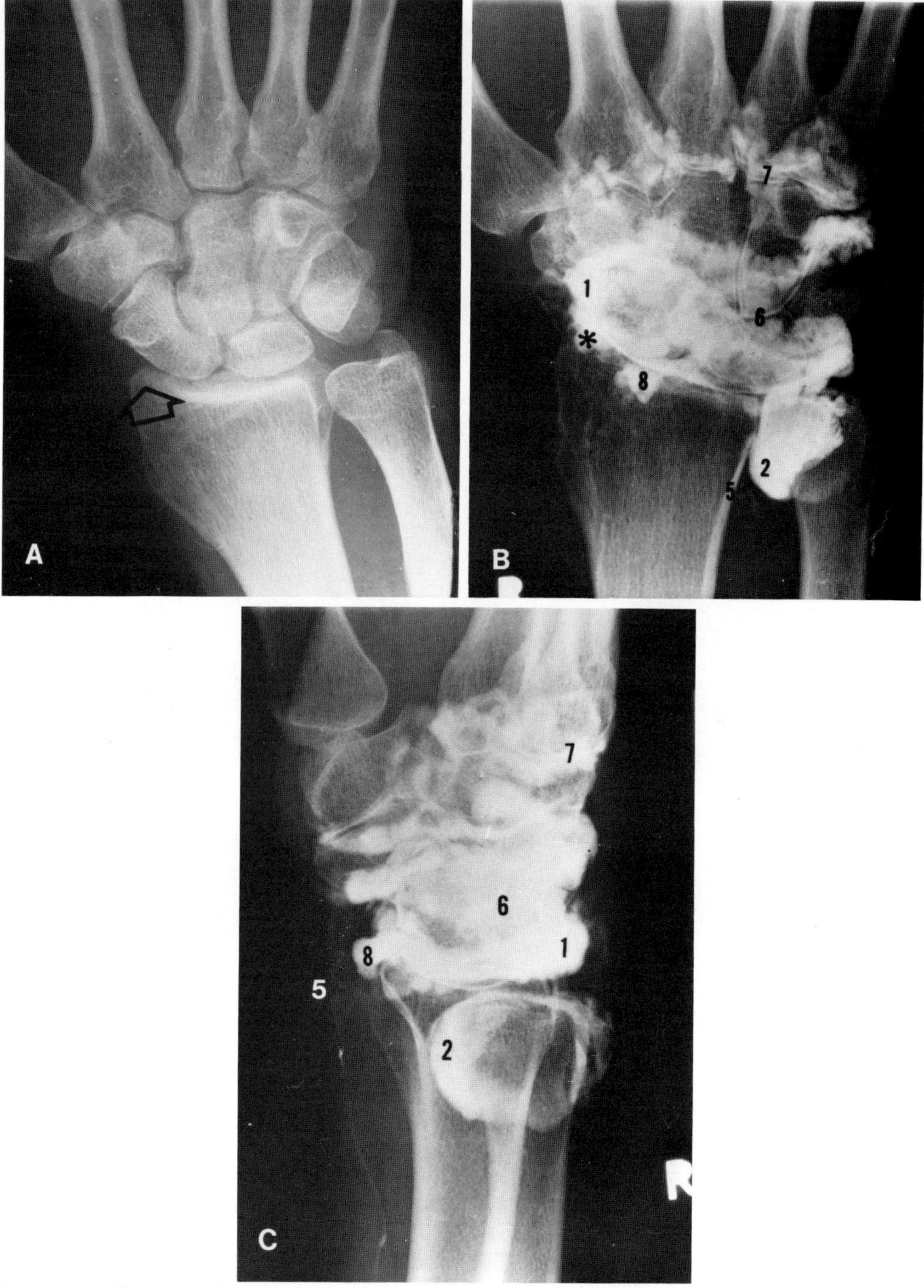

Figure 6.17. Rheumatoid arthritis. *A,* Posteroanterior plain radiograph reveals a small erosion of the radial styloid (*open arrow*) and osteoporosis. *B* and *C,* Posteroanterior and lateral arthrographic projections reveal severe synovial irregularity with corrugations (*asterisk*) typical of rheumatoid arthritis. The contrast medium extends from the radiocarpal compartment (*1*) through pathological communications to the inferior radioulnar (*2*), midcarpal (*6*), and common carpometacarpal (*7*) compartments. Opacification of volar lymphatic channels (*5*) has occurred. A prominent palmar radial recess (*8*) is present. (Reproduced with permission from D. Resnick: Radiology, *113:331–340, 1974.)*

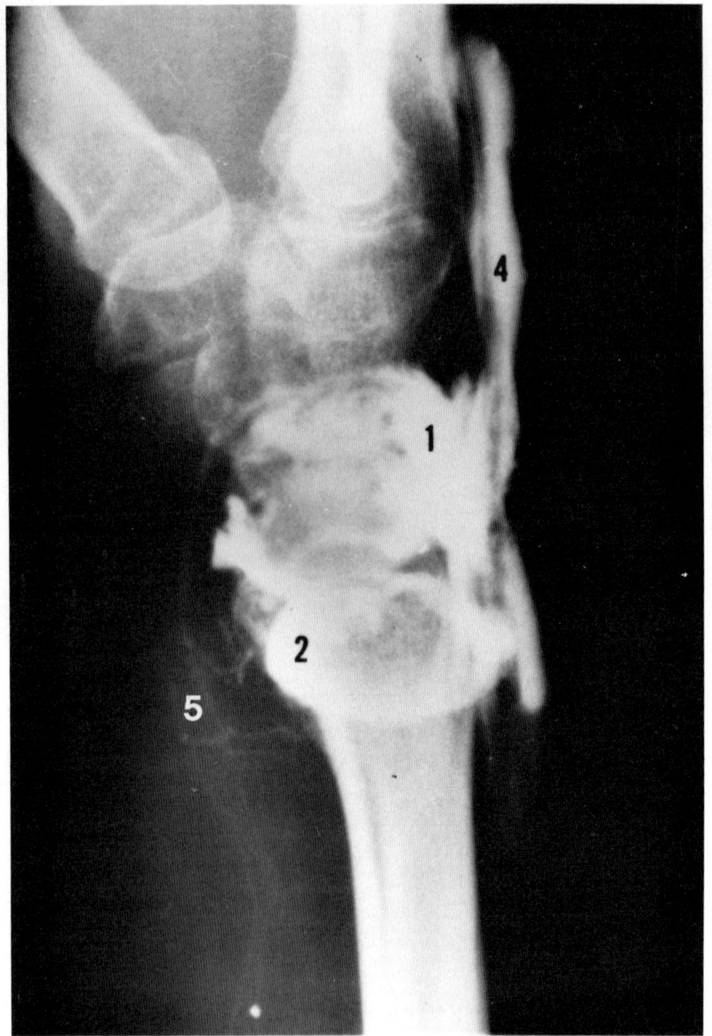

Figure 6.18. Rheumatoid arthritis. Lateral view reveals a corrugated synovium (1), communication with the inferior radioulnar compartment (2), opacification of extensor tendons (4), and lymphatic filling (5). (Courtesy of Donald Resnick, M.D., and Radiology, *113*:331–340, 1974.)

Arthrography is useful for locating the communication between a recurrent ganglion and the wrist joint, so that the communicating channel can be excised at its origin together with the ganglion, thus preventing further recurrence (Fig. 6.19). Most ganglia originate from the radiocarpal or midcarpal compartments, with the third most common site of origin being the carpometacarpal compartment of the thumb. The initial attempt at opacification should be made by injecting the compartment of the wrist nearest the ganglion. In the event of a dorsal ganglion, the contrast medium should be injected from the volar aspect of the wrist to avoid misinterpreting any extravasation of contrast medium at

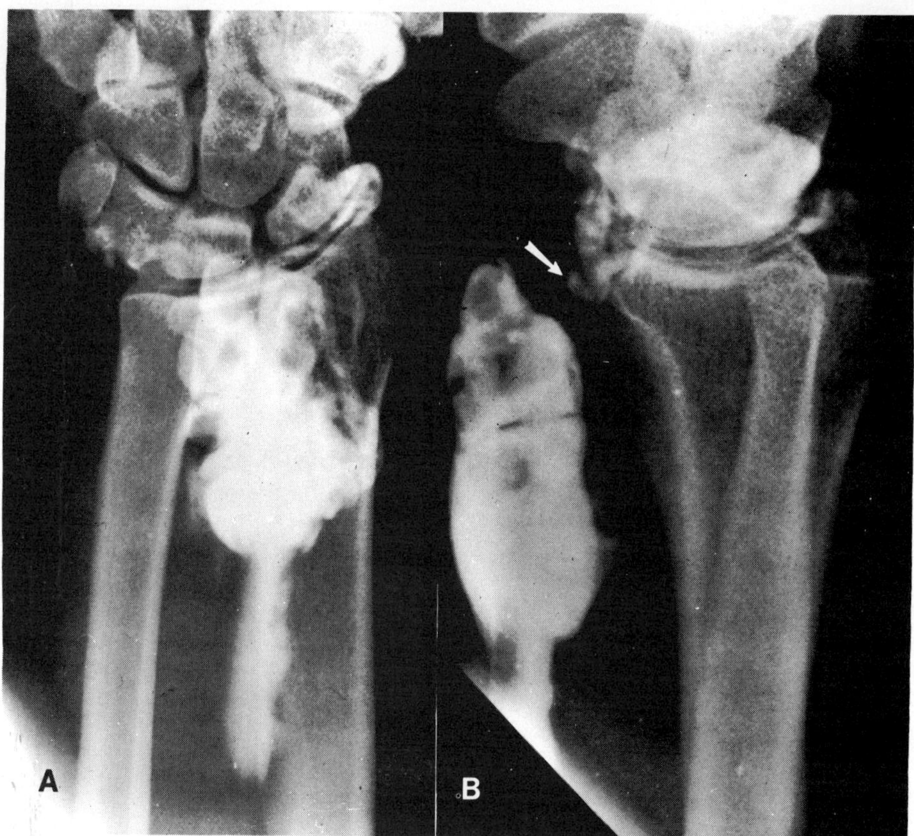

Figure 6.19. Large volar ganglion communicating with the radiocarpal compartment by way of a tortuous channel (*arrow*). Posteroanterior (*A*) and lateral (*B*) views. In order to prevent postoperative recurrence, excision should include not only the ganglion but the entire communicating channel as well. (Reproduced with permission from T. W. Staple, A. K. Poznanski: *The Hand in Radiologic Diagnosis*. W.B. Saunders, Philadelphia, 1974.)

the site of injection. Considerable distension of the injected compartment may be necessary to obtain opacification of the communicating stalk and ganglion. If the ganglion is very firm, aspiration of its viscous fluid contents may ease the entrance of the contrast medium.

References

Andrén, L., Eiken, O., Arthrographic studies of wrist ganglions. J Bone Joint Surg, *53A*:299–302, 1971.

Harrison, M.O., Freiberger, R.H., Ranawat, C.S., Arthrography of the rheumatoid wrist joint. AJR, *112:* 480–486, 1971.

Kessler, I., Silberman, Z., An experimental study of the radiocarpal joint by arthrography. Surg Gynecol Obstet, *112*:33–40, 1961.

Lewis, O.J., Hamshere, R.J., Bucknill, T.M., The anatomy of the wrist joint. J Anat, *106*:539–552, 1970.

Nelson, C.L., Burton, R.I., Upper extremity arthrography. Clin Orthop, *107*:62–72, 1975.

Nelson, C.L., Sawmiller, S., Phalen, G.S., Ganglions of the wrist and hand. J Bone Joint Surg, *54A*:1459–1464, 1972.

Ranawat, C.S., Freiberger, R.H., Jordan, L.R. Straub, L.R., Arthrography in the rheumatoid wrist joint: A preliminary report. J Bone Joint Surg, *51A*:1269–1281, 1969.

Resnick, D., Arthrography in the evaluation of arthritic disorders of the wrist. Radiology, *113*:331–340, 1974.

Resnick, D., Rheumatoid arthritis of the wrist: The compartmental approach. Med Radiogr Photogr, *52:* 50–88, 1976.

Resnick, D., Rheumatoid arthritis of the wrist: Why the ulnar styloid? Radiology, 112:29–35, 1974.

Resnick, D., Roentgenographic anatomy of the tendon sheaths of the hand and wrist: Tenography. AJR, 124:44–51, 1975.

Resnick, D., Niwayama, G., Goergen, T.G., Utsinger, P.D., Shapiro, R.F., Haselwood, D.H. Wiesner, K.B., Clinical, radiographic and pathologic abnormalities in calcium pyrophosphate dihydrate deposition disease (CPPD): Pseudogout. Radiology, 122:1–15, 1977.

Walmsley, R., Joints. In *Cunningham's Textbook of Anatomy*, Ed. 11, edited by G.J. Romanes. Oxford University Press, London, 1972.

Weigl, K., Spira, E. The triangular fibrocartilage of the wrist joint. Reconstr Surg Traumatol, 11:139–153, 1969.

Wirth, W., Arthrography. In *Roentgen Diagnosis*, Ed. 2, edited by H.R. Schinz et al., Vol. 1. Grune and Stratton, New York, 1968.

7

Arthrography of the Metacarpophalangeal and Interphalangeal Joint

R. D. Arndt, M.D.

The application of arthrography to metacarpophalangeal and interphalangeal joint disorders is limited to date but gathering some interest among radiologists and orthopedic surgeons.

Arthrography of these joints can be useful to diagnose radial and ulnar collateral ligament tears, especially in the thumb, search for loose bodies, and evaluate the condition of the articular cartilage in inflammatory as well as infectious or degenerative arthritis.

METHOD OF ARTHROGRAPHY

Arthrocentesis of the metacarpophalangeal joint of the thumb is performed with the palm flat on the x-ray table and the thumb abducted. After local anesthesia, the same 26-gauge needle is inserted perpendicular to the tabletop into the dorsal-radial aspect of the joint, under fluoroscopic guidance (Fig. 7.1). When resistance to injection of saline or lidocaine diminishes, indicating the needle tip to be intraarticular, 1 to 1.5 m of dilute diatrizoate meglumine (Renografin 60 diluted with an equal volume of sterile saline or water) is injected. Anteroposterior and a lateral film without stress is performed. Then, with the joint in full extension, an anteroposterior film under stress abduction is obtained. A comparison view of the contralateral uninjured thumb is obtained with abduction stress applied to the metacarpophalangeal joint.

In the case of the interphalangeal joints of the hand or foot, arthrocentesis is performed in the same way, with the palm or foot on the x-ray table and the joint in slight flexion. The point of entry is along the dorsal aspect of the joint, away from the site of pain. Anteroposterior, lateral, right and left oblique films are obtained with the joint extended, followed by a lateral film with the joint in flexion.

183

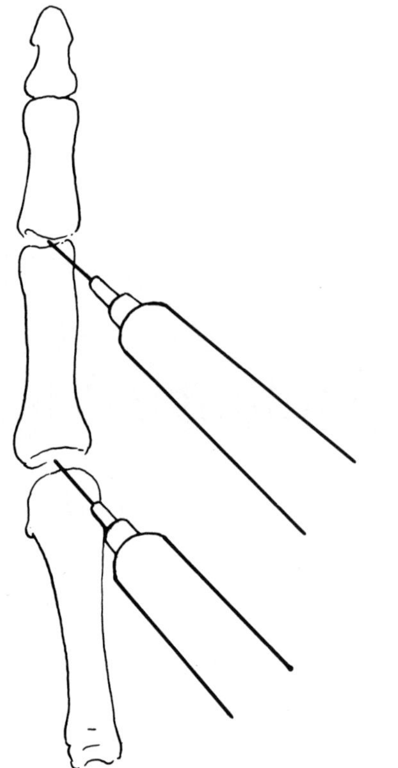

Figure 7.1. Sites of arthrocentesis for metacarpophalangeal and interphalangeal arthrography.

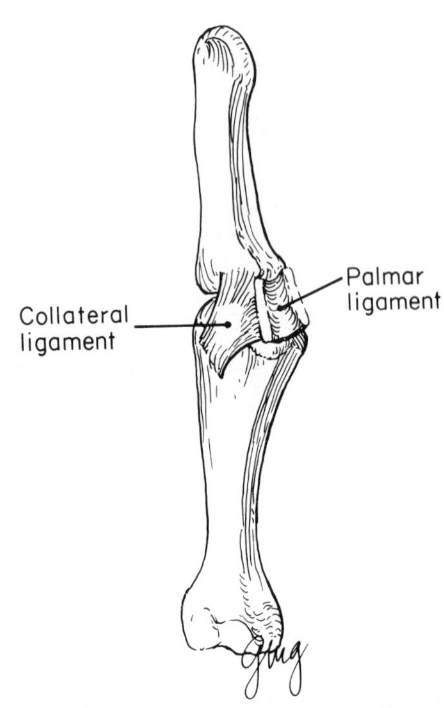

Figure 7.2. Ligamentous support of the metacarpophalangeal and interphalangeal joint. (Modified from Grant, J.C.B., *An Atlas of Anatomy*, Ed. 5 Williams & Wilkins, Baltimore, 1962.

Single contrast examination is the method of choice to detect a collateral ligament tear. If the arthrogram is performed to search for loose bodies or cartilaginous damage, the single contrast study usually suffices; however, occasionally a double contrast (0.5 m of iodinated contrast medium and 0.5 to 1 m of filtered room air) or air only arthrogram may be applied.

FUNCTIONAL ANATOMY AND NORMAL ARTHROGRAM

The metacarpophalangeal and interphalangeal joints are diarthrodial joints. The main movements of the interphalangeal joints are flexion and extension. The metacarpophalangeal joint, especially that of the thumb, also carries out abduction and adduction. The anatomical relationships and movement capabilities of these joints are similar in the hands and feet.

Stability for these joints is derived from ulnar and radial collateral ligaments, the fibrocartilagenous volar ligament or plate anteriorly, and the extensor expansions of the extensor muscles posteriorly (Fig. 7.2).

In the metacarpophalangeal joint, the synovial sac is attached to the head of

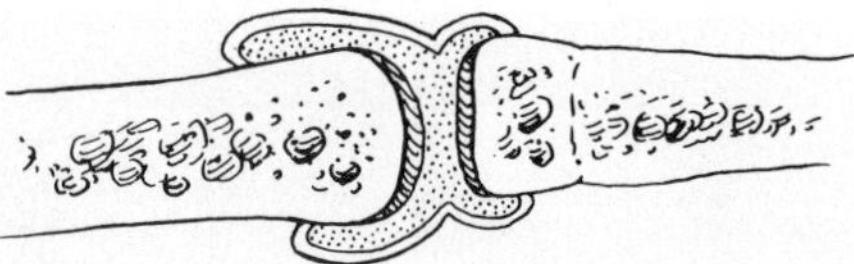

Figure 7.3. Schematic lateral, saggital view of the distended metacarpophalangeal and interphalangeal joint demonstrating that the greater portion of the synovial sac extends proximally. In the interphalangeal joint, the palmar recess is usually the largest.

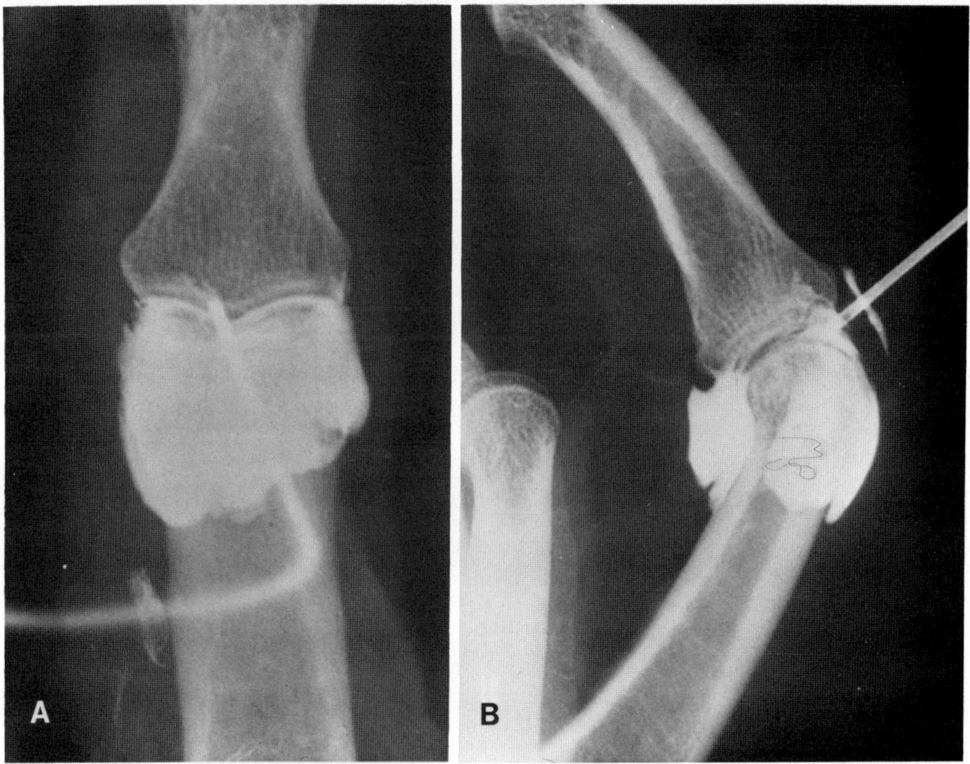

Figure 7.4. Normal proximal interphalangeal arthrogram. *A,* Anteroposterior projection showing articular cartilage and predominantly proximal extension of the joint capsule. *B,* Lateral projection reveals dorsal and palmar recesses. The small indentation on the palmar recess at the joint line is from the palmar ligament. (Reproduced with permission from W.J. Weston: Australas Radiol, 13:211–218, 1969.)

the metacarpal proximal to the joint line and to the base of the proximal phalanx immediately distal to the articular surface (Fig. 7.3). In the metacarpophalangeal arthrogram as described by Bowers and Hurst the synovial sac can be divided into a palmar recess, extending no more than 1 to 2 mm distal to the joint line on the proximal phalanx and 10 to 12 mm proximal to the joint line on the metacarpal head, and a dorsal recess extending no more than 5 mm distal to the joint line on the proximal phalanx and 10 to 20 mm proximal to the joint line over the metacarpal head. In the thumb the proximal portion of the dorsal

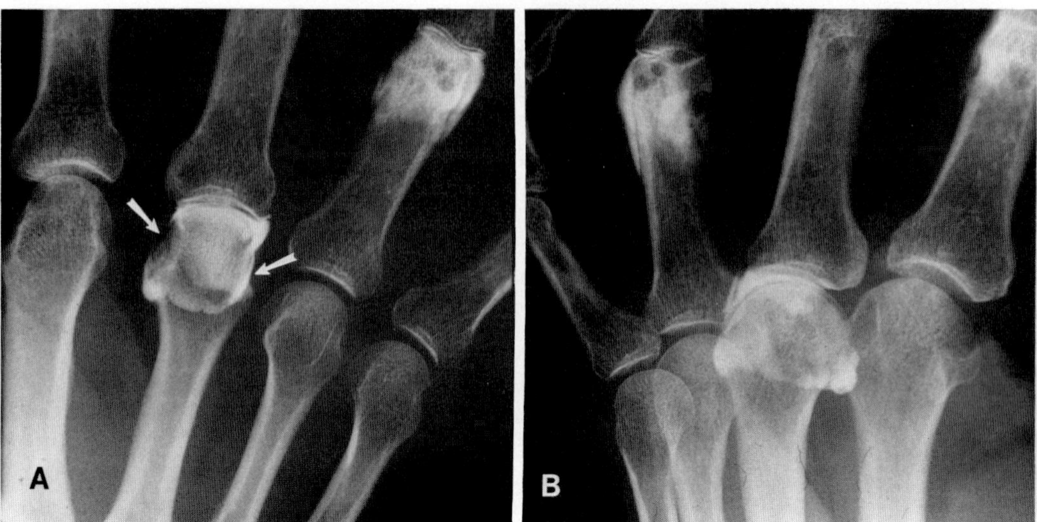

Figure 7.5. Normal metacarpophalangeal arthrogram. *A,* Anteroposterior view. The constriction of the synovial sac caused by the extrinsic compression of the radial and ulnar collateral ligaments is visible (*arrows*). *B,* Oblique lateral projection. As in the interphalangeal joints, the greater portion of the synovial sac extends proximally. (Reproduced with permission from W.J. Weston: Australas Radiol, *13*:211–218. 1969.)

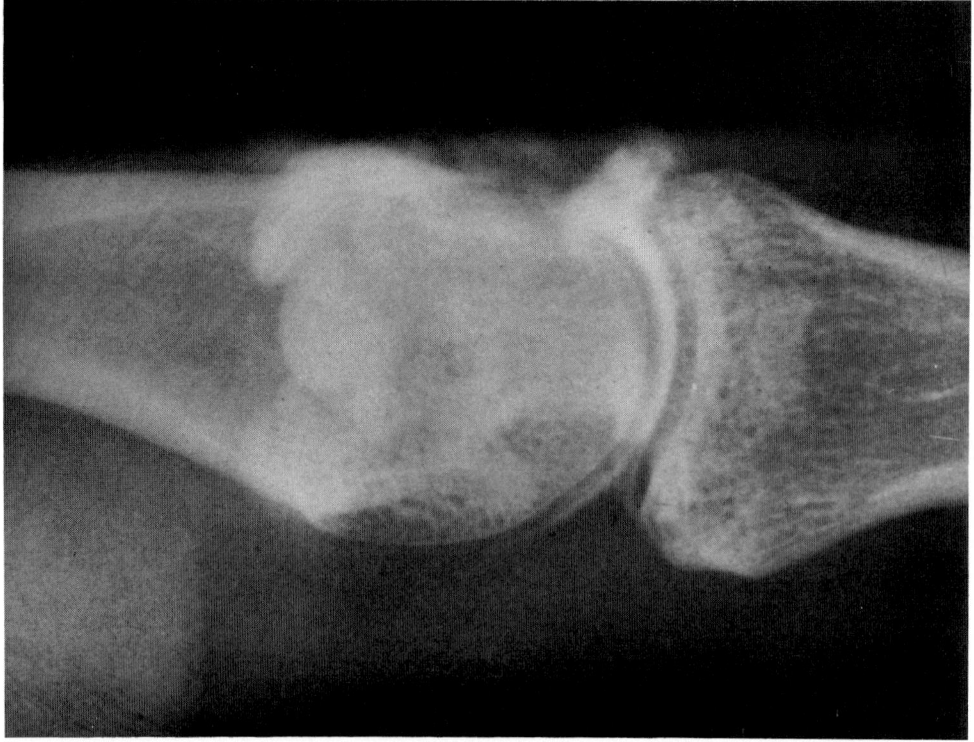

Figure 7.6. Normal metacarpophalangeal arthrogram. Lateral projection, reveals detail of the articular cartilage. Normal thickness is 1 to 1.5 mm.

recess is indented by the tendon of the extensor pollicis brevis which inserts on the capsule dorsally. In the interphalangeal joints, according to Weston (1969), these anatomical relationships are very similar except that the palmar recess is often larger than the dorsal recess, extending proximally on the more proximal phalanx (Fig. 7.4).

Laterally and medially the synovial sac is constricted at and proximal to the level of the joint line by the radial and ulnar collateral ligaments, respectively (Fig. 7.5). The margins of the synovial sac are smooth and regular. The usual volume of the joint distended with contrast is 1 to 1.5 m. The thickness of the articular cartilage is 1 to 1.5 mm (Fig. 7.6).

ABNORMAL METACARPOPHALANGEAL AND INTERPHALANGEAL ARTHROGRAM

Ligament Injuries—Gamekeeper's Thumb

A growing use for arthrography of the metacarpophalangeal and interphalangeal joints is in the evaluation of trauma to the ulnar and radial collateral ligaments. This is of particular importance in the thumb, where the arthrogram is useful for determining the presence of a tear in the ulnar collateral ligament complex, an entity known as "gamekeeper's thumb." This disability was first described by Campbell in Scottish gamekeepers who suffered repeated injury

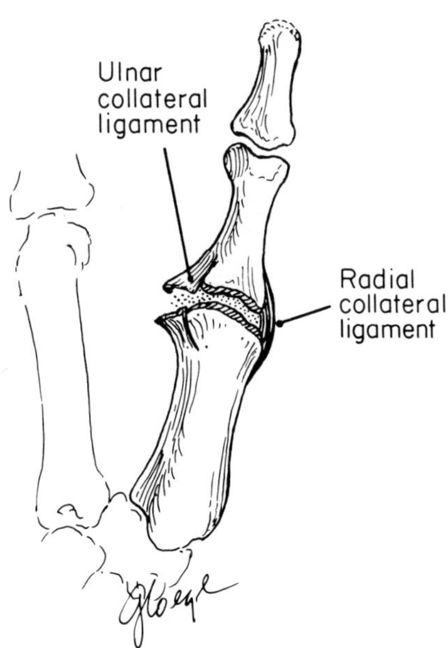

Figure 7.7. Gamekeeper's thumb. A tear of the ulnar collateral ligament complex is usually accompanied by a tear of the joint capsule. The latter allows demonstration of this injury by arthrography. Rupture of the collateral ligament is not always complete, and an avulsion fracture of its bony attachments may be part of the injury. In all cases a capsular tear is necessary to allow arthrographic diagnosis.

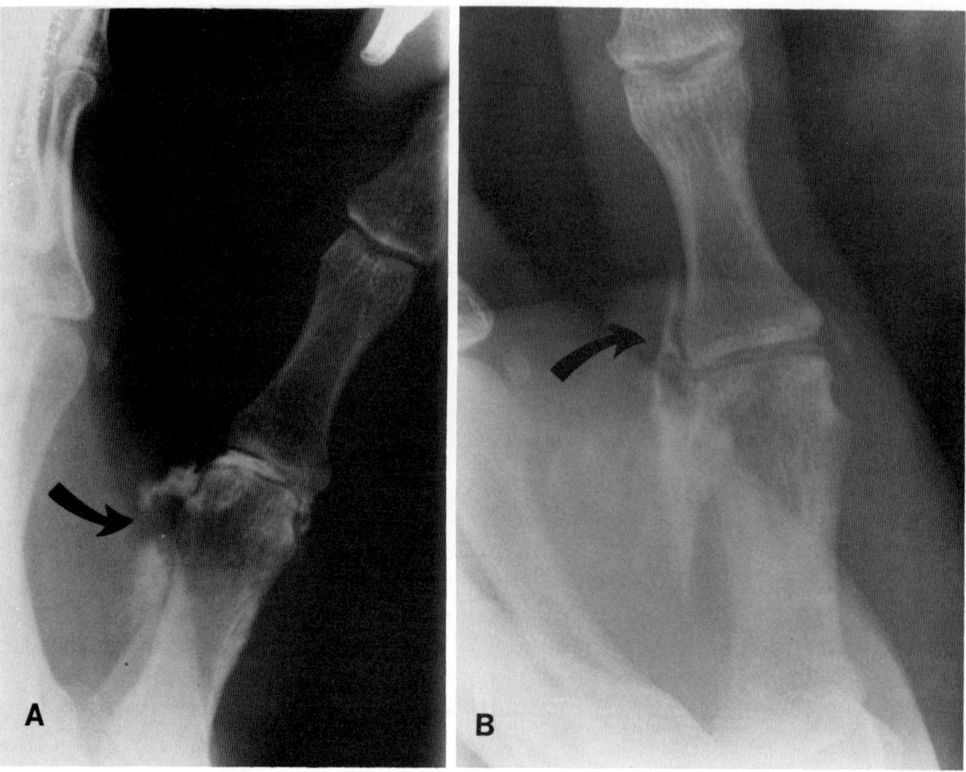

Figure 7.8. Abnormal metacarpophalangeal arthrogram of thumb. Gamekeeper's thumb. *A,* Contrast extravasation from dorsoulnar aspect of joint is readily visible (*arrows*), indicating a capsular leak secondary to a tear of the ulnar collateral ligament complex (proper ulnar collateral ligament and accessory ulnar collateral ligament). *B,* Another case. *Arrow* indicates contrast leaking through torn capsule and ruptured ulnar collateral ligament. (Reproduced with permission from W.H. Bowers, L.C. Hurst: J Bone Joint Surg, *59A*:519–524, 1977.

to this joint when killing rabbits by twisting and distracting the neck. A similar injury occurs in skiers during falls with ski poles in hand. In both cases, according to Resnick and Danzig, the injury consists of excessive abduction-extension movement of the thumb resulting in tears of the ulnar collateral ligament complex (Fig. 7.7). This may cause significant impairment in strength of grip and pinch, requiring plaster immobilization and on some occasions surgical repair.

Prior to arthrography of the metacarpophalangeal joint of the thumb, plain films with and without stress should be obtained to search for an avulsion fracture on the ulnar aspect of the base of the proximal phalanx which may accompany the injury. The anteroposterior abduction stress film with the joint in full extension is compared with an identical film of the uninjured thumb. According to Bowers and Hurst, an abduction arc greater than 30° or 10 ° more than the uninjured thumb is probably abnormal and suggests injury of the ulnar collateral ligament complex and hence "gamekeeper's thumb."

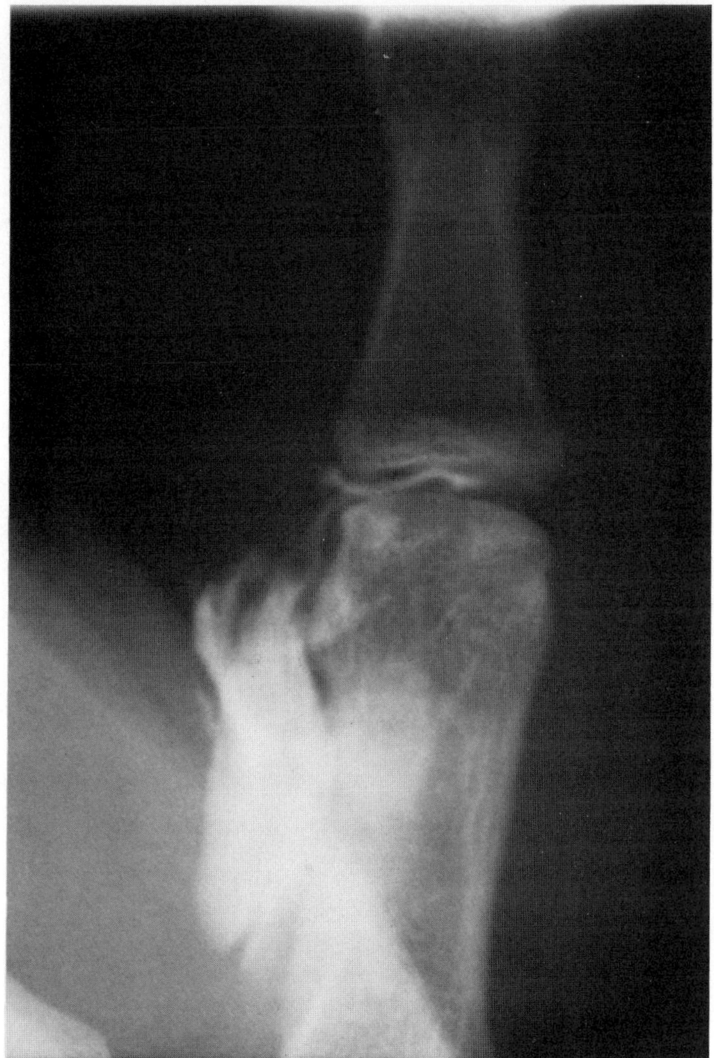

Figure 7.9. Abnormal metacarpophalangeal arthrogram of thumb. Skiing injury. There is frank contrast extravasation from the dorsoulnar aspect of the joint, indicating a capsular tear and implying injury of the ulnar collateral ligament complex. (Reproduced with permission from R. L. Linscheid: Clin Orthop, *103*:91, 1974)

This is confirmed on the arthrogram by noting leakage of contrast along the dorsoulnar aspect of the joint, verifying a tear of the capsule and ulnar collateral ligament (Figs. 7.8 to 7.10). As in ligamentous tears of other joints, the arthrogram should be performed within 3 days of the injury before healing seals the rent.

An arthrogram of the metacarpophalangeal or interphalangeal joint of the remaining digits may show collateral ligament injuries in a similar way, by demonstrating contrast extravasation along the radial or ulnar aspect of the

Figure 7.10. Abnormal metacarpophalangeal arthrogram of thumb: capsular tear. There is diffuse leak of contrast from a torn capsule. Contrast outlines the radial and ulnar collateral ligaments (*arrows*). These were felt to be intact because of normal abduction arcs on stress films. (Reproduced with permission from W.H. Bowers, L.C. Hurst: J Bone Joint Surg, 59:519–524, 1977)

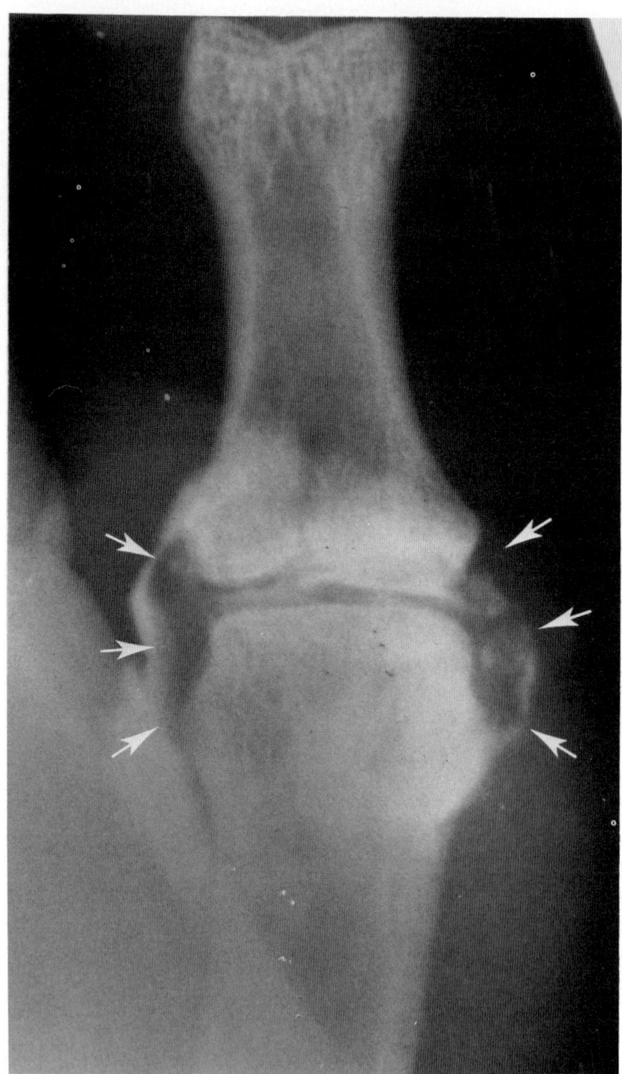

joint. In these joints the injury is not as disabling as in metacarpophalangeal joint of the thumb.

Arthritis

Arthrography may also be applied to help diagnose infectious and inflammatory arthritis. In infectious arthritis, one expects to find adhesive capsulitis with irregular, retracted margins of the synovial sac and diminished joint volume. This may be accompanied by thinned, damaged articular cartilage. If possible, joint fluid or contrast medium should be aspirated for bacteriological study.

The most consistent arthrographic finding of rheumatoid arthritis is an enlarged synovial sac with considerable increase in the joint volume (Fig. 7.11). The usual waist created by collateral ligaments is lost, and all margins of the synovial sac become convex. The filling defects of nodular synovial hypertrophy may be visible. Occasionally, contrast appears in periarticular lymphatics.

In degenerative arthritis, the synovial margins become moderately irregular, and there is thinning of the articular cartilage (Fig. 7.12).

Loose Bodies

Loose bodies, as in other joints, may be demonstrated with single, double contrast, or air arthrography. In the metacarpophalangeal and interphalangeal

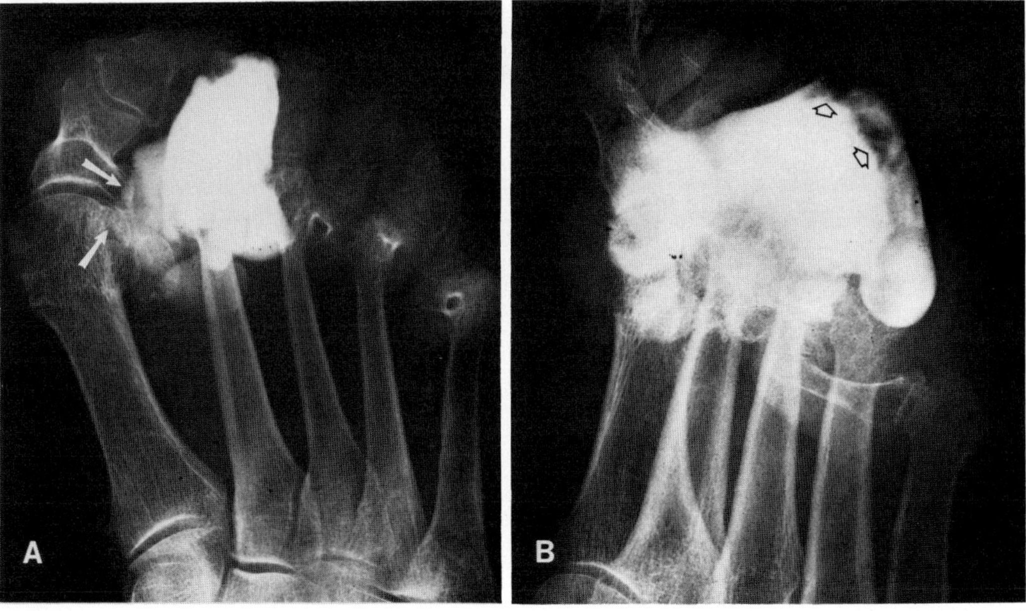

Figure 7.11. Abnormal metacarpophalangeal arthrogram right second toe: Rheumatoid arthritis. Anteroposterior (*A*) and oblique films (*B*) reveal a huge synovial sac with dissecting inflammatory cysts (*arrows*). In the distal portion of the enlarged bursa, nodular synovial hypertrophy is visible (*open arrows*). (Reproduced with permission from W.J. Weston, D.G. Palmer: *Soft Tissues of the Extremities, A Radiologic Study of Rheumatic Disease*, p. 117. Springer-Verlag, New York, 1978.)

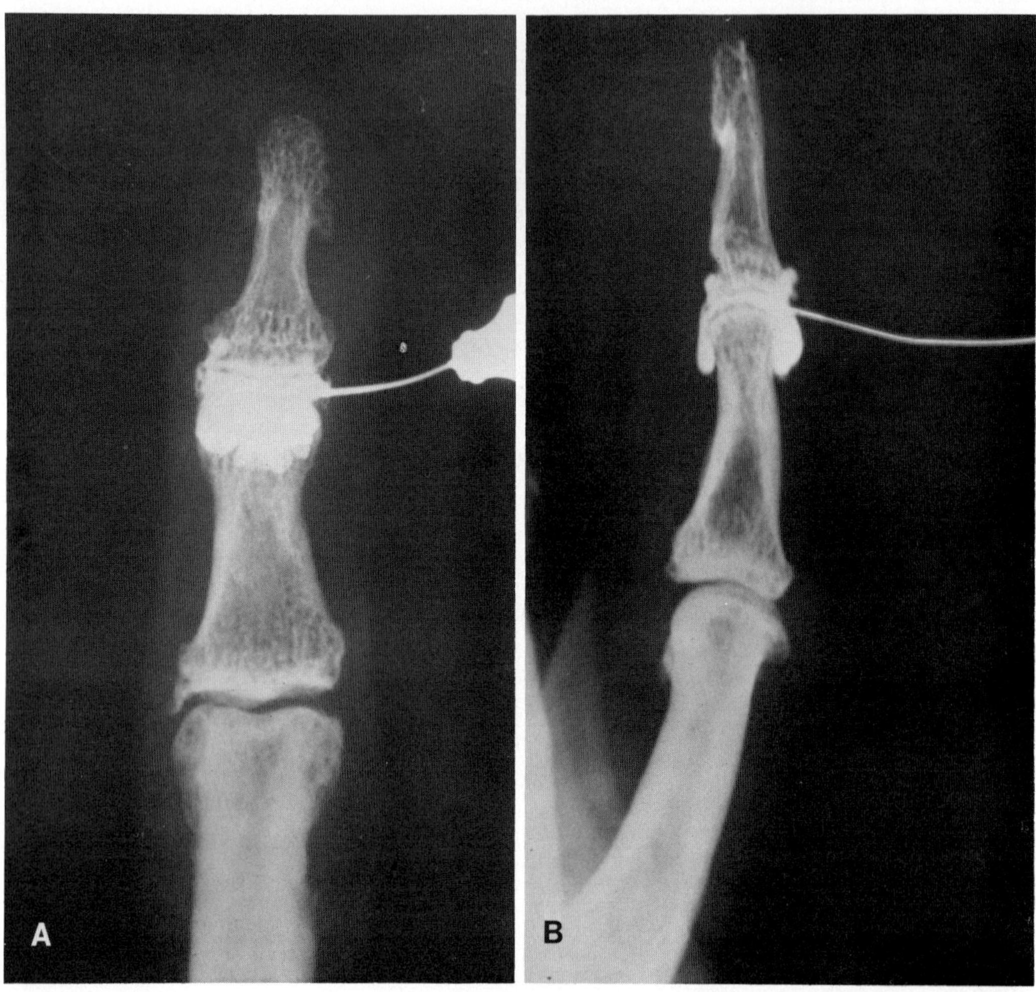

Figure 7.12. Distal interphalangeal joint arthrogram. Anteroposterior (*A*) and lateral (*B*) views. There is slight thinning of the articular cartilage secondary to degenerative arthritis. (Reproduced with permission from W.J. Weston: Australas Radiol, *13*:211–218, 1969.)

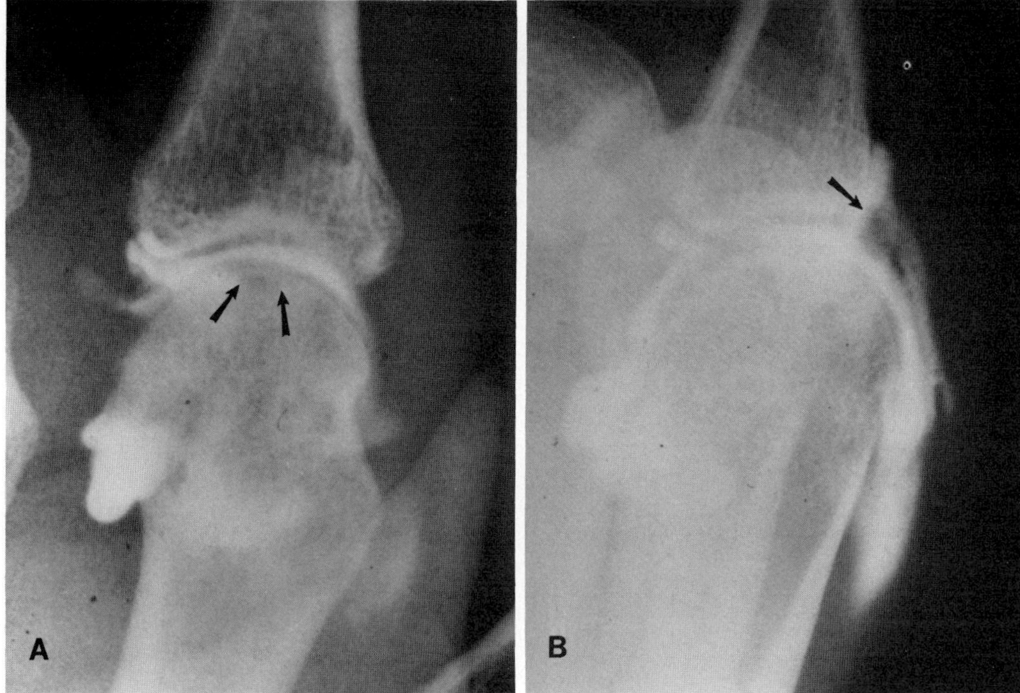

Figure 7.13. Abnormal metacarpophalangeal arthrogram of third finger: loose body. *A*, Anteroposterior view with slight obliquity suggests a filling defect near the joint line (*arrows*). *B*, Lateral view verifies the filling defect of a small cartilaginous loose body in the dorsal recess, at the joint line (*arrow*).

arthrogram, single contrast examination is usually sufficient. The loose bodies, which are generally fragments of bone or articular cartilage, are most commonly found in the dorsal and palmar recess on the lateral projection (Fig. 7.13).

References

Ahmad, I., De Palma, A.F., Treatment of gamekeeper's thumb by a new operation. Clin Orthop, *103*: 167–169, 1974.

Bowers, W.H., Hurst, L.C., Gamekeeper's thumb, evaluation by arthrography and stress roentgenography. J Bone Joint Surg, *59*:519–524, 1977.

Campbell, C.S., Gamekeeper's thumb. J Bone Joint Surg, *37B*:148–149, 1955.

Linscheid R.L., Arthrography of the metacarpophalangeal joint. Clin Orthop, *103*:91, 1974.

Nance, P.E., Kaye, J.J., Milek, M.A., Volar plate fracture. Radiology, *133*:61–64, 1979.

Resnick, D., Danzig, L.A., Arthrographic evaluation of injuries of the first metacarpophalangeal joint: Gamekeeper's thumb. AJR, *126*:1046–1052, 1976.

Schinz, H.R., et al., *Roentgen Diagnosis: The Skeleton*, Part 2, Edited by J. T. Case, Ed. 1, pp. 1218–1277. Grune and Stratton, New York, 1952.

Schultz, R.J., Fox, J.M., Gamekeeper's thumb: Result of skiing injuries. NY State J Med, *73*:2329–2331, 1973.

Weston, W.J., The normal arthrograms of the metacarpophalangeal, metatarsophalangeal and interphalangeal joints. Australas Radiol, *13*:211–218, 1969.

Weston, W.J., Rheumatoid arthritis in the hand, *Recent Advances in Radiology and Medical Imaging*, edited by T. Lodge and R.E. Steiner, No. 6, pp. 163–175. Churchill Livingstone, New York, 1979.

Weston, W.J., Palmer, D.G., *Soft Tissues of the Extremities: A Radiologic Study of Rheumatic Disease*, Ed. 1, pp. 117–119. Springer-Verlag, Berlin, 1978.

8

Arthrography of the Temporomandibular Joint

D. D. Blaschke, D.D.S.*

Arthrography of the temporomandibular joint (TMJ) is not, per se, a new procedure. It was introduced to the radiological literature in 1944 by Norgaard. Only in the past year or two, however, have radiologists expressed interest in the procedure on even a modest scale. The recent development of TMJ arthrography into a useful clinical diagnostic procedure (although still performed routinely at only a few institutions) is based on two principal factors: (1) There have been significant advancements in the understanding of TMJ soft tissue anatomy and function in the last few years. (2) Fluoroscopy and tomography have greatly improved the feasibility and technical quality of the procedure. Thus, in areas where TMJ surgical treatment is actively practiced, requests for TMJ arthrography can be expected to increase in the years ahead.

Patients referred for the procedure typically demonstrate clinical signs of TMJ soft tissue dysfunction, i.e., clicking, popping, or locking TMJs. The disability is usually unilateral, although in time contralateral signs may present. Since patients generally have painful limitation of jaw opening, the clinical presentation may be characterized simply as "TMJ pain and dysfunction." Prearthrographic plain radiographs and tomograms are typically normal except for some retrusion of the condyle within the articular fossa of the joint. In cases where significant temporomandibular degenerative joint disease is present radiographically, an arthrogram may show positive findings but the information has less unique clinical value.

TMJ arthrography can provide, in indicated cases, critical diagnostic information obtainable in no other way except by direct surgical inspection. Specifically, the examination can and should demonstrate: (1) the anteroposterior position of the joint articular disc (meniscus) relative to the articulating bony

* The author sincerely thanks Irene Petravisius for the drawings, Dick Friske and Catherine Boris for the clinical photography, and the Word Processing Center, Mrs. Rhoda Freeman, Supervisor, for the final preparation of this manuscript.

surfaces; (2) the morphology of the disc as seen on lateral view; and (3) the presence or absence (but not the specific location) of disc perforations or tears.

FUNCTIONAL ANATOMY

In light of recent investigations of human TMJs obtained at autopsy, the TMJ anatomy displayed in most general anatomy texts is incomplete and often misleading. The articular disc of the TMJ is now known to be a biconcave wafer interposed between the bony convexities of the anterosuperior surface of the mandibular condyle and the articular eminence of the temporal bone. There are two separate, noncommunicating, joint spaces: the upper, situated between the disc and the temporal bone surface; and the lower, between the disc and the condylar surface.

Figure 8.1A displays these structures as they would be seen in vivo in sagital section. The illustration is of a normal, decalcified TMJ taken from a young human subject at autopsy. Notice particularly the biconcavity of the articular disc, with the thin, central portion situated between the bony convexities. The physiological position of the disc is apparently always between the bony articulating convexities, where loading pressures on the joint are greatest, regardless of whether the jaws are closed, partially open or fully open. Also, in Figure 8.1A, the thin radiolucent slivers bordering the disc and its posterior attachment are the two joint spaces, here seen in their nondistended, physiological state. A line drawing of the same joint (Fig. 8.1B), shows with greater clarity the relationship between the disc, its ligamentous posterior attachment, and the joint bony components.

In opening and closing movements of the jaws, a hinge type of movement occurs in the lower joint compartment of the TMJ, (i.e., between the disc and the condyle), whereas a gliding type of movement predominates in the upper compartment.

METHOD OF ARTHROGRAPHY

Fluoroscopy is necessary for the performance of TMJ arthrography. Tomographic capability in the same radiology room greatly facilitates the examination, in that the patient need not be moved during the procedure. The patient lies on a radiology table with the TMJ of interest up, head slightly rotated (about 20°) toward the side of interest. The central x-ray beam for fluoroscopy and plain radiography is directed cranially through the TMJ at an angulation approximately 25° from the vertical.

Following disinfection of the preauricular soft tissues and the placement of a sterile plastic drape, local anesthesia is obtained in the soft tissues superficial to the joint. The site of skin puncture is approximately 1 cm anterior to the tragus of the ear. It is wise, however, to palpate the lateral rim of the articular fossa and enter the skin at a point just inferior to this rim. Local anesthetic solution is injected through a 25-gauge needle into the soft tissues down to the lateral condyle pole. The needle is then withdrawn and is exchanged (on the local anesthetic syringe) for a 1-in, 22-gauge angiocatheter.

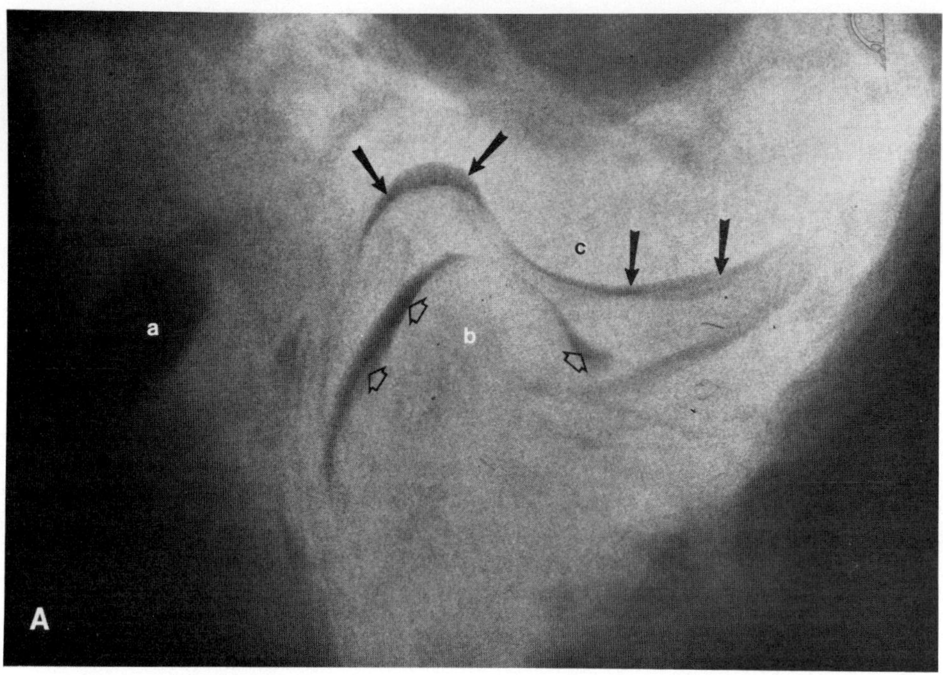

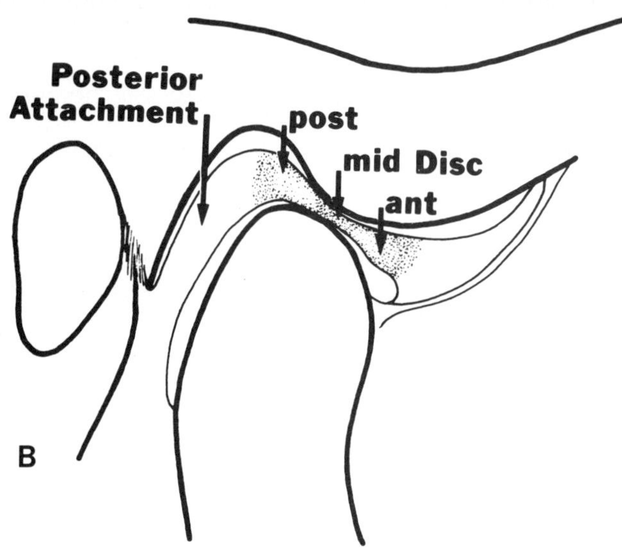

Figure 8.1. Anatomy. *A,* Autopsy specimen in lateral view. A human TMJ obtained at autopsy and subsequently decalcified is seen with the joint soft and hard tissues at comparable radiographic densities. To the posterior is the external ear canal (*a*). Interposed between the condyle (*b*) and articular eminence (*c*) is the biconcave articular disc. The curvilinear radiolucencies separating the soft tissue from the bony surfaces are the upper (*arrows*) and lower (*open arrows*) joint spaces. (Reproduced with permission from D.D. Blaschke: *Temporomandibular Joint Problems: Biological Diagnosis and Treatment,* edited by W.K. Solberg, G.T. Clark. Quintessenz, Berlin, 1980.) *B,* Line drawing of above illustration. Between the bony surfaces, the joint soft tissue component is subdivided into the posterior attachment and the articular disc (stippled). The disc has relatively thick posterior and anterior rims and a much thinner middle portion, which serves as the articulating or stress-bearing part. The upper and lower joint spaces (not labeled) do not communicate with each other; each has a posterior and an anterior recess. (Reproduced with permission from D.D. Blaschke, W.K. Solberg, B. Sanders: J Am Dent Assoc, *100*:388–395, 1980, ©American Dental Association, Chicago.)

The local anesthesia occasionally causes sluggishness of the patient's eyeblink reflex on the side of interest, through involvement of the facial nerve superior branches. If this happens, the patient should be reassured about the cause of and the transiency of the effect. The affected eyelid should be taped closed if it cannot be blinked by the patient with effort. When this side effect does present, it usually completely resolves by the time the patient is dismissed at the termination of the examination.

The lower joint space is catheterized first since its subsequent infusion and opacification is crucial to the examination's interpretation. The 22-gauge angio-catheter-syringe instrument is directed through the skin at the local anesthetic puncture site (Fig. 8.2A) and under intermittent fluoroscopic guidance is advanced to the posterosuperior aspect of the condyle surface. The angiocatheter should be virtually perpendicular to the skin surface until the bone surface is reached. After the needle contacts the condyle, the tip is "walked" around to the posterior surface where it should enter the posterior recess of the lower joint space. It is important to keep the needle tip near the superior aspect of the bone, not down on the condylar neck. If 0.5 cc of local anesthetic solution can be injected easily at this point, the needle tip is likely in the proper intraarticular position.

Following opacification of the lower space (description follows), catheterization of the upper joint space is begun with slight modifications from the procedure just described. The patient's mouth is opened moderately wide, in order to move the articular disc anteriorly, out of the line of possible needle puncture. From a skin puncture site 1 to 2 mm anterior to the lower catheter, the upper angiocatheter instrument is directed toward the posterior slope of the articular eminence with slight superior and anterior inclinations (Fig. 2C). The angiocatheter is advanced until the bony fossa is reached, at which point the hub of the instrument will be at or nearly at the skin surface. (Occasionally, for added catheter length, a 1¼-in, 20-gauge angiocatheter must be used).

Filling of the two joint spaces with radiopaque contrast medium follows their individual successful catheterizations. The operator first connects a stopcock and connecting tubing to the lower angiocatheter hub and initiates opacification of the lower joint space (Fig. 2B). Under fluoroscopic monitoring, 0.5 to 0.7 cc of water-soluble contrast medium such as Reno-M-60 is slowly injected. The operator should be alert at this point for inadvertant opacification of the upper joint space. Following catherization of the upper joint space, 0.5 to 0.8 cc of contrast medium is specifically injected into that space. The infusion of either the upper or lower space is made easier by moderate mouth opening during the actual injection. It is emphasized that rarely is it necessary to inject more than 0.7 cc of contrast medium into either of the joint spaces. Overinjection of fluid may damage the joint capsule or internal soft tissues and result in considerable discomfort to the patient after the local anesthesia resolves. Gross overinjection is also counterproductive to the interpretation of the exam.

Tomography of the opacified joint spaces commences as soon as possible after joint space filling. Because of the rapid dispersion of contrast medium into the synovium of the joint, noticeable deterioration of the radiographic image occurs within 5 to 10 minutes of the injections. The radiography should therefore be expedited. Ordinarily, tomograms are made at sagital planes 1½ to 3 cm below the skin surface, and with the jaws closed, halfway open and opened to their maximal extent. The examination is then terminated.

The angiocatheters are pulled and the skin puncture site is covered with a small bandage. The patient is advised to intermittently apply an icebag to the preauricular area for the remainder of the day. Two short-term postarthrographic effects are generally observed. It is common for the patient to notice an altered bite (occlusion), especially with regard to the posterior teeth on the side of the arthrogram. In addition, following resolution of the local anesthesia, mild to moderate discomfort in the joint will typically ensue. A moderate analgesic may be prescribed. Both the altered dental occlusion and the joint discomfort resolve within a day or two of the procedure.

NORMAL TMJ ARTHROGRAM

Interpretation of the TMJ arthrogram requires the radiologist to make at least four important judgments, concerning (in order of importance): (1) the posteroanterior position of the articular disc; (2) the limit of anterior translation of the mandibular condyle; (3) the possibility of perforation in the disc or its posterior attachment; (4) the shape of the disc. Figure 8.3 demonstrates normal appearances for these interpretative considerations in drawing form.

Upon normal opening of the jaws, the condyle and articular disc both translate anteriorly and counterclockwise around the articular eminence. The position of the disc is highly regulated in both closed and open mouth sequences, especially with respect to the bony convexities. At any given point of joint function, the thin, central part of the disc intervenes between the convex, bony articulating surfaces. The thicker, posterior rim of the disc is normally positioned either directly superior to or slightly posterior to the condyle articulating surface, depending on whether the jaws are closed or in some stage of opening. On fluoroscopic observation, the paired movements of disc and condyle occur smoothly and harmoniously, with no sense of hesitation or jerkiness.

The condyle should translate anteriorly past the crest of the articular eminence and slightly on to the latter's anterior slope. This degree of forward movement will normally be observed fluoroscopically upon commanding the patient to open his jaws as widely as possible. Another radiographic sign of normal condyle and disc anterior translation is obliteration of the opacified anterior recesses of the joint spaces. In normal TMJ arthrography, forward movement of the condyle and disc hydraulically force contrast medium from the anterior recesses into the posterior recesses (Fig. 8.4). However, the finding of normal wide open condyle translation may be seen in cases of clicking TMJ dysfunction, so the degree of condyle movement or nonmovement is not per se as sensitive a diagnostic finding as is the actual position of the disc.

The disc should maintain its biconcave shape at all stages of joint function. The integrity of the disc and its posterior attachment may be presumed if contrast does not escape from the lower joint space into the upper, or vice versa, when the first space is opacified.

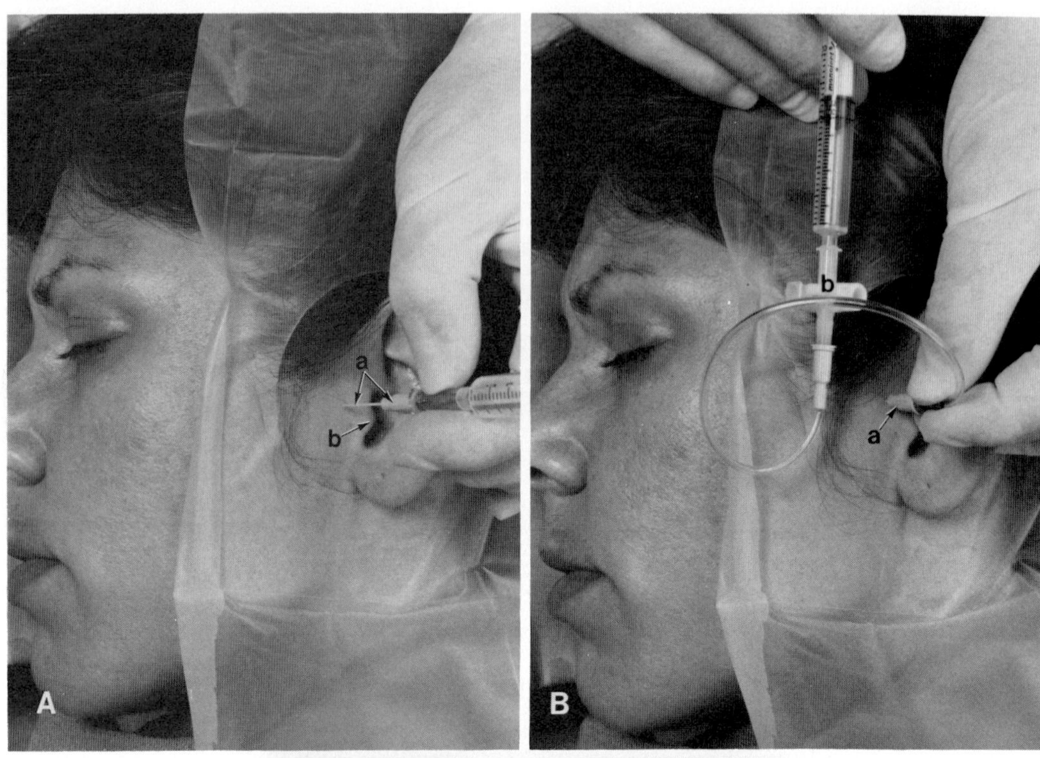
a
b
A
b
a
B

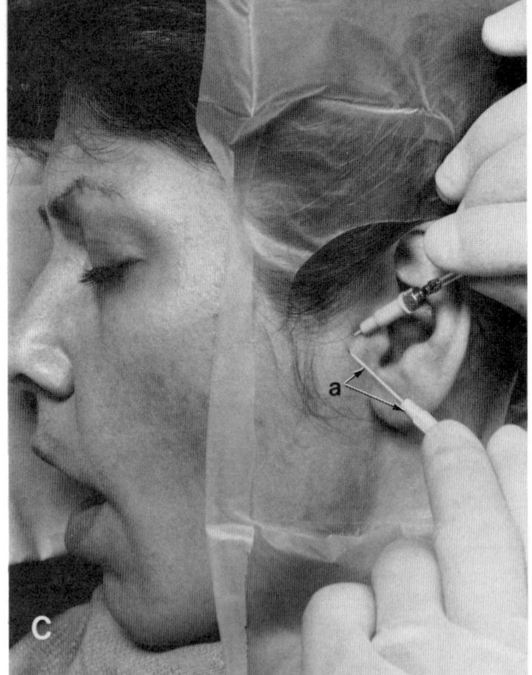
a
C

ABNORMAL TMJ ARTHROGRAM

The principal abnormality revealed by TMJ arthrography is anterior displacement of the articular disc. This finding has been corroborated by direct inspection of dysfunctional TMJs at surgical exploration (see Wilkes and Dolwick, et al.). In actuality, the anteriorly displaced disc is often found at surgical exploration to be *medially* displaced as well, although this finding is not apparent on lateral fluoroscopy or lateral TMJ arthrotomography. In positive cases of anteriorly displaced TMJ discs, several secondary arthrographic findings having

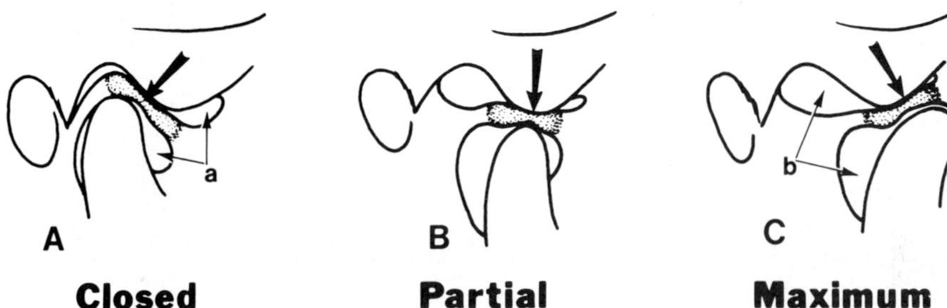

Figure 8.3. Normal TMJ arthrographic features. *A*, Jaws closed. The condyle is seated in the joint's articular fossa. The disc (*stippled*) is normally positioned superior and slightly anterior to the condyle, such that the thin, middle portion of the disc (*arrow*) intervenes between the anterosuperior part of the condyle and the posterior slope of the articular eminence. Note the slight bulging of the anterior recesses (*a*) distended with contrast fluid (compare with the nondistended state seen in Fig. 1B). *B*, Upon partial opening of the mouth, condyle and disc both translate anteriorly in a smooth, harmonious manner. Of critical diagnostic importance, the thin, midportion of the disc (*arrow*) remains positioned between the bony articulating surfaces. *C*, Maximal jaw opening. The condyle has translated past the crest of the articular eminence. The disc has moved less anteriorly in the absolute sense but the thin part (*arrow*) is still found between the narrowest point of the bony articulation. The anterior joint space recesses have been obliterated as the contrast has been hydraulically forced to the posterior recesses (b). (Reproduced with permission from D.D. Blaschke, W.K. Solberg, B. Sanders: J Am Dent Assoc, *100*:388–395, 1980, ©American Dental Association, Chicago.)

Figure 8.2. Technique. *A*, Lower joint space catheterization. Following disinfection of the preauricular skin site, placement of a sterile drape (shown), and the administration of local anesthesia, a 22-gauge, 1-in angiocatheter (*a*) connected to a 3-cc syringe is brought to position. The instrument punctures the skin approximately 1 cm anterior to the tragus (*b*) of the external ear. The jaws are closed or very slightly open. Fluoroscopy is utilized to guide the instrument to the posterosuperior surface of the mandibular condyle. *B*, Lower joint space contrast filling. The needle (stylet) of the angiocatheter has been withdrawn, the plastic catheter (*a*) is slightly advanced into the lower joint space, and the syringe containing lidocaine is replaced with one containing Reno-M-60 contrast medium. A stopcock (*b*) and a short connecting tube are also used. Under fluoroscopic observation, 0.5 to 0.7 cc of contrast is slowly injected. *C*, Upper joint space catherization. Following lower space contrast filling and initial radiography, the operator places a second 1-in, 22-gauge angiocatheter (*a*) into the preauricular tissue. Occasionally a 1¼-in, 20-gauge instrument is needed for added length. The placement technique is similar to that for the lower space except that the mouth is opened moderately wide and the instrument is directed slightly superiorly and anteriorly, toward the posterior slope of the articular eminence. The upper space will hold slightly more contrast than the lower, although rarely is more than 0.8 cc necessary. TMJ tomography follows successful upper space filling.

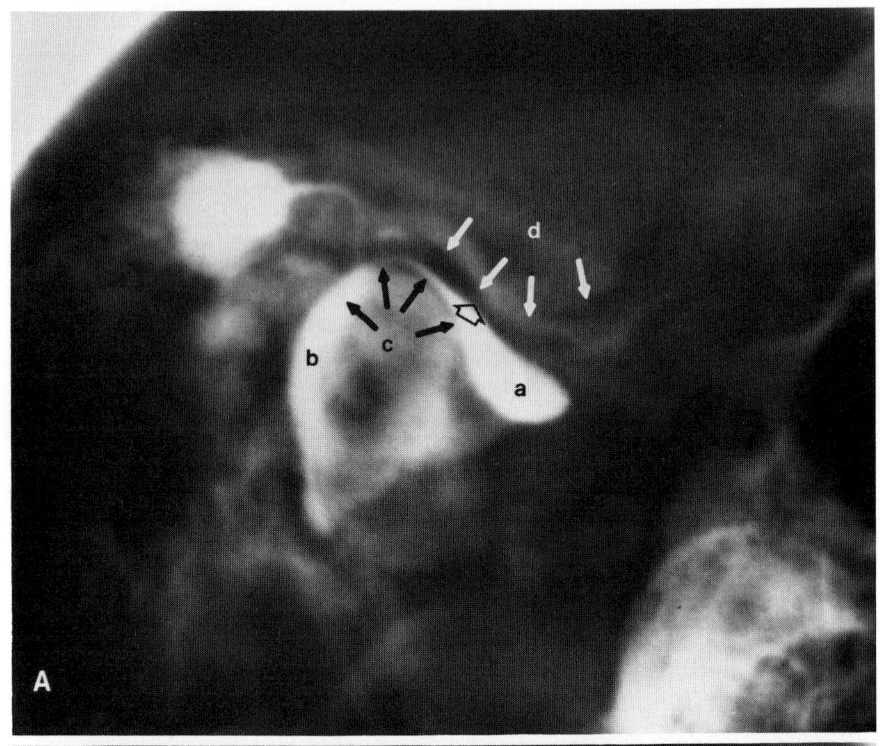

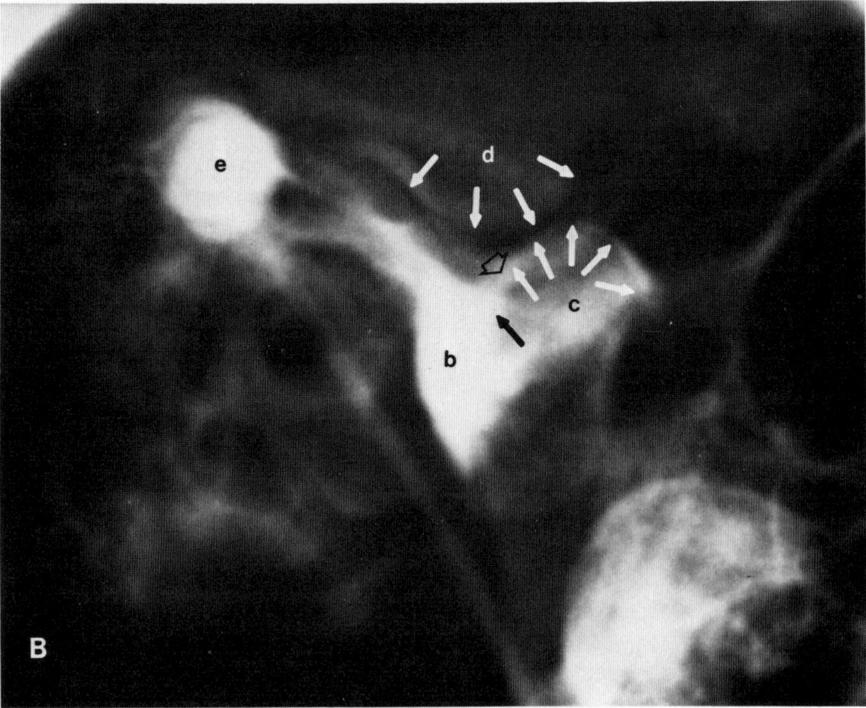

clinical importance are sometimes also found. These findings concern: (1) whether the anterior disc displacement reduces during condyle movement; (2) whether both joint spaces simultaneously opacify following injection into only one space; and (3) the severity and/or chronicity of the displacement as evidenced by morphological changes in disc shape. Among these, arthrographic differentiation on the basis of whether a reduction of the anterior displacement takes place or not is especially important to most referring clinicians.

Anterior Displacement of Disc, with Reduction

The term "anterior displacement of the disc" is defined as that state in which the entire disc, including the thicker posterior rim, is positioned anterior to the articulating surface of the condyle, i.e., the bony surface approximating the posterior, crestal, or anterior surface of the articular eminence as the jaws are closed, partially open, or fully open. Figure 8.5 graphically displays a reducing anterior disc displacement as it typically presents arthrographically. The point of reduction of the displacement usually occurs shortly after mouth opening

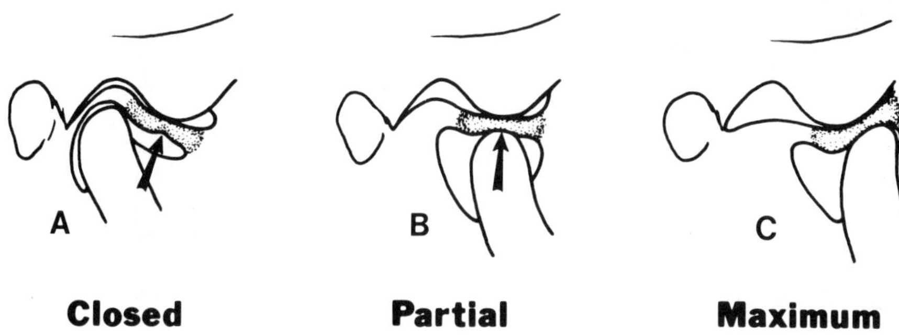

Figure 8.5. Anterior displacement of the disc *with* reduction. *A*, The closed mouth arthrogram image carries the most critical diagnostic information. The disc (*stippled*) is displaced anterior to the condylar articulating surface. Instead of the thin, midportion of the disc (*arrow*) interposed in this narrow, stress-bearing part of the joint, the posterior attachment tissue has been pulled into the area. With early jaw opening, the disc will stick or hesitate, while the condyle will tend to pop forward and under the thickened posterior rim of the disc. *B*, At partial jaw opening, the condyle has achieved a normal positional relationship with the disc (thin part of disc (*arrow*) at point of bony articulation) and moves harmoniously with it through the remainder of the anterior translation. *C*, Maximal jaw opening finds the condyle and disc both translated to their normal maximal limits, with a normal relationship in their positions. (Reproduced with permission from D.D. Blaschke, W.K. Solberg, B. Sanders: J Am Dent Assoc, 100:388–395, 1980, ©American Dental Association, Chicago.)

Figure 8.4. Normal TMJ Arthrogram. The condyle (*c*) and articular eminence (*d*) are outlined by small *arrows* to aid visibility. *A*, With the jaws closed, contrast medium fills the anterior (*a*) and posterior (*b*) recesses of the lower joint space. The thin, articulating portion of the disc (*open arrow*) is seen very slightly anterior to the condyle articulating surface, while the posterior rim of the disc lies over the condyle superior surface. *B*, On wide jaw opening, the condyle has translated anterior to the articular eminence. Contrast medium has been extruded to the posterior recess (*b*). Although the superior aspect of the disc is not seen, the lower joint space contour reveals the normal position of the disc's posterior (*open arrow*) portion. Contrast medium in the catheter hub is seen at *e*.

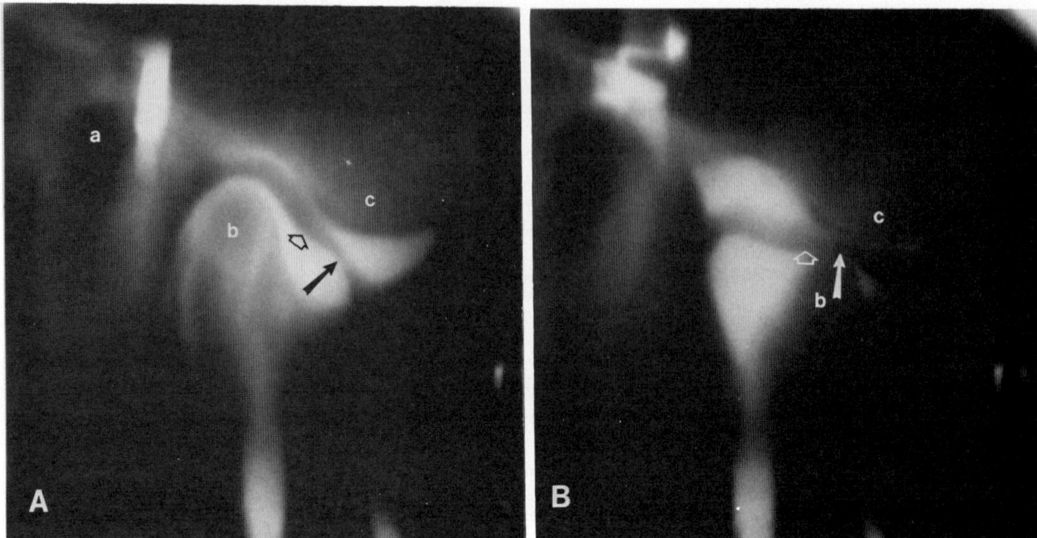

Figure 8.6. Disc displacement with reduction—arthrogram image. *A,* The external ear canal (*a*), condyle (*b*), and articular eminence (*c*), are labeled. With the jaws closed, the condyle is seated in its fossa. Notice, however, that the thin part of the disc (*arrow*) does not intervene between the condyle and posterior slope of the articular eminence but is anterior and inferior to the bony articulation. Note the disc's relatively thick posterior rim (*open arrow*). *B,* The patient has opened her mouth slightly, has felt a popping sensation in the joint, and has heard a click. The arthrogram image is consistent with these clinical phenomena by showing that the condyle has popped under the thick posterior rim (*open arrow*) of the disc. The midportion is again noted by an *arrow*. From this point on, the opening sequence in the TMJ was normal.

begins. The malpositioned disc remains fairly stable in position while the condyle passes just below the thick posterior disc rim. Once the condyle is normally seated in the inferior concavity of the disc the displacement is said to be "reduced" (Fig. 8.6). During the remainder of the opening jaw movement, the anterior translations of condyle and disc are harmonious and physiological.

On the fluoroscope monitor, the observer will see the initial reducing movements of condyle and disc occurring suddenly, as if spring-loaded. Either the condyle snaps or pops into position below the disc or the latter recoils back over the condyle. The radiographic event occurs at the same instant that the patient hears an audible click within the joint. On closing the jaws, a second, reciprocal popping phenomenon typically occurs within the joint, this time as the disc displaces forward of the condyle as the latter becomes seated within its articular fossa.

In most cases, disc anterior displacement with reduction is not a clinically or pathologically severe condition. This is reflected arthrographically by the common preservation of the normal biconcave shape of the disc and the absence of signs of disc perforation.

Anterior Displacement of Disc, without Reduction

If, during opening movements of the jaws, the condyle absolutely cannot move anteriorly past the thick posterior rim of the disc, the anterior displacement of the disc is said to be "nonreducing." Figure 8.7 illustrates this situation with artistic renditions. When such a nonreducing disc anterior displacement is found, the closed-mouth projection usually shows the displacement to be more severe (i.e., the disc more anteriorly positioned) than the corresponding displacement in which there *is* reduction on condyle movement. Another indication of a relatively severe anterior disc displacement is that the lower anterior recess is said to be especially prominent and elongated.

The articular disc in this pathological situation becomes, in essence, a mechanical obstruction to the normal range of anterior condyle translation. On the wide open projection of the TMJ, the disc is seen as a mass situated between the two anterior pools of contrast. It does not budge anteriorly, even as the condyle abuts against its posterior surface (Figs. 8.8 and 8.9). This picture of joint obstruction usually presents before the condyle has reached the crest of the articular eminence in its translatory path.

Another finding having major clinical pertinence is the simultaneous filling of both upper and lower joint spaces following injection of contrast into only one. This indicates, with few exceptions, that either the disc or its posterior attachment is perforated or torn. Any communication between the two joint spaces is considered to be pathological. Thus, following double joint space filling, the arthrographer may confidently advise of a perforation with only one disclaimer: anterior displacement of the disc *without reduction* must also be present (unless bony degenerative joint changes are prominent). Perforations are rarely observed, either arthrographically or surgically, in joints *not* having some degree of nonreducing disc anterior displacement. On the other hand, when major bony degenerative changes are present, discs are commonly perforated even without evidence of displacement.

Some deformation of the disc is usually discerned on well-made tomograms

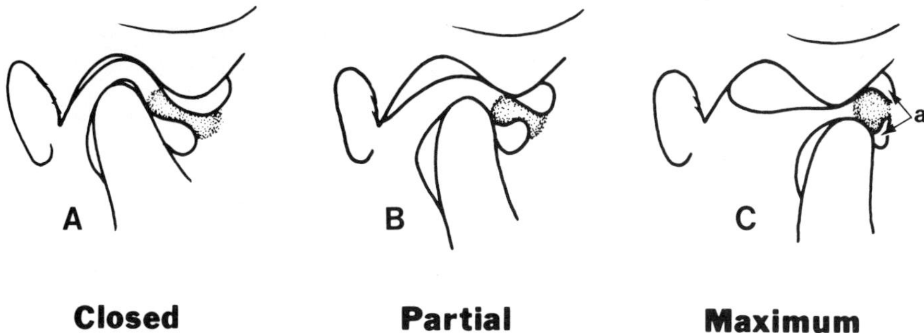

Figure 8.7. Anterior displacement of the disc *without* reduction. *A,* With the jaws closed, the disc (*stippled*) is considerably anterior to the condyle. *B,* At the stage of partial jaw opening, the disc continues to be anteriorly displaced, i.e., the displacement has not been *reduced.* Instead, the disc shows moderate deformation in shape due to the compressive force of the condyle, itself pulled anteriorly by muscle action. *C,* The condyle, shown at the point of maximal jaw opening, remains limited in terms of normal anterior excursion. The disc, severely compressed into a round radiolucent mass, remains anteriorly displaced. It acts as a mechanical obstruction to further condyle translation. Note the residual contrast in the anterior joint space recesses (*a*), another reflection of the limited condyle translation. (Reproduced with permission from D.D. Blaschke, W.K. Solberg, B. Sanders: J Am Dent Assoc, *100*:388–395, 1980, ©American Dental Association, Chicago.)

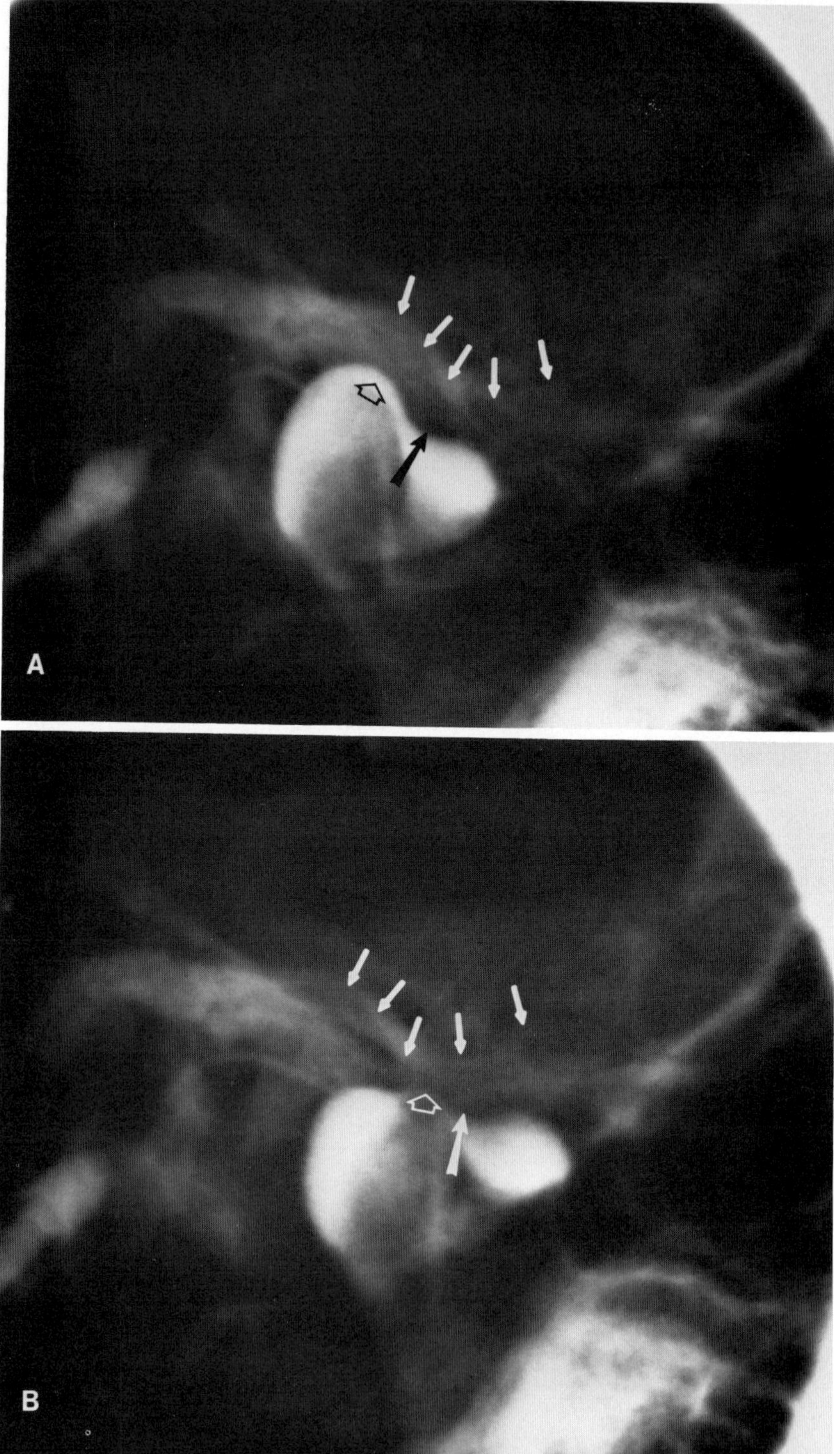

Figure 8.8. Disc displacement without reduction—arthrogram image. The articular eminence is outlined by small *arrows*. *A*, Plain radiograph, jaws closed. The thick, posterior rim of the disc (*arrow*) is positioned decidedly anterior to the articulating surface (*open arrow*) of the mandibular condyle. Only the lower joint space is opacified. *B*, Plain radiograph, maximum (but limited) jaw opening. The condyle articulating surface (*open arrow*) is blocked in its anterior excursion by the posterior rim (*arrow*) of the disc. *C* and *D*, Closed and open tomograms. Same sequence is seen following opacification of the upper joint space in addition to the lower joint space. The external ear canal (*a*), condyle (*b*), and articular eminence (*c*) are marked. The anterior displacement of the disc (posterior rim indicated by *arrow*) is seen in both views. Notice in *D* that the obstruction to condyle anterior movement has not reduced at maximal jaw opening.

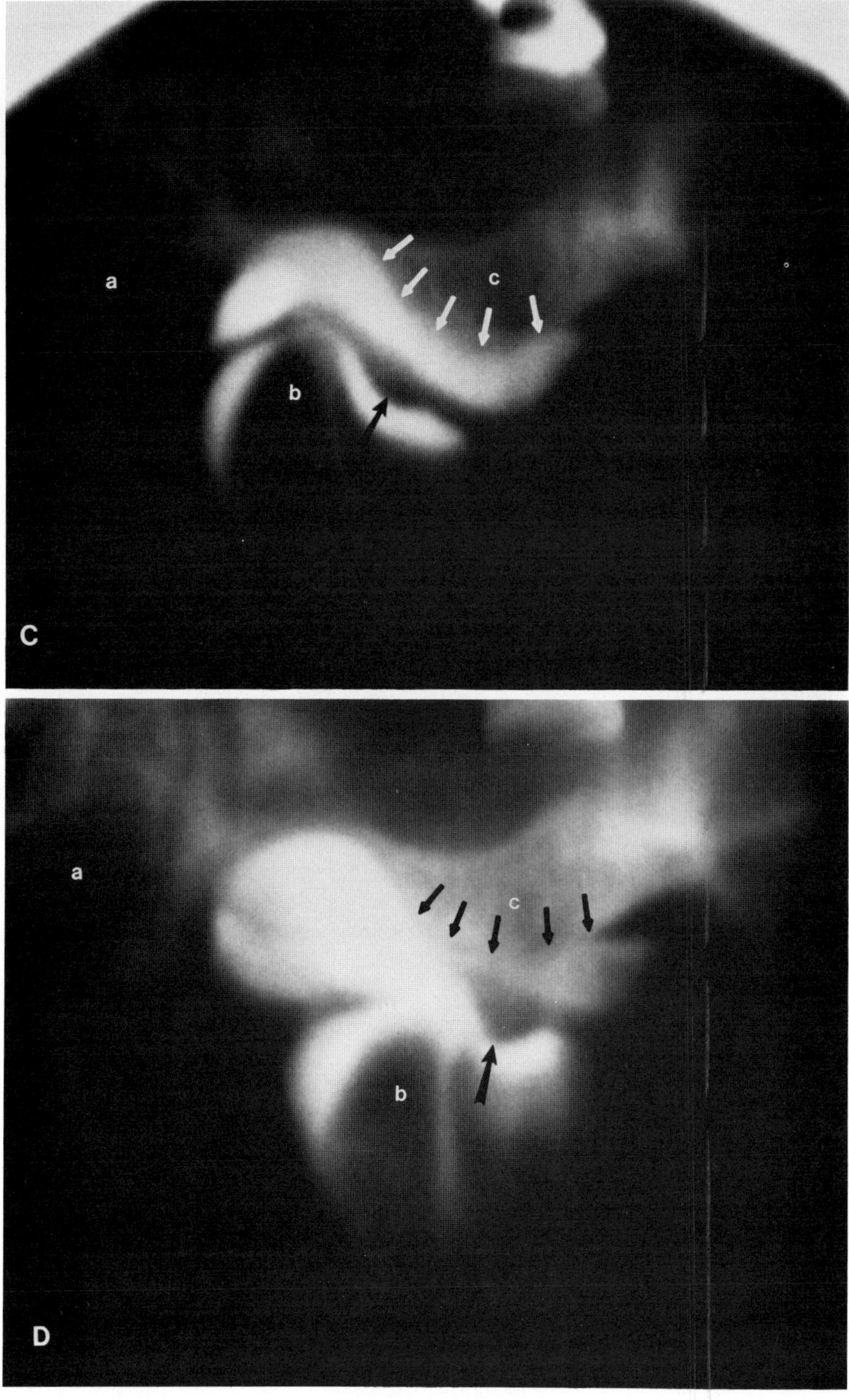

Figure 8.8 (*C* and *D*)

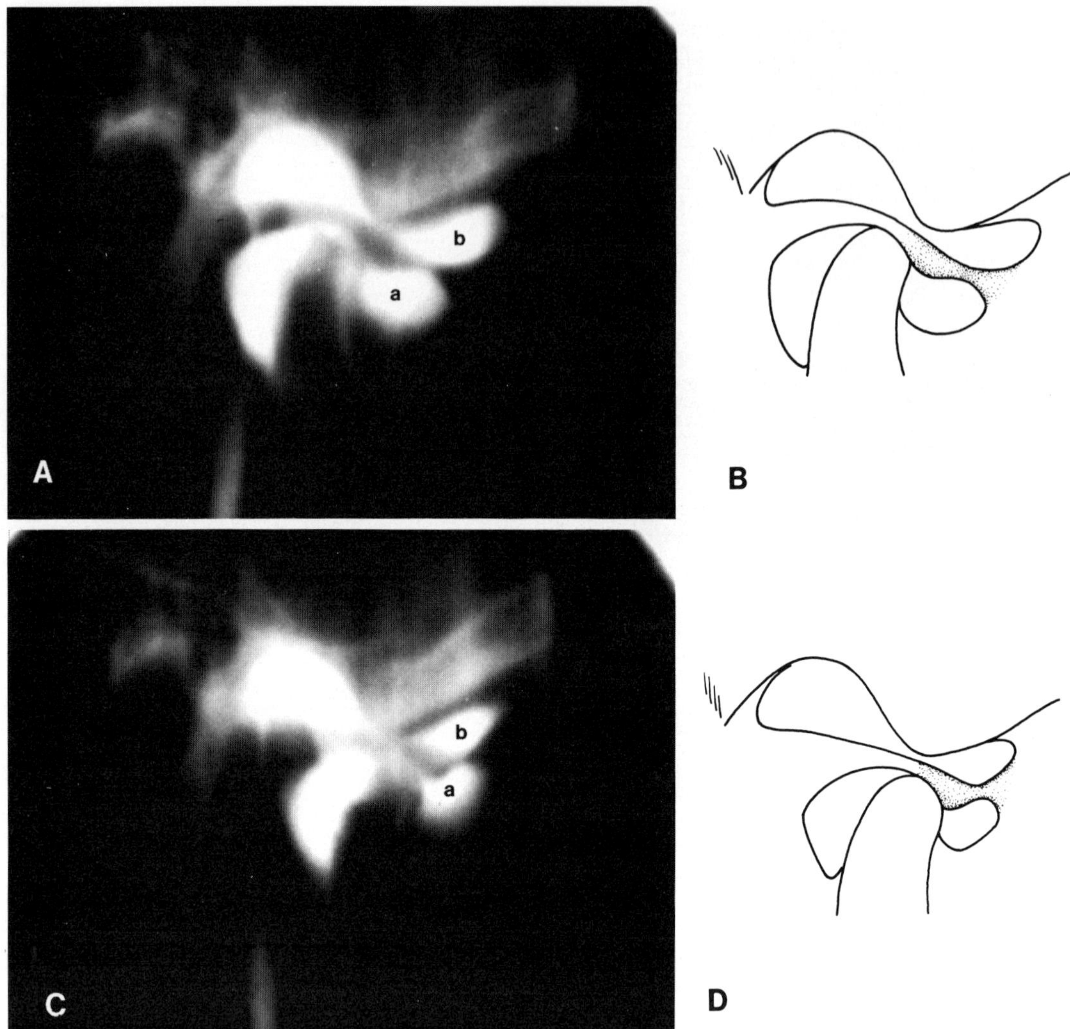

Figure 8.9. Anterior disc displacement without reduction—tomograms and line drawings. *A,* At partial (approximately 1 fingerbreadth between anterior teeth) opening of jaws, the radiolucent, biconcave (butterfly-shaped) disc is clearly anterior to the condyle. Anterior recesses of the lower (*a*) and upper (*b*) joint spaces are indicated. *B,* Line drawing of same, with disc (*stippled*). *C,* At slightly greater (2 fingerbreadths) jaw opening, the condyle has approached the crest of the articular eminence. *D,* Line drawing. Note the early compression of the disc, caused by the anterior shearing force of the condyle. *E,* Maximal jaw opening (2½ fingerbreadths). The disc has been forced sufficiently anteriorly and superiorly to obliterate the anterior recess of the upper joint space. The disc displacement has, however, prevented the complete translation of the condyle, which would have resulted in obliteration of the lower space's anterior recess (*a*). *F,* Line drawing of same.

in cases of nonreducing anterior disc displacement. Clinical importance may be attached to the radiologist's impression of whether there is a pliable rounding or "balling-up" of the disc as opposed to rigid deformation as the condyle exerts compressive force against the disc. Consider the milder situation: In the closed-

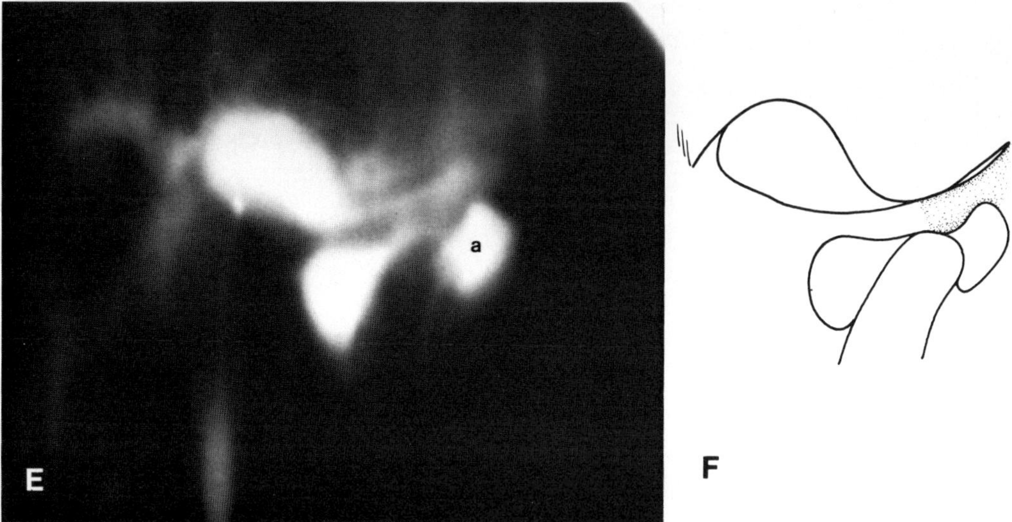

Figure 8.9 (*E* and *F*)

mouth view, the pliable disc commonly retains its normal biconcave shape despite being anteriorly displaced, whereas on opening it is subject to a plastic deformation. This situation advises the surgeon that the disc probably has retained its functional anatomy when not subject to compression. On the other hand, if arthrographic tomograms show the disc to be rigidly altered in shape in both closed and open views, the supposition is that considerable scarring has taken place over a long period of time and that the disc will likely have to be removed at surgery. Such a fibrotic disc has a "hard," fairly unalterable, shape on all arthrographic images, appearing often like a rectangular block or log.

References

Blaschke, D.D., Arthrography of the temporomandibular joint. In *Temporomandibular Joint Problems: Biological Diagnosis and Treatment*, edited by W.K. Solberg, G.T. Clark. Quintessenz, Berlin, 1980.

Blaschke, D.D., Solberg, W.K., Sanders, B., Arthrography of the temporomandibular joint—review of status. J Am Dent Assoc, *100*:388–395, 1980.

Dolwick, M.F., Katzberg, R.W., Helms, C.A., Bales, .J., Arthrotomographic evaluation of the temporomandibular joint. J Oral Surg *37*:793–799, 1979.

Farrar, W.B., McCarty, W.L., Inferior joint space arthrography and characteristics of condylar paths in internal derangements of the TMJ. J Prosthet Dent, *41*:548–555, 1979.

Katzberg, R.W., Dolwick, M.F., Bales, D.J., Helms, C.A., Arthrotomography of the temporomandibular joint: New technique and preliminary observations. AJR, *161*:100–105, 1979.

Lynch, T.P., Chase, D.C., Arthrography in the evaluation of the temporomandibular joint. Radiology, *126*:667–672, 1978.

Norgaard, F., Arthrography of the mandibular joint. Acta Radiol 25:679–685, 1944.

Norgaard, F., *Temporomandibular Arthrography.* Einar Munksgaard, Copenhagen, 1947.

Toller, P.A., Opaque arthrography of the temporomandibular joint. Int J Oral Surg, *3*:17–28, 1974.

Wilkes, C.H., Arthrography of the temporomandibular joint in patients with the TMJ pain-dysfunction syndrome. Minn Med, *61*:645–652, 1978.

Index